ENGLISH–SPANISH
SPANISH–ENGLISH
MEDICAL DICTIONARY

DICCIONARIO MÉDICO
INGLÉS–ESPAÑOL
ESPAÑOL–INGLÉS

ENGLISH–SPANISH
SPANISH–ENGLISH
MEDICAL DICTIONARY

DICCIONARIO MÉDICO
INGLÉS-ESPAÑOL
ESPAÑOL-INGLÉS

Second Edition

Glenn T. Rogers, M.D.

McGraw-Hill
HEALTH PROFESSIONS DIVISION

New York   St. Louis   San Francisco   Auckland
Bogotá   Caracas   Lisbon   London   Madrid
Mexico City   Milan   Montreal   New Delhi
San Juan   Singapore   Sydney   Tokyo   Toronto

McGraw-Hill

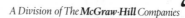

A Division of The **McGraw·Hill** Companies

ENGLISH-SPANISH SPANISH-ENGLISH MEDICAL DICTIONARY, 2/e

123456789   DOCDOC   987

ISBN   0-07-053680-5

This book was set in Times Roman.
The editor was Gaii Gavert; the production supervisor was Bob Laffler. R. R. Donnelley and Sons Company was printer and binder.

This book is printed on acid-free paper.

Library of Congress Cataloging-in-Publication Data

Rogers, Glenn T.
 English-Spanish Spanish-English medical dictionary = Diccionario médico, inglés-español, español-inglés Glenn T. Rogers.–2nd ed.
      p. cm.
 ISBN 0-07-053680-5
 1. Medicine–Dictionaries.   2. English language–Dictionaries–Spanish.
3. Medicine–Dictionaries–Spanish.   4. Spanish language–Dictionaries–
English.
 [DNLM: 1. Dictionaries, Medical–Spanish.   W 13 R726e 1997]
R121.R626   1997
610'. 3–dc21
DNLM/DLC
for Library of Congress   96-50377
                                                                CIP

CONTENTS / MATERIAS

PREFACE TO THE SECOND EDITION

This edition contains 3,000 additional entries while remaining faithful to the original goal of providing only those words which could conceivably be needed in a conversation between a health professional and a patient. Several trends in healthcare over the last five years contributed to the need for the new entries.

As documented in the New England Journal of Medicine, patients are more likely to seek alternative forms of healthcare than they were five years ago, and I have added the names of commonly used herbs as well as terms like "acupressure," "holistic," and "reflexology." Nutrition has become increasingly important, particularly with developments relating to cholesterol and tight control of diabetes, and I have added the names of common foods as well as foods believed to possess special properties relating to health. With patients taking a greater part in their own healthcare nowadays, I find that many prefer to know the precise name of the procedure or surgery they will be undergoing, and I have added a number of terms that might have seemed too technical at the time of this book's first printing.

Not included in this work are terms used strictly in the medical literature or in technical discussions between health professionals—terms like "leukocytogenesis" or "ureterocystoneostomy." A complete listing of such terms would require a book the size of Stedman's, and by omitting them I have been able to produce a book which fits in the pocket of a typical doctor's coat. Strictly technical terms are generally easy to translate anyway, because of their derivation from Latin (cf., *leucocitogenesis* and *ureterocistoneostomía*.)

Besides adding new terms I reviewed the complete text and refined many of the previous translations with the goal of providing the most concise, accurate and generally helpful translations possible. I also made a point of adding terms and phrases relevant to the allied health professions, so that healthcare workers treating Latin patients in any capacity should find this book useful.

As with the original edition, many people contributed to this work. Special thanks go to my wife, Cynda Valle, for the cover art, and to Dr. Jose de la Torre, who proofed the entire work prior to publication.

PREFACE TO THE FIRST EDITION

Good medicine requires a good history. Few experiences are more frustrating for the health practitioner than to greet a patient and realize that the practitioner and the patient have no common language. For the patient, the experience must be equally frustrating and also frightening. Stories abound regarding the mishaps that occur due to ineffective communication. One such story, which appeared in the Oakland Tribune, involves an Oakland woman who returned to her native Mexico to die, believing she had leukemia. In fact, her doctors had told her she was anemic.

The rapid growth of the Spanish-speaking population presents a special challenge to health workers in the United States. Courses in medical Spanish are now available at many medical centers, and more than a dozen books have been published which offer medical Spanish instruction in the form of sample phrases, exercises, and the like. Notably absent has been a comprehensive medical Spanish dictionary to reinforce these other efforts. This dictionary is the first of its kind.

With over fourteen thousand entries, this dictionary contains virtually every health-related term likely to occur in a conversation between a health worker and a Spanish-speaking patient. There are technical terms which could be important to certain patients (e.g., "white blood cell count," "glucose monitor"), common terms (e.g., "stomachache," "to go to the bathroom"), recently coined terms, colloquialisms, and slang. The colloquialisms form an important feature of this dictionary, as they are used frequently by Latins to describe their ailments and can be quite frustrating when offered in response to the practitioner's carefully-crafted textbook Spanish. Many of these colloquialisms are recorded here for the first time.

Another unique feature of this dictionary is its focus on Spanish as it is spoken in the United States. The great majority of Spanish-speaking people in this country come from Mexico, Central America, Cuba, Puerto Rico, and the Dominican Republic, and translations have been chosen which will be best understood by the people of these areas. Terms peculiar to a particular country carry regional labels.

Over thirty doctors from eleven Spanish American countries assisted with the extensive verification and editing of this dictionary. Four Latin dentists reviewed the dental terms. Translations are based on current usage at major Spanish American medical centers and in the Spanish American medical literature. Multiple revisions were made to ensure completeness and accuracy.

Many people helped with various aspects of the production of this book. I would like to thank my wife Cynda Valle Rogers for her patience, Richard Blum for his help with the data management, and my parents for wiring me money to pay my Mexico City hotel bill when my credit card was suddenly and inexplicably declined. I would also like to thank Peter Beren, José de la Torres, Victor Guerrero, Antonio Gutiérrez, Gabriel Lerman, Camilo Leslie, Victor Marrero, Allan Ortejarai, Dan Poynter, Rolando Valdez, Gustavo Valero, and Vicente Valero.

PRÓLOGO A LA 2.ª EDICIÓN

Esta edición incluye 3.000 vocablos adicionales y le será útil a los que, en el campo de salud, laboran con pacientes de habla inglesa o a los que deseen un alcance completo a la literatura médica. Aquellos que se proponen hacer su práctica en los Estados Unidos encontrarán que este volumen es indispensable ya que contiene virtualmente todos los términos vinculados a la medicina que puedan surgir en una conversación con un paciente. Los que deseen leer en inglés textos o publicaciones médicas, también encontrarán este libro de gran valor ya que contiene muchos términos técnicos además de los vocablos más comunes (que suelan ser los más difíciles de reconocer porque no son de origen latín.) En esta obra no se incluyen términos que se usan exclusivamente entre los profesionales de salud: términos como "leucocitogenesis" o "ureterocistoneostomía." Las traducciones de estos términos no se diferencian mucho del español y su exclusión ha permitido la producción de un libro liviano, a un precio módico, que cabe en el bolsillo de la típica bata de doctor.

Los nuevos términos abarcan los nombres de procedimientos médicos y quirúrgicos, las medicinas recientemente asequibles, las hierbas de uso común, términos relacionados a la medicina alternativa, y los alimentos comunes al igual que los alimentos que se cree tienen propiedades especiales vinculadas a la salud. Al incorporar los nuevos términos, el texto se revisó en su totalidad y muchas de las traducciones anteriores se perfeccionaron para proveer la traducción más concisa, atinada y en general, de lo más útil posible. Se hizo un gran esfuerzo para incluir términos y ejemplos de frases pertinentes a las profesiones afiliadas con la salud; así todos los que ejercen en el campo de salud podrán encontrar este libro provechoso.

Al igual que en la edición original, muchas personas han contribuido a esta obra. En particular, quiero agradecer a mi esposa, Cynda Valle, por la pintura de la portada, y al doctor José de la Torre, que revisó la obra en su totalidad previo a la publicación.

PRÓLOGO A LA 1.ª EDICIÓN

La mayoría de la literatura médica de importancia aparece en inglés y el estudiante de medicina, médico u otro practicante de la salud que quiere acceder a ella debe saber inglés médico básico. Un obstáculo a esta meta ha sido la falta de un práctico diccionario médico bilingüe. Hasta ahora no ha existido ninguno suficientemente extenso, preciso, económico y de tamaño conveniente. Este diccionario viene a llenar ese espacio vacío.

Abarcando más de 14.000 términos, este diccionario contiene la mayoría de los términos que se encuentran en artículos médicos. Además, contiene muchos modismos, los cuales podrían ser muy útiles para los que quieren practicar su profesión en Los Estados Unidos o que tienen contacto con pacientes de habla inglesa. Las formas irregulares de los plurales, comparativos, superlativos, pretéritos y participios pasados aparecen al igual que indicaciones de las funciones gramaticales y del nivel lingüístico. Para aquellos médicos que intentan presentarse al "FLEX" o a los "National Boards" este diccionario será indispensable.

Más de treinta médicos y otros especialistas han asistido en la redacción de este diccionario para asegurar la exactitud de las traducciones. Su tamaño conveniente lo hace ideal para ser llevado al hospital o a la biblioteca. Los principiantes del inglés médico podrán usar el diccionario para aumentar su vocabulario, mientras que los estudiantes más avanzados lo podrán usar como referencia. El propósito de este diccionario es llegar a servir como una autoridad para todo lo vinculado a la traducción médica.

Muchos me han ayudado en la realización de esta obra. Quisiera dar gracias en particular a mi esposa Cynda Valle Rogers por su paciencia, a Richard Blum por su consejo sobre computadoras, y a mis padres por haberme enviado con prontitud dinero para pagar la cuenta de mi hotel en México, D.F., cuando mi tarjeta de crédito fue repentina e inexplicablemente rechazada. Quiero dar gracias también a Peter Beren, José de la Torres, Victor Guerrero, Antonio Gutiérrez, Gabriel Lerman,

Camilo Leslie, Victor Marrero, Allan Ortejarai, Dan Poynter, Rolando Valdez, Gustavo Valero, y Vicente Valero.

HOW TO USE THIS DICTIONARY

Terms are listed in alphabetical order. In Spanish the letter *ñ* is a separate letter from *n* and follows it alphabetically. *Ch* and *ll* are no longer considered separate letters and are alphabetized as they would be in English.

Terms consisting of more than one word and phrases are listed either as individual entries or as run-ons under the key word of the term or phrase. When the entry word is repeated in a run-on, it is replaced by a dash (———). "Rigor mortis," "tardive dyskinesia," and "nonsteroidal antiinflammatory drug (NSAID)" are examples of terms which are listed as individual entries. By contrast, "nerve block" is listed as a run-on under "nerve," "pernicious anemia" is listed as a run-on under "anemia," and "to give birth" is listed as a run-on under "birth." For the convenience of the reader, many phrases are listed under more than one word. All chemicals, including medications, acids, and oils, are listed according to the first word of the term.

Entries are followed by an indication of the part of speech. In the Spanish-English section, noun entries are followed by *m* if they are masculine, by *f* if they are feminine, and by *mf* if they vary according to context, as with *cardiólogo -ga, doctor -ra,* and *adolescente (el adolescente* or *la adolescente).* The indication *m&f* applies to a few Spanish nouns, such as *azúcar,* which may be considered either masculine or feminine.

In the English-Spanish section, the same indications of gender noted above follow translated nouns save in the following cases where the gender is considered to be obvious: masculine nouns ending in *-o* or modified by an adjective ending in *-o,* and feminine nouns ending in *-a* or modified by an adjective ending in *-a.*

For a given entry, translations are listed in order of preference according to accuracy, level of usage, and likelihood of being understood by a broad range of Latins. When a term has more than one meaning, only those meanings relevant to healthcare are translated. Synonymous translations are separated by commas, while translations with distinct meanings are separated by semicolons.

Abbreviations for region, level of usage, and field of medicine appear in italics between parentheses. When they precede a translation, they apply to the entry term; when they follow a translation, they apply to the translation. This same principle applies to parenthetical explanations. The label "(*fam*)" applies to colloquial terms used frequently in speech and rarely in writing. Some of these terms could seem overly familiar or inappropriate, particularly to a highly educated or aristocratic Latin when used on first meeting. On the other hand, such a term may be the only term understood by a less educated Latin and should be tried when a more formal term fails to make the point. Terms labeled "(*form*)" will not be understood by many Latins. The label "(*vulg*)" applies to slang terms, including drug jargon, and to terms considered by most people to be crude. They will be used from time to time, particularly by male patients with little education, but should rarely if ever be used by the health practitioner.

The reflexive "se" following an infinitive is enclosed in parentheses when it is optional or dependent on context. For example, "bathe" is translated as "*vt, vi* bañar(se)." In this situation "se" would be used with the intransitive form of the verb, but not the transitive form.[*]

---

[*] Recall that a transitive verb form takes an object, while an intransitive verb form does not. Consider the two example sentences: "The nurse will bathe your baby," and, "Use a mild soap when you bathe." In the first sentence "bathe" is transitive ("your baby" is the object); in the second it is intransitive (there is no object).

USO DE ESTE DICCIONARIO

Los artículos se presentan en orden alfabético. Términos que tienen más de una palabra, al igual que frases, se encuentran como anotaciones individuales o a continuación de la palabra más importante. Cuando la anotación se repite en una continuación, se la reemplaza con un guión largo (———). "Rigor mortis," "discinesia tardía," y "colangiopancreatografía retrógrada endoscópica" son ejemplos de términos que se encuentran como anotaciones individuales. En cambio, "trabajo de parto" se encuentra a continuación de "parto," "en polvo" se encuentra a continuación de "polvo," y "enfermedad de Graves" se encuentra a continuación de "enfermedad." Para los vocablos que tienen varios significados, solo los pertinentes a la salud se han traducido. Sinónimos se separan con coma; significados que son distintos se separan con punto y coma.

Las abreviaturas de región, nivel lingüístico, y campo aparecen entre paréntesis en letra cursiva. Cuando aparecen antes de la traducción, quiere decir que modifican la anotación; cuando aparecen después de la traducción, quiere decir que modifican la traducción misma. Lo mismo se aplica a las frases aclaradoras que están entre paréntesis. La etiqueta "(*fam*)" se aplica a los términos que se usan mucho al hablar, raras veces al escribir, y que a veces podrían ser inapropiados, especialmente al utilizarse en el primer encuentro con un paciente mayor o muy formal. Traducciones denotadas como "(*form*)" serán desconocidas para algunas personas. La etiqueta "(*vulg*)" se aplica a la jerga y a los términos que la mayoría de la gente considera ofensivos.

MEDICAL SPANISH TIPS

- The most important advice I can give to anyone learning a foreign language is to try to master the pronunciation at an early stage. This has a double benefit. Not only will you be understood more easily, but you will be better able to identify and retain words and phrases of the foreign language as you hear them. This will greatly accelerate the learning process. As you hear the foreign language being spoken by a native speaker, repeat key phrases over and over in your mind—or even aloud if possible—comparing your pronunciation to the immediate memory of the correctly spoken sounds. Experiment with your tongue, lips, and palate to create sounds which may be unfamiliar to you. Take a deep breath and pronounce the soft "i" of "sin," then slowly modulate it to the "ee" of "seen." Go back and forth between these two sounds. Somewhere in between is the *i* as it sounds in Spanish, for example in *cinco*. Pronounce the English "d" sound over and over again and gradually modulate it to the "th" of "the." Somewhere in between is the Spanish *d*. Pronounce the English "h" sound over and over again and gradually modulate it to the English "k." Somewhere in between is a close facsimile of the Spanish *j*. Exercises like these will improve your pronunciation rapidly.

- On the subject of pronunciation, note that Spanish vowels are short and pure. Never linger on a vowel as in English. Say the sentence, "No way!" with feeling and notice how the vowel sounds are drawn out. This rarely happens in Spanish; Spanish is much more staccato in its delivery. Note also that there is no schwa sound in Spanish. The schwa sound is the "uh" sound so often given to unaccented syllables in English. For example the first, third, and possibly fifth syllables of **acetaminophen** are schwa sounds. In Spanish, vowels retain their characteristic sounds whether or not they are accented. *Acetaminofén* is pronounced ah-ceh-tah-mee-noh-FEHN, not uh-ceh-tuh-mee-nuh-FEHN. It is often helpful first to practice a word without consonants. ***Acetaminofén*** without consonants would be *ah-eh-ah-ee-oh-EH*. When you have mastered the vowel changes for a given word, it is usually a simple matter to fill in the consonants. Learn to say *cah-BEH-sah*, not *cuh-BEH-suh*; *meh-dee-SEE-nah*, not *meh-duh-SEE-nuh*.

■ When referring to a part of the body in Spanish, it is common to use the definite article instead of the possessive adjective, provided it is clear whose body is involved. The Spanish definite articles, recall, are *el* and *la*. *Me duele la cabeza* is the best translation of "My head hurts." *Me duele mi cabeza* is redundant in Spanish.

■ The indirect object[*] is used much more often in Spanish than in English. Health workers are frequently doing things to patients and this often involves the use of *le* or, in familiar speech, *te*.

> *Quiero tomarle el pulso*...I want to take your pulse.
> *Voy a escucharle el corazón*...I'm going to listen to your heart.
> *Tenemos que operarte la pierna*...We need to operate on your leg.

This phrasing often sounds less brusque than *Quiero tomar su pulso, Voy a escuchar su corazón,* etc.

■ English-speaking people are often confused by the choices available for the direct object in Spanish. *Te* is always correct when speaking informally, for instance to a child.

> *Voy a examinarte, hijo.*.I'm going to examine you, son.

---

[*] Recall that a *direct* object may be any type of object and receives the direct action of the verb, while the *indirect* object is always a person (or other living being) *to* whom or *for* whom the action is being performed.

When speaking formally, most Spanish Americans use *lo* for males and *la* for females.

> *Voy a examinarlo, señor*..I'm going to examine you, sir.
> *Voy a examinarla, señora*..I'm going to examine you, ma'am.

There are a few exceptions to this rule; for instance, the verb *pegar*, when it means "to hit" takes *le* for a direct object.

> *¿Le pegó?*..Did it hit you?

Some Spanish Americans will use *le* for *all* (formal) second person direct objects, male or female.

> *Voy a examinarle, señor*..I'm going to examine you, sir.
> *Voy a examinarle, señora*..I'm going to examine you, ma'am.

This style is common in Mexico.

- Some verbs require that the subject and object be inverted when translating between English and Spanish. The Spanish student is likely to encounter this for the first time when learning to translate the verb "to like." "I like coffee" would be *Me gusta el café*. The subject and object are inverted. This particular construction is a stumbling block to fluency and even advanced students often have to think for a couple seconds in order to conjugate the verb correctly and choose the correct object pronouns.

> *Me falta el aire*..I am short of breath.
> *Les falta el aire*..They are short of breath.
> *Le salieron los dientes*..His teeth came in.
> *Me dieron náuseas*..I got nauseated.
> *¿Le salieron moretones?*..Did you get bruised?
> *Te falta hierro*..You're low on iron.

Notice that the English subject corresponds to the Spanish *indirect* object in all these cases.

- Many Spanish verbs are used in the reflexive form when applied to medicine. The use of the reflexive pronoun *se* in some way turns the action of the verb back on the verb's subject.

    Orinó..He urinated.
    Se orinó..He urinated on himself.

    Corté el pan..I cut the bread.
    Me corté el dedo..I cut my finger.

    Puede vestirla..You can dress her.
    Puede vestirse..You can get dressed (literally "dress your-self").

    La enfermera le va a inyectar..The nurse will give you an injection.
    La enfermera le va a enseñar como inyectarse..The nurse will teach you how to inject yourself.

    A reflexive construction is often used when an English-speaking person would use the past participle preceded by "to get," "to be," or "to become."

    Tiene que internarse..You need to be admitted.
    Se cansa..He gets tired..He becomes tired.
    Ud. se curó..You were cured..You got cured.
    Se mejoró..She got better.
    Se dislocó..It became dislocated.
    Se infectó..It became infected..It got infected.

- Most Spanish nouns which end in *-o* are masculine and most which end in *-a* are feminine, however there are some important exceptions in medical Spanish. For instance, most Spanish words which end in *-ma* are derived from Greek and retain their original masculine gender.

> *un problema médico*..a medical problem
> *el electrocardiograma*..the electrocardiogram

Other medical terms which end in *-a* and are masculine include *aura, día, cólera* (the disease), *herbicida, insecticida, pesticida, raticida, espermaticida* and *vermicida*.

The word *mano*, which comes from the Latin *manus*, retains its original feminine gender——despite the fact it ends in *-o*.

> *Tengo las manos frías*..My hands are cold.

A source of confusion to Spanish students is the construction "*el agua*." Although *agua* is feminine (and requires feminine modifiers), *el* is used instead of *la* to avoid the awkward double "*ah*" sound of "*la agua*." This rule applies to any word which begins with an accented *ah* sound.

> *el agua fría*..the cold water
> *terapista del habla*..speech therapist

This rule also applies to the indefinite article.

> *un afta*..a canker sore
> *un arma blanca*..a sharp weapon

This rule does not apply to plural forms, since the double "*ah*" sound is then broken up by an *s* sound.

> *las aguas frías*..the cold waters
> *unas aftas*..some canker sores

Other medical Spanish terms which begin with an accented *ah* sound include *ámpula, área, asma,* and *hambre*.

- When comparing quantities, use *de*.

    más de dos pastillas..more than two pills
    menos de una taza..less than a cup

In all other situations use *que*.

    más alto que tu hermano..taller than your brother
    más que pesabas hace dos meses..more than you weighed
       two months ago
    menos que siempre..less than usual
    menos que nunca..less than ever

- Health practitioners should be aware that the Spanish word *alcohol*
  is often considered a synonym for "hard liquor." Many Latin beer
  and wine drinkers will answer no in all sincerity to the question
  ¿Toma alcohol? A broader question would be *¿Acostumbra tomar
  bebidas alcohólicas?* To avoid all misunderstandings, you could
  then follow a negative answer with *¿Cerveza?..¿Vino?*

SPANISH PRONUNCIATION

a   Like the English **a** in **father** (e.g., *padre*, *cama*).

b   Similar to the English **b**. At the beginning of a breath group or following an *m* or *n*, the Spanish *b* sounds like the **b** in **bite** (e.g., *boca*, *embarasada*). In all other situations the Spanish *b* lies somewhere between the English **b** and the English **v** (e.g., *tubo*, *jarabe*). Allow a little air to escape between slightly parted lips as you make this latter sound.

c   Like the English **c**. Before *a*, *o*, or *u* it is hard (e.g., *cara*); before *e* or *i* it is soft (e.g., *ácido*). (In Castilian Spanish, *c* preceding **e** or **i** is pronounced like the **th** in **bath**, but this form of Spanish is rarely spoken by Spanish Americans.) The Spanish *ch* sounds like the English **ch** in **child**.

d   Similar to the English **d**. At the beginning of a breath group or following *l* or *n*, the Spanish *d* sounds like the English **d** in **dizzy** (e.g., *dosis*, *venda*). In all other situations the Spanish *d* lies somewhere between the English **d** and the **th** in **this** (e.g., *mudo*, *nacido*). Allow a little air to escape between the tip of your tongue and upper teeth as you make the latter sound.

e   Similar to the **ey** in **they** (e.g., *peso*, *absceso*), unless followed by a consonant in the same syllable, in which case it is closer to the **e** in **sepsis** (e.g., *esperma*, *recto*).

f   Like the English **f**.

g   When followed by *a*, *o*, *u*, or a consonant, the Spanish *g* is similar to the English **g** in **gout** (e.g., *gota*, *grasa*). Allow a little air to escape between your tongue and palate as you make this sound.

When followed by *e* or *i*, the Spanish *g* is similar to the **h** in **hot** shaded slightly toward the English **k** (e.g., *gen*, *gingiva*).

h   Silent (e.g., *hombre*, *almohada*).

i   Like the **i** in **saline** or **latrine** (e.g., *orina*, *signo*, *sífilis*). Preceding another vowel, the Spanish *i* sounds like the English **y**. *Siesta* is pronounced *SYES-tah*, *sodio* is pronounced *SO-dyoh*, *viudo* is pronounced *VYOO-doh*, etc. Following another vowel, *i* forms individual diphthongs: *ai* sounds like the **y** in **cry** (e.g., *aire*, *aislar*); *ei* sounds like the **ay** in **tray** (e.g., *aceite*, *afeitar*); *oi* sounds like the **oy** in **boy** (e.g., *toxoide*, *coloide*); and *ui* sounds like the **ui** in **suite** (e.g., *cuidado*, *ruido*).

j   The Spanish *j* is pronounced the same as the Spanish *g* followed by *e* or *i* (e.g., *jugo*, *bajar*). See above.

k   Like the English **k**. (*k* is not included in the Spanish alphabet and appears only in foreign words.)

l   Similar to the English **l** (e.g., *lado*, *pelo*). The Spanish *l* is articulated rapidly, never drawn out as in English. The Spanish *ll* is prounounced somewhere between the **ll** of **million** and the **y** of **yes**.

m   Like the English **m**.

n   Like the English **n**.

ñ   Like the **ni** in **bunion** (e.g., *baño*, *sueño*).

o   Similar to the English **o** in **coma**.

p   Like the English **p** in **spit**. Hold your hand in front of your mouth as you say **spit** and then **pit**. Note that less air is expelled in pronouncing **spit**. The Spanish *p* is not aspirated, which means little air should be expelled. It is a shorter, more explosive sound than the English **p**.

q Like the English **k**. The Spanish *q* is always followed by *u*, but lacks the **w** sound of the English **qu**. *Quinina* is pronounced *kee-NEE-nah*, not *kwee-NEE-nah*. The **kw** sound of **quit** is represented in Spanish by *cu*, as in *cuarto*, *cuidado*, etc.

r Similar to the **tt** of **butter**. At the beginning of a word the Spanish *r* is trilled. The Spanish *rr* is always trilled.

s Like the English **s**. Before voiced consonants, the Spanish *s* sounds like the English **z** (e.g., *rasgar*, *espasmo*).

t Like the English **t** in **stent**. Hold your hand in front of your mouth as you say **stent** and then **tent**. Note that less air is expelled in pronouncing **stent**. The Spanish *t* is not aspirated, which means little air should be expelled. It is a shorter, more explosive sound than the English **t**, made by quickly tapping the tip of the tongue against the back of the upper front teeth.

u Like the English **u** in **flu** or **rule**. Be sure not to pronounce it like **you** (unless it follows an *i*—see below). The Spanish *u* has a **w** sound when it precedes another vowel (e.g., *agua*, *cuello*), except in the case of *gue*, *gui*, *que*, and *qui*, when it is silent (e.g., *inguinal*, *quebrar*). The **w** sound is retained in *güe* and *güi* (e.g., *agüita*, *ungüento*). The diphthong *au* sounds like the **ow** of **brow** (e.g., *aura*, *trauma*). The diphthong *iu* sounds like the **u** in **acute** or **use** (e.g., *viudo*, *diurético*).

v Identical to the Spanish *b*. See above.

x Like the English **x** in **flex**. Before consonants, the Spanish *x* is often pronounced like the English **s** (e.g., *extra*, *expediente*).

y Similar to the English **y** (e.g., *yeso*, *yodo*). An exception is the word *y* (= **and**), which is pronounced like the **ee** in **see**.

z Like the English **s** (e.g., *nariz*, *brazo*).

ABBREVIATIONS / ABREVIATURAS

abbr	abbreviation	abreviatura
adj	adjective	adjetivo
adv	adverb	adverbio
anat	anatomy	anatomía
Ang	Anglicism	anglicismo
ant	antiquated	antiguo
arith	arithmetic	aritmética
bot	botany	botánica
CA	Central America	Centroamérica
card	cardiology	cardiología
Carib	Caribbean	caribe
chem	chemistry	química
comp	comparative	comparativo
Cub	Cuba	Cuba
dent	dentistry	odontología
derm	dermatology	dermatología
ES	El Salvador	El Salvador
esp	especially	especialmente
f	feminine	femenino
fam	familiar	familiar
fig	figurative	figurado
form	formal	formal
fpl	feminine plural	femenino plural
frec	frequently	frecuentemente
ger	gerund	gerundio
gyn	gynecology	ginecología
m	masculine	masculino
Mex	Mexico	México
micro	microbiology	microbiología
mpl	masculine plural	masculino plural

n	noun	nombre *o* sustantivo
neuro	neurology	neurología
Nic	Nicaragua	Nicaragua
npl	noun plural	nombre plural
obst	obstetrics	obstetricia
ortho	orthopedics	ortopedia
path	pathology	patología
ped	pediatrics	pediatría
pharm	pharmacology	farmacología
physio	physiology	fisiología
pl	plural	plural
pp	past participle	participio pasado
PR	Puerto Rico	Puerto Rico
prep	preposition	preposición
pret	preterit	pretérito
psych	psychology	psicología
SA	South America	Sudamérica
SD	Santo Domingo	Santo Domingo
super	superlative	superlativo
surg	surgery	cirugía
US	United States	Estados Unidos
V.	See	Véase
vi	verb, intransitive	verbo intransitivo
vr	verb, reflexive	verbo reflexivo
vt	verb, transitive	verbo transitivo
vulg	slang	vulgar

ENGLISH-SPANISH

INGLÉS-ESPAÑOL

A

AA V. Alcoholics Anonymous.

abdomen n abdomen m, estómago (fam)

abdominal adj abdominal

ability n (pl -ties) habilidad f, capacidad f, facultad f

abnormal adj anormal

abnormality n (pl -ties) anormalidad f

abort vt, vi abortar

abortion n aborto (esp inducido); **accidental** —— aborto accidental; **habitual** —— aborto habitual; **incomplete** —— aborto incompleto; **spontaneous** —— aborto espontáneo; **therapeutic** —— aborto terapéutico; **threatened** —— amenaza de aborto; **to have an** —— tener un aborto, abortar

abrasion n abrasión f (form), raspón m, raspadura

abrasive adj & n abrasivo

abscess n absceso, (dent) postemilla (Mex, CA)

absence n ausencia, falta

absent adj ausente

absent-minded adj distraído, olvidadizo

absorb vt absorber

absorbable adj absorbible

absorbent adj absorbente

absorption n absorción f

abstain vi abstenerse; **to** —— **from sex** abstenerse del sexo

abstinence n abstinencia

abuse n abuso; **child** —— abuso infantil, abuso de niños; **substance** —— abuso de drogas o alcohol; vt abusar

abuser n abusador -ra mf; **drug** —— toxicómano -na mf (form), drogadicto -ta mf

acarbose n acarbosa

access n acceso; **wheelchair** —— acceso para sillas de rueda

accident n accidente m, (automobile) choque m

accident-prone adj propenso a sufrir accidentes

accumulate vt, vi acumular(se)

accuracy n exactitud f, precisión f

accurate adj exacto, preciso

acetaminophen n acetaminofén m, paracetamol m

acetazolamide n acetazolamida

acetic acid n ácido acético

acetone n acetona

achalasia n acalasia

ache n dolor m, dolor persistente; vi doler

achondroplasia n acondroplasia

acid adj & n ácido; **fatty** —— ácido graso; **gastric** —— ácido gástrico

acidity n acidez f

acne n acné f

acoustic adj acústico

acquire vt adquirir

acromegaly n acromegalia

acrophobia n acrofobia

acrylic adj acrílico

act n acto; vi (to behave) comportarse; **to** —— **out** (psych) expresar impulsos reprimidos en conducta sin inhibiciones

ACTH abbr **adrenocorticotropic hormone.** V. hormone.

actinomycosis n actinomicosis f

action n acción f

activate vt activar

activator n activador m

active adj activo

activity n actividad f; **strenuous** —— actividad fuerte

acuity n agudeza; **visual** —— agudeza visual

acupressure *n* acupresión *f*

acupuncture *n* acupuntura

acute *adj* agudo

acyclovir *n* aciclovir *m*

Adam's apple *n* manzana de Adán

adapt *vt, vi* adaptar(se)

adaptation *n* adaptación *f*

add *vt* agregar; (*arith*) sumar; **Add a teaspoon of salt**..Agregue una cucharadita de sal.

addict *n* adicto -ta *mf*, vicioso -sa *mf*; **drug** —— farmacodependiente *mf* (*form*), drogadicto -ta *mf*; *vt* enviciar; **to become addicted** enviciarse, volverse adicto

addiction *n* adicción *f*

addictive *adj* adictivo, que crea hábito

additive *adj & n* aditivo

address *n* dirección *f*, domicilio

adenitis *n* adenitis *f*

adenocarcinoma *n* adenocarcinoma *m*

adenoidectomy *n* (*pl* -mies) adenoidectomía

adenoiditis *n* adenoiditis *f*

adenoids *npl* vegetaciones *fpl* adenoides, adenoides *fpl*

adenoma *n* adenoma *m*; **villous** —— adenoma velloso

adequate *adj* adecuado, suficiente

adhesion *n* adherencia

adhesive *adj* adhesivo; —— **tape** tela *or* cinta adhesiva

adjust *vt* ajustar, modificar

adjustable *adj* ajustable

adjustment *n* ajuste *m*, corrección *f*, modificación *f*

adjuvant *adj* adyuvante, coadyuvante

administration *n* administración *f*

admission *n* (*to the hospital*) admisión *f*, ingreso

admit *vt* (*pret & pp* admitted; *ger* admitting) (*to the hospital*) internar, ingresar; **to be admitted** internarse, ingresarse; **She was admitted yesterday**..Fue internada ayer...**You need to be admitted**..Ud. necesita ser internado.

Admitting *n* Admisión *f*, Ingresos

adolescence *n* adolescencia

adolescent *adj & n* adolescente *mf*

adopt *vt* adoptar

adoption *n* adopción *f*

adoptive *adj* adoptivo

adrenaline *n* adrenalina

adsorbent *adj* adsorbente

adult *adj & n* adulto -ta *mf*

advance *n* avance *m*

advance directive *n* (*US*) documento que indica de antemano la atención médica deseada en caso de coma u otra incapacidad para expresarse

advantage *n* ventaja

aerobic *adj* aeróbico; *npl* aeróbicos

aerosol *n* aerosol *m*

aerosolized *adj* en aerosol

affect *n* (*psych*) afecto; *vt* afectar

affection *n* afecto, cariño

affectionate *adj* afectuoso, cariñoso

affinity *n* (*pl* -ties) afinidad *f*

affliction *n* mal *m*, achaque *m*

afraid *adj* **to be** —— tener miedo; **Are you afraid of injections?**..¿Tiene miedo a las inyecciones?

afterbirth *n* (*fam*) placenta, secundinas (*fam*)

afternoon *n* tarde *f*

aftertaste *n* sabor *m* que queda después de tomar un medicamento o alimento

agammaglobulinemia *n* agammaglobulinemia

age *n* edad *f*; **bone** —— edad ósea; **middle** —— edad madura *or* mediana; **old** —— vejez *f*

agency *n* (*pl* -cies) agencia

agent *n* agente *m*

aggravate *vt* agravar

aggression *n* agresión *f*

aggressive *adj* agresivo

agile *adj* ágil

aging *n* envejecimiento

agitate *vt* agitar; **to become agitated** agitarse

agitated *adj* agitado

ago *adj* hace; atrás; **two weeks ago**..hace dos semanas..dos semanas atrás

agoraphobia *n* agorafobia

aid *n* ayuda, auxilio; *vt* ayudar, asistir

aide *n* asistente *mf*, ayudante *mf*, auxiliar *mf*; **nurse's** —— asistente de enfermera

AIDS *abbr* acquired immunodeficiency

syndrome. *V.* **syndrome.**

ailment *n* mal *m,* achaque *m,* padecimiento

air *n* aire *m*

air conditioning *n* aire acondicionado

airsickness *n* mareo (*en avión*)

airway *n* vía aérea

alanine *n* alanina

albinism *n* albinismo

albino *adj* albino; *n* (*pl* -nos) albino -na *mf*

albumin *n* albúmina

albuterol *n* albuterol *m*

alcaptonuria *See* **alkaptonuria.**

alcohol *n* alcohol *m,* bebidas alcohólicas (*incluyendo vino y cerveza*); **Do you drink alcohol?**..¿Toma Ud. bebidas alcohólicas? **denatured** —— alcohol desnaturalizado; **rubbing** —— alcohol para fricciones

alcoholic *adj & n* alcohólico -ca *mf*

Alcoholics Anonymous (AA) *n* Alcohólicos Anónimos

alcoholism *n* alcoholismo

aldosterone *n* aldosterona

aldosteronism *n* aldosteronismo

alendronate *n* alendronato

alert *adj* alerta

alfalfa *n* (*bot*) alfalfa

algae *npl* algas

alienated *adj* aislado emocionalmente, incapaz de establecer relaciones con los demás

alienation *n* aislamiento emocional, incapacidad *f* para establecer relaciones con los demás

align *vt, vi* alinear(se)

alignment *n* alineamiento

alimentary *adj* alimentario

alive *adj* vivo, con vida

alkali *n* álcali *m*

alkaline *adj* alcalino; —— **phosphatase** fosfatasa alcalina

alkalosis *n* alcalosis *f*

alkaptonuria *n* alcaptonuria

allergen *n* alergeno

allergic *adj* alérgico; **Are you allergic to any medicine?**..¿Es Ud. alérgico a algún medicamento?

allergist *n* alergólogo -ga *mf,* especialista *mf* en alergias

allergy *n* (*pl* -**gies**) alergia

alleviate *vt* aliviar

allopathic *adj* alopático

allopurinol *n* alopurinol *m*

aloe *n* áloe *m*

alpha *n* alfa; —— **fetoprotein** alfa feto proteína; —— **methyldopa** alfa metildopa

alprazolam *n* alprazolam *m*

alternate *adj* alterno; —— **days** días alternos; *vt, vi* alternar

altitude *n* altitud *f*

aluminum *n* aluminio

alveolus *n* (*pl* -**li**) alveolo *or* alvéolo

amalgam *n* (*dent*) amalgama

Amanita Amanita

amantadine *n* amantadina

ambidextrous *adj* ambidextro

ambulance *n* ambulancia

ambulatory *adj* ambulatorio

ameba *n* (*pl* -**bas** *o* -**bae**) amiba *or* ameba

amebiasis *n* amibiasis *or* amebiasis *f*

amebic *adj* amibiano *or* amebiano

amenorrhea *n* amenorrea

American *adj* americano, norteamericano, estadounidense; *n* americano -na *mf,* norteamericano -na *mf*

amikacin *n* amikacina

amiloride *n* amilorida

amino acid *n* aminoácido

aminoglycoside *n* aminoglucósido

aminophylline *n* aminofilina

amitriptyline *n* amitriptilina

ammonia *n* amoniaco *or* amoníaco

amnesia *n* amnesia

amniocentesis *n* (*pl* -**ses**) amniocentesis *f*

amnionitis *n* amnionitis *f*

amoxacillin *n* amoxacilina

amphetamine *n* anfetamina

amphotericin B *n* anfotericina B

ampicillin *n* ampicilina

ampule *n* ampolleta, ámpula

amputate *vt* amputar

amputation *n* amputación *f*

amylase *n* amilasa

amyloidosis *n* amiloidosis *f*

amyotrophic lateral sclerosis *n* esclerosis lateral amiotrófica

anabolic *adj* anabólico

anaerobic *adj* anaerobio
anal *adj* anal
analgesia *n* analgesia
analgesic *adj* & *n* analgésico
analysis *n* (*pl* -ses) análisis *m*
analyst *n* (*fam*) psicoanalista *mf*
analyze *vt* analizar
anaphylactic *adj* anafiláctico
anaphylaxis *n* anafilaxis *f*
anatomical, anatomic *adj* anatómico
anatomy *n* anatomía
ancestor *n* antepasado
androgen *n* andrógeno
anemia *n* anemia; **aplastic** —— anemia aplásica; **hemolytic** —— anemia hemolítica; **iron deficiency** —— anemia ferropriva (*form*), anemia por deficiencia de hierro; **pernicious** —— anemia perniciosa; **sickle cell** —— anemia de células falciformes, anemia drepanocítica; **sideroblastic** —— anemia sideroblástica
anemic *adj* anémico
anencephaly *n* anencefalia
anergy *n* anergia
anesthesia *n* anestesia; **general** —— anestesia general; **local** —— anestesia local; **regional** —— anestesia regional
anesthesiologist *n* anestesiólogo -ga *mf*
anesthesiology *n* anestesiología
anesthetic *adj* & *n* anestésico
anesthetist *n* anestesista *mf*
anesthetize *vt* anestesiar
aneurysm *n* aneurisma *m*; **dissecting** —— aneurisma disecante; **micotic** —— aneurisma micótico
angel dust *n* polvo de ángel (*Ang*)
angelica *n* (*bot*) angélica
anger *n* ira, enojo
angiitis *n* angiitis *f*
angina *n* angina (*de pecho*); **Prinzmetal's** —— angina de Prinzmetal; **unstable** —— angina inestable
angiodysplasia *n* angiodisplasia
angioedema *n* angioedema *m*
angiogram *n* angiograma *m*, angiografía
angiography *n* angiografía
angioma *n* angioma *m*
angioplasty *n* (*pl* -ties) angioplastia; **per-**

cutaneous transluminal coronary —— angioplastia transluminal percutánea coronaria
angiosarcoma *n* angiosarcoma *m*
angle *n* ángulo
angry *adj* enojado; **to get** —— enojarse
aniline *n* anilina
animal *n* animal *m*; —— **fat** grasa de animal
ankle *n* tobillo
anklebone *n* hueso del tobillo
ankylosis *n* anquilosis *f*
annoying *adj* molesto, fastidioso
annual *adj* anual
annular *adj* anular
anointing of the sick *n* santos óleos
anomaly *n* (*pl* -lies) anomalía
anorexia *n* anorexia; —— **nervosa** anorexia nerviosa
anovulation *n* anovulación *f*
anovulatory *adj* anovulatorio
ant *n* hormiga
antacid *adj* & *n* antiácido
anterior *adj* anterior
anthelminthic *adj* & *n* antihelmíntico
anthrax *n* ántrax *m*
antiarrhythmic *adj* & *n* antiarrítmico
antibacterial *adj* antibacteriano
antibiotic *adj* & *n* antibiótico; **broad spectrum** —— antibiótico de amplio espectro
antibody *n* (*pl* -dies) anticuerpo
anticholinergic *adj* anticolinérgico
anticoagulant *adj* & *n* anticoagulante *m*
anticoagulate *vt* anticoagular
anticonvulsant *adj* & *n* anticonvulsivo, anticonvulsivante *m*
antidepressant *adj* & *n* antidepresivo; **tricyclic** —— antidepresivo tricíclico
antidiarrheal *adj* antidiarreico
antidote *n* antídoto
antiemetic *adj* & *n* antiemético
antifreeze *n* anticongelante *m*
antigen *n* antígeno
antihistamine *n* antihistamínico
antihypertensive *adj* & *n* antihipertensivo
antiinflammatory *adj* antiinflamatorio
antimicrobial *adj* & *n* antimicrobiano
antiperspirant *n* antitranspirante *m*

antipsychotic *adj & n* antipsicótico
antipyretic *adj & n* antipirético
antiseptic *adj & n* antiséptico
antiserum *n* (*pl* **-ra** *o* **-rums**) antisuero
antisocial *adj* antisocial
antispasmodic *adj & n* antiespasmódico, antiespástico
antitoxin *n* antitoxina
anus *n* (*pl* **anus** *o* **anuses**) ano
anxiety *n* ansiedad *f*, desesperación *f*, nervios (*fam*)
anxious *adj* ansioso
aorta *n* aorta
aortic *adj* aórtico
apathetic *adj* apático
apathy *n* apatía, indiferencia
Apgar score *n* índice *m* or valoración *f* de Apgar
aphasia *n* afasia
apnea *n* apnea; **sleep** —— apnea del sueño
apparatus *n* (*pl* **-tus** *o* **-tuses**) aparato
appearance *n* apariencia, aspecto
appendectomy *n* (*pl* **-mies**) apendicectomía
appendicitis *n* apendicitis *f*
appendix *n* (*pl* **-dixes** *o* **-dices**) apéndice *m*
appetite *n* apetito
apple *n* manzana
applesauce *n* puré *m* de manzana
application *n* aplicación *f*
applicator *n* aplicador *m*
apply *vt* (*pret & pp* **applied**) aplicar; **to** —— **to oneself** aplicarse
appointment *n* cita
appropriate *adj* adecuado, apropiado (*Ang*)
approximately *adv* aproximadamente
apraxia *n* apraxia
apron *n* delantal *m*; **lead** —— delantal de plomo
aptitude *n* aptitud *f*
aqueous *adj* acuoso; —— **humor** humor acuoso
ARC *abbr* **AIDS-related complex.** V. **complex.**
arch *n* arco; —— **of the foot** arco del pie; *vt, vi* arquear(se)
ARDS *abbr* **adult respiratory distress syndrome.** V. **syndrome.**
area *n* área, zona

Argentine, Argentinean *adj & n* argentino -na *mf*
arginine *n* arginina
arm *n* brazo
armpit *n* axila, sobaco (*fam*)
arnica *n* (*bot*) árnica
arouse *vt* (*from sleep*) despertar; (*sexually, etc.*) excitar
arrest *n* paro; **cardiac** —— paro cardiaco; **respiratory** —— paro respiratorio
arrhythmia *n* arritmia
arsenic *n* arsénico
arterial *adj* arterial
arteriosclerosis *n* arteriosclerosis *f*
arteriovenous *adj* arteriovenoso
arteritis *n* arteritis *f*; **temporal** *o* **giant cell** —— arteritis temporal
artery *n* (*pl* **-ries**) arteria; **brachial** —— arteria braquial; **carotid** —— arteria carótida; **coronary** —— arteria coronaria; **femoral** —— arteria femoral; **iliac** —— arteria iliaca; **radial** —— arteria radial; **subclavian** —— arteria subclavia
arthritic *adj* artrítico
arthritis *n* artritis *f*; **juvenile** —— artritis juvenil; **rheumatoid** —— artritis reumatoide
arthrogram *n* artrograma *m*, artrografía
arthrography *n* artrografía
arthroscopy *n* (*pl* **-pies**) artroscopia *or* (*esp spoken*) artroscopía
artificial *adj* artificial, postizo
asbestos *n* asbesto
ascariasis *n* ascariasis *f*, ascaridiasis *f*
Ascaris Ascaris
ascending *adj* ascendente
ascites *n* ascitis *f*
ascorbic acid *n* ácido ascórbico
ASD *abbr* **atrial septal defect.** V. **defect.**
aseptic *adj* aséptico
asleep *adj* dormido; **to fall** —— dormirse; **My foot fell asleep.**.Se me durmió el pie.
asparagine *n* asparagina
asparagus *n* espárrago
aspergillosis *n* aspergilosis *f*
asphyxia *n* asfixia
asphyxiate *vt, vi* asfixiar(se)
aspirate *vt* aspirar

aspiration *n* aspiración *f*; **joint** —— aspiración articular; **needle** —— aspiración con aguja

aspirin *n* aspirina

assault *n* asalto; *vt* asaltar

assist *vt* asistir

assistant *n* asistente *mf*, ayudante *mf*, auxiliar *mf*; **nursing** —— asistente de enfermera

associate *n* socio -cia *mf*

association *n* asociación *f*

astemizole *n* astemizol *m*

asthma *n* asma

asthmatic *adj* & *n* asmático -ca *mf*

astigmatism *n* astigmatismo

astringent *adj* & *n* astringente *m*

asylum *n* asilo; **insane** —— (*ant*) manicomio

ataxia *n* ataxia

ataxic *adj* atáxico

ate *pret de* eat

atenolol *n* atenolol *m*

atherosclerosis *n* aterosclerosis *f*

athlete *n* atleta *mf*; **athlete's foot** pie *m* de atleta

athletic *adj* atlético

athletic supporter *n* suspensorio

atmosphere *n* atmósfera

atopic *adj* atópico

atrial *adj* auricular

atrioventricular (A-V) *adj* auriculoventricular (AV)

atrium *n* (*pl* **atria**) (*of the heart*) aurícula

atrophy *n* atrofia; *vi* (*pret* & *pp* -**phied**) atrofiarse

atropine *n* atropina

attach *vt* ligar

attack *n* ataque *m*, acceso; **heart** —— ataque cardiaco *or* al corazón; **transient ischemic** —— isquemia cerebral transitoria; *vt* atacar

attend *vt* (*a clinic, class, etc.*) asistir a

attention *n* atención *f*

attenuated *adj* atenuado

attitude *n* actitud *f*

atypical *adj* atípico

audiogram *n* audiograma *m*

audiologist *n* audiólogo -ga *mf*

audiology *n* audiología

audiometer *n* audiómetro

audiometry *n* audiometría

audition *n* audición *f*

auditory *adj* auditivo; —— **tube** conducto auditivo

aunt *n* tía

aura *n* aura

autism *n* autismo

autist *n* (*form*) autista *mf*

autistic *adj* autístico; *n* autista *mf*

autoclave *n* autoclave *m*

autoimmune *adj* autoinmune

autoimmunity *n* autoinmunidad *f*

autologous *adj* autólogo

automobile *n* automóvil *m*

autopsy *n* (*pl* -**sies**) autopsia

autosomal *adj* autosómico

autumn *n* otoño

A-V *V.* atrioventricular.

available *adj* disponible

average *adj* **the** —— **height** el promedio de altura; *n* promedio; **on** —— como promedio

aversion *n* aversión *f*

avocado *n* aguacate *m*

avoid *vt* evitar; **You should avoid salt**..Debe evitar la sal.

awake *adj* despierto

axilla *n* (*pl* -**lae**) axila

axillary *adj* axilar

axis *n* (*pl* **axes**) eje *m*

azathioprine *n* azatioprina

azithromycin *n* azitromicina

B

babble n (*sounds made by baby*) balbuceo; vi balbucear

baby n (*pl* -**bies**) bebé m, criatura

baby-sitter n persona que cuida niños, niñera

bacillus n (*pl* -**li**) bacilo; **Calmette-Guérin** —— (**BCG**) bacilo de Calmette-Guérin (BCG)

bacitracin n bacitracina

back adj de atrás; adv atrás; n espalda; (*of the hand*) dorso; **the back of**..la parte de atrás de; **lower** —— parte baja de la espalda

backache n dolor m de espalda

backbone n columna vertebral, espina dorsal, columna (*fam*)

backup n respaldo

backward adv hacia atrás

bacon n tocino

bacteria pl de **bacterium**

bacterial adj bacteriano

bactericidal adj bactericida

bacterium n (*pl* -**ria**) bacteria (*en inglés se emplea casi siempre la forma plural:* **bacteria**); **Bacteria cause disease**..Las bacterias causan enfermedades.

Bacteroides Bacteroides

bad adj (*comp* **worse**; *super* **worst**) malo; **Salt is bad for you**..La sal le hace mal...**a bad cold**..un resfriado fuerte; —— **for one's health** malo or nocivo para la salud

bag n bolsa; —— **of waters** fuente f, bolsa de las aguas; **bags under one's eyes** bolsas bajo los ojos; **doctor's** —— maletín del médico; **hot-water** —— bolsa de agua caliente

bake vt cocer al horno, hornear

baker n panadero -ra mf

balance n (*equilibrium*) equilibrio

balanced adj balanceado, equilibrado

balanitis n balanitis f

bald adj calvo

baldness n calvicie f

balloon n (*of a Foley catheter, etc.*) balón m

balls npl (*vulg*) testículos, huevos (*vulg*), cojones mpl (*vulg*)

balm n bálsamo; **lip** —— crema para los labios

banana n plátano

band n cinta, banda, faja

bandage n vendaje m, (*material*) venda; **Mr. Mata's bandage is dirty**..El vendaje del señor Mata está sucio...**We need a new bandage**..Necesitamos una nueva venda; **adhesive** —— venda adhesiva; **butterfly** —— cinta de mariposa; **elastic** —— venda elástica

Band-Aid n Curita m&f (*Both terms are trademarks. Los dos términos son marcas.*)

bands npl frenos, frenillos

barbecue vt asar a la parrilla

barbed wire n alambre m de púas

barber n peluquero -ra mf, barbero

barbiturate n barbitúrico

barefoot adj descalzo, sin zapatos

barf (*vulg*) n vómito; vt, vi arrojar, devolver, deponer (*Mex*), tener basca, vomitar

barium n bario

bark n (*bot*) corteza

barrel n (*of a syringe*) barril m

barrier n barrera

basal ganglia npl ganglios basales

base n (*chem, pharm, etc.*) base f; **oil-based** a base de aceite; **water-based** a base de agua

baseball n béisbol m

baseline adj basal; n (*behavior, physical*

exam) estado habitual (*para el paciente*); (*lab value*) nivel habitual

bashful *adj* tímido

basic *adj* básico

basin *n* palangana, vasija; **emesis** —— riñón *m*, riñonera, escupidera

basketball *n* baloncesto, basketball *m* (*Ang*)

bassinet *n* moisés *m*

bat *n* (*zool*) murciélago

bath *n* baño (*de tina*); **sitz** —— baño de asiento; **sponge** —— baño de esponja; **steam** —— baño de vapor; **to take a** —— bañarse

bathe *vt, vi* bañar(se)

bathroom *n* baño; **to go to the** —— ir al baño

bathtub *n* tina (de baño), bañera, bañadera (*Cub*)

BCG *abbr* **Calmette-Guérin bacillus. V. bacillus.**

beam *n* (*light, X-ray, etc.*) rayo

beans *npl* frijoles *mpl*

bear *vt* (*pret* **bore**; *pp* **borne** *o* **born**) (*to give birth to*) dar a luz, parir (*esp Carib, fam*); (*to endure*) tolerar, aguantar, soportar; *vi* **to** —— **down** pujar; **Bear down as if you were having a bowel movement..** Puje como si estuviera defecando.

bearable *adj* tolerable, soportable

beard *n* barba

beat *n* (*of the heart*) latido; *vi* (*pret* **beat**; *pp* **beaten** *o* **beat**) latir

beclomethasone *n* beclometasona

bed *n* cama; (*sickbed, deathbed, fig*) lecho; **to stay in** —— guardar cama, quedarse en cama; **vascular** —— lecho vascular

bedbug *n* chinche *f*

bedclothes *npl* ropa de cama

bedding *n* ropa de cama

bedpan *n* bacinilla, pato, cómodo (*Mex*)

bedrail *n* barandal *m*, baranda

bedridden *adj* postrado en cama

bedroom *n* cuarto, dormitorio, recámara

bedside *n* lado de la cama

bedsore *n* llaga (*debida a permanecer mucho tiempo sin cambiar de posición*)

bed-wetting *n* enuresis *f* (*form*); (el) orinarse en la cama

bee *n* abeja; **Africanized** *o* **killer** —— abeja africanizada *or* asesina

beef *n* carne *f* de res, res *f*

beefsteak *n* bistec *m*

beeper *n* bíper *m* (*Ang*)

beer *n* cerveza

beginning *n* comienzo, principio

behavior *n* conducta, comportamiento; —— **modification** modificación de la conducta

behind *n* (*fam*) trasero

belch *vi* eructar

belief *n* creencia

belladonna *n* belladona

Bell's palsy *n* parálisis *f* de Bell, parálisis facial

belly *n* (*pl* **-lies**) vientre *m*, barriga, panza, estómago (*fam*)

bellyache *n* dolor *m* de barriga

bellybutton *n* (*fam*) ombligo

belt *n* cinto, cinturón *m*, correa

benazepril *n* benazepril *m*

bend *n* curva, ángulo; *vt* (*pret & pp* **bent**) doblar; **Bend your knee..**Doble la rodilla; **to** —— **one's head down** bajar *or* agachar la cabeza; **Bend your head down..** Baje la cabeza; *vi* doblarse; **to** —— **over** *o* **down** doblarse; **Bend over..**Dóblese.

bends *n* enfermedad *f* por descompresión

beneficial *adj* benéfico

benefit *n* bien *m*, beneficio; **for your** —— por su bien

benign *adj* benigno

bent *pret & pp de* **bend**

benzedrine *n* bencedrina

benzene *n* benceno

benzodiazepine *n* benzodiacepina

benzoin *n* benzoína, benjuí *m*

benzoyl peroxide *n* peróxido de benzoílo

beriberi *n* beriberi *m*

beta *n* beta; —— **blocker** beta bloqueador *m*

beta-hemolytic *adj* beta hemolítico

better *adj & adv* (*comp de* **good** *y* **well**) mejor; **to get** —— mejorarse

bib *n* babero

bicarbonate *n* bicarbonato

biceps *n* bíceps *m*

bicuspid *adj & n* bicúspide *m*

bicycle n bicicleta; **stationary** —— bicicleta fija; **to ride a** —— ir or montar en bicicleta

bifocal adj bifocal; npl (fam) lentes mpl bifocales, bifocales mpl (fam)

big adj (comp **bigger**; super **biggest**) grande; **How big was it?**..¿Qué tan grande era? **to get bigger** crecer, ponerse más grande

bile n bilis f

biliary adj biliar

bilingual adj bilingüe

bilirubin n bilirrubina

bill n (charges) cuenta, cobro

bind vi (clothing, etc.) apretar

binder n faja, faja abdominal

binge n borrachera (esp por varios días seguidos)

biochemical adj bioquímico

biochemistry n bioquímica

biodegradable adj biodegradable

biofeedback n biorretroalimentación f

biological, biologic adj biológico

biology n biología

biopsy n (pl **-sies**) biopsia; **needle** —— biopsia con aguja; **open** —— biopsia abierta

biorhythm n ritmo biológico

biostatistics n bioestadística

bipolar adj bipolar

bird n pájaro

birth n nacimiento; (childbirth) parto, alumbramiento; —— **canal** canal m del parto; —— **certificate** certificado or acta de nacimiento; —— **control** control m de la natalidad, método anticonceptivo; **Do you use birth control?**..¿Usa algún método anticonceptivo?; ——**control pill** píldora anticonceptiva; **natural** —— parto or alumbramiento natural; **to give** —— dar a luz, aliviarse (Mex, fam); **She gave birth to a baby girl**..Dio a luz una niña.

birthday n cumpleaños m; **Happy birthday!**..¡Feliz cumpleaños!

birthing n parto natural

birthmark n marca de nacimiento, lunar m

birthweight n peso al nacimiento, peso al nacer

bisexual adj bisexual

bismuth n bismuto

bite n mordida, mordedura; (insect) piquete m, picadura; vt, vi (pret **bit**; pp **bitten** o **bit**) morder; (insect) picar; **Bite down, please**..Apriete los dientes, por favor.

bitter adj amargo

black adj negro; n (person) negro -gra mf, moreno -na mf; **to** —— **out** desmayarse, perder el conocimiento

black-and-blue adj amoratado, moreteado

black eye n ojo morado

blackhead n espinilla

blackout n (faint) desmayo; (lapse of memory) laguna mental

black widow n viuda negra

bladder n vejiga

blade n hoja

bland adj (food) no picante, sin sabor fuerte

blanket n frazada, cobija (Mex), friza (PR, SD); **electric** —— frazada or cobija eléctrica, cobertor eléctrico

blastomycosis n blastomicosis f

bleach n blanqueador m, cloro

bled pret & pp de **bleed**

bleed n hemorragia, sangrado, (cerebral) derrame m; vi (pret & pp **bled**) sangrar

bleeding adj sangrante; —— **ulcer** úlcera sangrante; n hemorragia, sangrado

bleomycin n bleomicina

blepharitis n blefaritis f

blew pret de **blow**

blind adj ciego

blindness n ceguera; **color** —— daltonismo (form), dificultad f para diferenciar ciertos colores; **night** —— ceguera nocturna

blink n parpadeo; vi parpadear

blister n ampolla, vesícula; **fever** —— fuego, ampolla en los labios (debida al herpes)

bloated adj hinchado; (stomach) hinchado, inflado (del estómago); **She looks bloated**..Se ve hinchada...**Do you get bloated after you eat?**..¿Se le hincha el estómago después de comer?

block n bloqueo; **bundle branch** —— bloqueo de rama; **heart** —— bloqueo cardiaco; vt (pharm, physio) bloquear; (anat, surg) obstruir (form), tapar (fam)

blockage *n* obstrucción *f*

blocked *adj* obstruído (*form*), tapado

blocker *n* bloqueador *m*; **beta** —— beta bloqueador; **calcium channel** —— bloqueador de los canales de calcio; **H₂-blocker** bloqueador de los receptores H₂

blond *adj* rubio, güero (*Mex*); *n* rubio, güero

blonde *n* rubia, güera (*Mex*)

blood *n* sangre *f*; —— **flow** flujo sanguíneo (*form*), circulación *f*; —— **poisoning** envenenamiento de la sangre; —— **pressure** presión *f* arterial (*form*), presión sanguínea, presión (*de la sangre*) (*fam*); —— **pressure cuff** esfigmomanómetro, baumanómetro, tensiómetro, aparato para medir la presión (*fam*); —— **type** grupo sanguíneo (*form*), tipo de sangre; —— **vessel** vaso sanguíneo; **arterial** —— **gas** gasometría, gases *mpl* arteriales

blood bank *n* banco de sangre

blood-borne *adj* transmitido a través de la sangre

bloodshot *adj* rojos (*los ojos*)

bloodstream *n* torrente sanguíneo

blood thinner *n* (*fam*) anticoagulante *m*

bloody *adj* sanguinolento, con mucha sangre

bloody nose *n* (*fam*) sangrado por la nariz, hemorragia nasal

bloody show (*obst*) *n* sangrado vaginal (*antes de la expulsión del feto*)

blot *vt* (*pret & pp* **blotted**; *ger* **blotting**) secar por presión con material absorbente

blotch *n* mancha, roncha, grano

blouse *n* blusa

blow *n* (*stroke*) golpe *m*; *vt* (*pret* **blew**; *pp* **blown**) **to** —— **one's nose** sonarse *or* soplarse (*Carib*) la nariz; *vi* (*to breathe out air forcefully*) soplar; **Blow as hard as you can**..Sople lo más fuerte que pueda.

blue *adj* azul; (*fam, sad*) triste; *n* **the blues** (*fam*) tristeza, melancolía

bluish *adj* azulado

blur *vi* (*pret & pp* **blurred**; *ger* **blurring**) (*one's vision*) empañarse *or* borrarse (*la vista*)

blurred *adj* empañado, borroso; —— **vision** vista empañada, visión borrosa; **Do you get blurred vision?**..¿Se le empaña la vista?

blurry *adj* empañado, borroso

BM *abbr* bowel movement. *V.* bowel.

body *n* (*pl* **bodies**) cuerpo; —— **heat** calor *m* corporal; —— **image** imagen *f* corporal; —— **language** lenguaje *m* corporal

bodybuilder *n* fisicoculturista *mf*

boil *n* furúnculo (*form*), absceso (*de la piel*), nacido (*esp Carib*); *vt* (*water*) hervir, hacer hervir; (*meat, etc.*) cocer, hacer cocer; *vi* hervir

boiled *adj* hervido; —— **water** agua hervida

Bolivian *adj & n* boliviano -na *mf*

bomb *n* bomba; **atomic** —— bomba atómica

bond (*psych, obst*) *n* vínculo, enlace *m*; *vi* formar un vínculo *or* enlace (con)

bonding (*psych, obst*) *n* formación *f* de un vínculo *or* enlace, enlazamiento (*form*)

bone *adj* óseo; —— **marrow** médula ósea; *n* hueso

booklet *n* folleto

booster *adj* de refuerzo; —— **shot** revacunación *f*, inyección *f* de refuerzo

boot *n* bota

booze *n* (*vulg*) bebida alcohólica

border *n* (*edge, margin*) borde *m*, margen *m*

bore *vt* aburrir; **to become bored** aburrirse

bore *pret de* bear

boric acid *n* ácido bórico

born (*pret & pp de* **bear**) *adj* nacido; **to be** —— nacer

borne *pp de* bear

bother *vt* molestar; **Is your neck bothering you?**..¿Le molesta el cuello?

bottle *n* botella; (*for pills*) frasco, pomo; **hot-water** —— bolsa de agua caliente; **nursing** —— *o* **baby's** —— biberón *m*, mamadera, pacha (*CA*)

bottom *n* fondo; (*fam, buttocks*) nalgas, trasero, sentaderas

botulism *n* botulismo

bout *n* ataque *m*, episodio

bovine *adj* bovino

bowel *n* intestino, tripa (*frec pl*); —— **movement (BM)** defecación *f* (*form*), evacuación *f*, deposición *f* (*SA*); **large** —— intestino grueso; **small** —— intestino delgado; **to have a** —— **movement** defecar (*form*) evacuar (*form*), hacer del baño (*fam*), obrar (*esp Mex, CA*), hacer popó *or* pupú (*fam, esp ped*), dar del cuerpo (*Carib, fam*); **When did you have your last bowel movement?**..¿Cuándo fue la última vez que defecó (evacuó, hizo del baño, etc.)?

bowlegged *adj* con las piernas arqueadas, zambo

boy *n* niño, muchacho

boyfriend *n* novio, amigo íntimo, amigo

bra *V.* **brassiere**.

brace *n* aparato ortopédico (*para estabilizar una articulación*)

braces *npl* frenos, frenillos

bradycardia *n* bradicardia

Braille *n* Braille *m*

brain *n* cerebro; —— **wave** onda cerebral

brainstem *n* tallo cerebral

bran *n* salvado, afrecho

branch *n* rama

brand *n* marca

brassiere *n* brassiere *m*, sostén *m*, ajustador *m* (*Cub*)

Brazilian *adj & n* brasileño -ña *mf*

bread *n* pan *m*

break *n* (*ortho*) fractura, quebradura; (*chromosome*) rompimiento; *vt, vi* (*pret* **broke**; *pp* **broken**) (*ortho*) fracturar(se), quebrar(se), romper(se) (*esp Carib*), partir(se) (*Cub*); **My foot broke**..Se me quebró el pie...**I broke my foot**..Me quebré el pie...**How did you break your foot?**..¿Cómo se quebró el pie? **to** —— **down** (*degrade*) degradar; **to** —— **out** (*one's skin*) salirle granos *or* barros; **When did your skin break out?**..¿Cuándo le salieron granos?

breakdown *n* colapso; **nervous** —— choque *or* colapso nervioso, crisis nerviosa

breakfast *n* desayuno; **to have** —— desayunar(se)

breast *n* mama, seno, pecho

breastbone *n* esternón *m* (*form*), hueso del pecho

breast-feed *vt* amamantar (*form*), dar pecho, dar de mamar; **Are you breast-feeding**

him?..¿Le está dando pecho?

breast-feeding *n* lactancia maternal, (el) dar pecho

breast pump *n* extractor *m* de leche, saca-leche *m*, tiraleche *m*

breath *n* aliento; **bad** —— mal aliento; **shortness of** —— falta del aire, sensación *f* de ahogo; **to be short of** —— faltarle la respiración *or* el aire; **Are you short of breath?**..¿Le falta la respiración?...**Do you get short of breath when you walk?**..¿Le falta el aire cuando camina?...**How many blocks can you walk before you get short of breath?**..¿Cuántas cuadras puede caminar antes que le falte el aire? **to hold one's** —— detener *or* aguantar la respi-ración; **Hold your breath**..Detenga la respiración; **to take a deep** —— respirar profundo, hacer una respiración profunda; **Take a deep breath**..Respire profundo.

breathe *vt, vi* respirar; **to** —— **in** inspirar (*form*), respirar (*fam*), tomar aire (*fam*); **Breathe in**..Respire..Tome aire; **to** —— **out** expulsar el aire (*form*), sacar aire (*esp Mex, CA; fam*), botar aire (*esp Carib, SA; fam*)

breech presentation *n* presentación pélvica (*form*), presentación de nalgas

bridge *n* (*dent, etc.*) puente *m*

brief *adj* breve

bring *vt* **to** —— **on** (*pain, etc.*) provocar, causar

bristle *n* (*of a brush*) cerda

broil *vt* asar, asar a la parrilla

broke *pret de* **break**

broken (*pp de* break) *adj* quebrado, roto

bromocriptine *n* bromocriptina

bronchial *adj* bronquial

bronchiectasis *n* bronquiectasia

bronchiole *n* (*pl* -**li**) bronquiolo

bronchiolitis *n* bronquiolitis *f*

bronchitis *n* bronquitis *f*

bronchodilator *n* broncodilatador *m*

bronchogenic *adj* broncogénico *or* bron-cógeno

bronchopneumonia *n* bronconeumonía

bronchoscope *n* broncoscopio

bronchoscopy *n* (*pl* -**pies**) broncoscopia *or*

(*esp spoken*) broncoscopía

bronchospasm *n* broncospasmo *or* bronco-espasmo

bronchus *n* (*pl* -**chi**) bronquio

broth *n* caldo

brother *n* hermano

brother-in-law *n* (*pl* **brothers-in-law**) cuñado

brow *n* frente *f*

brown *adj* café, marrón

brucellosis *n* brucelosis *f*

bruise *n* contusión *f* (*form*), moretón *m*, morete *m*, magulladura, lastimadura; *vt* causar moretones; *vi* hacerse moretones; **Do you bruise easily?**..¿Se le hacen moretones fácilmente?...**Did you bruise your hand?**..¿Se hizo un morete en la mano?

bruised *adj* (*one place*) que tiene moretón, (*all over*) amoratado, moreteado

brunette *adj* moreno, trigueño; *n* morena, trigueña

brush *n* cepillo; *vt* cepillar; **to ―― one's hair** cepillarse el pelo; **to ―― one's teeth** cepillarse los dientes

brushing *n* cepillado

bruxism *n* bruxismo

bubble *n* burbuja

bubo *n* (*pl* **buboes**) bubón *m*

bubonic *adj* bubónico

buckle *n* hebilla; *vt* abrochar(se)

buckteeth *n* dientes salidos

buffer *n* tampón *m*, amortiguador *m*, buffer *m*; **―― solution** solución amortiguadora

bug *n* insecto, bicho; (*fam*) microbio, virus *m*

build *n* físico, complexión *f*; *vt* **to ―― up** (*one's strength, muscles, etc.*) fortalecer; (*one's resistance*) aumentar (*las defensas*); *vi* **to ―― up** acumularse

buildup *n* depósito, acumulación *f*

bulb *n* bulbo

bulb syringe *n* perilla, pera

bulimia *n* bulimia

bulimic *adj* bulímico

bullet *n* bala

bumetanide *n* bumetanida

bump *n* protuberancia (*form*), bola, bolita, pelota, (*due to trauma, esp about the head*) chichón *m*

bunion *n* juanete *m*

burdock *n* (*bot*) bardana

burn *n* quemadura; *vt* (*pret & pp* **burned** *o* **burnt**) quemar; **Did you burn your hand?**..¿Se quemó la mano? **to ―― oneself** *o* **to get burned** quemarse; **Did you burn yourself?**..¿Se quemó? *vi* arder; **Does it burn when your urinate?**..¿Le arde al orinar?

burning *adj* ardiente, quemante; *n* ardor *m*

burp *vt* (*a baby*) sacar el aire, hacer eructar; **You should burp your baby after each meal**..Debe sacarle el aire a su bebé después de cada comida; *vi* eructar

burr *n* (*plant*) espina, cadillo; (*metal*) rebaba, astilla (*de metal*)

bursa *n* bolsa

bursitis *n* bursitis *f*

burst *vt, vi* (*pret & pp* **burst**) reventar(se)

buspirone *n* buspirona

bust *n* busto

busulfan *n* busulfán *m*

butcher *n* carnicero -ra *mf*

butt *n* (*vulg*) nalgas

butter *n* mantequilla

buttock *n* glúteo, nalga (*fam*)

button *vt* (*también* **to ―― up**) abotonar(se), abrochar(se)

buzz *n* zumbido; *vi* zumbar

buzzing *n* zumbido

bypass *n* puente coronario, derivación *f*, bypass *m* (*Ang*)

C

cactus *n* (*pl* **-tuses** *o* **-ti**) cacto, cactus
cadaver *n* cadáver *m*
cadmium *n* cadmio
caffeine *n* cafeína
calamine *n* calamina
calcify *vt, vi* (*pret & pp* **-fied**) calcificar(se)
calcitonin *n* calcitonina
calcium *n* calcio; —— **carbonate** carbonato de calcio; —— **channel blocker** bloqueador *m* de los canales de calcio; —— **gluconate** gluconato de calcio
calf *n* (*pl* **calves**) (*anat*) pantorrilla
calibrate *vt* calibrar
calisthenics *n* calistenia
call, on de guardia
callus *n* (*pl* **-luses**) callo, (*thin*) callosidad *f*
calm *adj* tranquilo, quieto; *n* calma; *vt* calmar; *vi* **to** —— **down** calmarse
calomel *n* calomel *m*
calorie *n* caloría
campaign *n* campaña
camphor *n* alcanfor *m*
Campylobacter Campylobacter
can *n* lata, bote *m*
canal *n* canal *m*, conducto; **auditory** —— canal auditivo; **birth** —— canal del parto; **semicircular** —— conducto semicircular
cancel *vt* (*pret & pp* **-celed** *o* **-celled**; *ger* **-celing** *o* **-celling**) cancelar
cancer *n* cáncer *m*; **breast** —— cáncer de la mama (*form*), cáncer del seno *or* pecho; **lung** ——, **prostate** ——, **etc.** cáncer del pulmón, cáncer de la próstata, etc.
cancerous *adj* canceroso
Candida Candida
candidiasis *n* candidiasis *f*
candy *n* (*pl* **-dies**) (*one piece*) dulce *m*, (*collective*) dulces
cane *n* bastón *m*

canker sore *n* afta, pequeña úlcera en la boca
cannula *n* cánula; **nasal** —— cánula nasal
cap *n* (*of a bottle*) tapa; (*of a needle*) protector *m* (*para una aguja*); (*dent*) corona; (*head covering*) gorro; **bathing** *o* **shower** —— gorro de baño; **cervical** —— capuchón *m* cervical; **safety** —— tapa de seguridad
capable *adj* capaz
capacity *n* (*pl* **-ties**) capacidad *f*
capillary *n* (*pl* **-ries**) capilar *m*
capsule *n* cápsula
captopril *n* captopril *m*
car *n* coche *m*, carro
carat *n* quilate *m*; **14** —— **gold** oro de 14 quilates
carbamazepine *n* carbamazepina *o* carbamacepina
carbidopa *n* carbidopa
carbohydrate *n* carbohidrato
carbon *n* (*element*) carbono; —— **dioxide** bióxido *or* dióxido de carbono; —— **monoxide** monóxido de carbono; —— **tetrachloride** tetracloruro de carbono
carbonate *n* carbonato
carbonated *adj* carbonatado
carbuncle *n* carbunco
carcinoembryonic antigen *n* antígeno carcinoembriónico
carcinoid *adj & n* carcinoide *m*
carcinoma *n* carcinoma *m*; **basal cell** —— carcinoma basocelular; **oat cell** —— carcinoma de células en avena; **small cell** —— carcinoma de células pequeñas; **squamous cell** —— carcinoma espinocelular *or* de células escamosas
card *n* (*hospital, business, etc.*) tarjeta
cardiac *adj* cardiaco *or* cardíaco

cardiogenic *adj* cardiogénico *or* cardiógeno

cardiologist *n* cardiólogo -ga *mf*

cardiology *n* cardiología

cardiomyopathy *n* cardiomiopatía; **dilated** —— cardiomiopatía dilatada; **hypertrophic** —— cardiomiopatía hipertrófica; **restrictive** —— cardiomiopatía restrictiva

cardiopulmonary *adj* cardiopulmonar; —— **resuscitation (CPR)** resucitación *f or* reanimación *f* cardiopulmonar (RCP)

cardiovascular *adj* cardiovascular

cardioversion *n* cardioversión *f*

carditis *n* carditis *f*

care *n* cuidado, atención *f*; **health** —— atención médica, servicios médicos; **intensive** —— cuidados intensivos, terapia intensiva; **prenatal** —— atención prenatal; **primary** —— atención primaria *or* del primer nivel; **tertiary** —— atención del tercer nivel; **to take** —— cuidar a, atender a; **Who takes care of your mother at home?**..¿Quién cuida a su madre en casa? **to take** —— **of oneself** cuidarse; **You should take care of yourself better**..Debe cuidarse más; *vi* **to** —— **for** cuidar a, atender a

careful *adj* **to be** —— tener cuidado; **Be careful with this medicine**..Tenga cuidado con esta medicina.

caregiver *n* cuidador -ra *mf*

careless *adj* descuidado

carelessness *n* descuido

caretaker *n* cuidador -ra *mf*

caries *n* caries *f*

carotid *adj* carótido

carpal *adj* carpiano

carpenter *n* carpintero

carrier *n* portador -ra *mf*

carrot *n* zanahoria

carsickness *n* mareo (*en un vehículo*)

cartilage *n* cartílago

cascara sagrada *n* (*bot*) cáscara sagrada

case *n* caso; **nine out of ten cases**..nueve de diez casos; **just in** —— por si acaso, para estar seguro, por precaución

cast *n* (*ortho*) yeso; **urinary** —— cilindro urinario

castor oil *n* aceite *m* de ricino

castrate *vt* castrar

castration *n* castración *f*

cat *n* gato

CAT *abbr* **computerized axial tomography.** *V.* **tomography.**

cataract *n* catarata

catatonia *n* catatonía

catatonic *adj* catatónico

catch *vt* (*pret & pp* **caught**) (*a disease*) darle (*a uno*), pegarle (*a uno*), coger; **I caught a cold**..Me dio un catarro; **to** —— **one's breath** recobrar *or* recuperar el aliento

catching (*fam*) *adj* contagioso

caterpillar *n* oruga

catgut *n* catgut *m*

catheter *n* catéter *m*, sonda; **Foley** —— sonda Foley; **Hickman** —— catéter Hickman; **Tenckhoff** —— catéter Tenckhoff

catheterization *n* cateterismo; **cardiac** —— cateterismo cardiaco

caught *pret & pp de* **catch**

cauliflower *n* coliflor *f*

causalgia *n* causalgia

cause *n* causa; *vt* causar

caustic *adj* cáustico

cauterization *n* cauterización *f*

cauterize *vt* cauterizar

cavity *n* (*pl* -ties) cavidad *f*; **You have a cavity**..Tiene un diente picado..Tiene una cavidad...**You have cavities**..Tiene caries.

cc. *V.* **cubic centimeter.**

cecum *n* (*pl* **ceca**) ciego

cefaclor *n* cefaclor *m*

cefadroxil *n* cefadroxil *m*

cefixime *n* cefixima

cefotaxime *n* cefotaxima

cefprozil *n* cefprozil *m*

ceftriaxone *n* ceftriaxona

cefuroxime axetil *n* acetilcefuroxima

celery *n* apio

celiac *adj* celiaco *or* celíaco

celibate *adj* que no tiene relaciones sexuales

cell *n* célula; **B** —— célula B; **plasma** —— célula plasmática; **red blood** —— glóbulo rojo; **T** —— célula T; **white blood** —— glóbulo blanco

cellulite *n* celulitis *f*

cellulitis *n* celulitis *f*

center *n* centro; **day-care** —— guardería infantil (*esp para niños de madres que trabajan durante el día*); **healthcare** —— centro de salud

centigrade *adj* centígrado

centimeter (cm.) *n* centímetro (cm.); —— **cubed** *o* **cubic** —— (**cc.**) centímetro cúbico (cc.)

centipede *n* ciempiés *m*

central *adj* central; —— **line** catéter *m* central

cephalexin *n* cefalexina

cephalic *adj* cefálico

cephalosporin *n* cefalosporina

cephalothin *n* cefalotina

cerclage *n* cerclaje *m*

cereal *n* cereal *m*

cerebellum *n* (*pl* -**la**) cerebelo

cerebral *adj* cerebral; —— **palsy** parálisis *f* cerebral

cerebrovascular *adj* cerebrovascular

cerebrum *n* (*pl* -**brums** *o* -**bra**) cerebro

certificate *n* certificado, partida; **birth** —— certificado *or* acta de nacimiento; **death** —— certificado de defunción

cervical *adj* cervical

cervicitis *n* cervicitis *f*

cervix *n* (*pl* -**vixes** *o* -**vices**) cérvix *f*, cuello de la matriz

cesarean section *n* operación cesárea

chafe *n* rozadura; *vt, vi* rozar(se)

chair *n* silla

chalazion *n* (*pl* -**zia**) chalazión *m*

chamber *n* cámara

chamomile *n* (*bot*) manzanilla

chancre *n* chancro; **soft** —— chancro blando

chancroid *n* chancroide *f*

change *n* cambio; —— **of life** cambio de vida; *vt, vi* cambiar

chap *vi* agrietarse, partirse (*debido a la resequedad*)

chapped *adj* agrietado, partido (*debido a la resequedad*)

Chap Stick *n* (*marca*) crema para los labios, lápiz *m* para labios partidos

characteristic *adj* característico; *n* carac-

terística

charcoal *n* carbón *m*; **activated** —— carbón activado

charge *n* costo, cobro

charity *n* caridad *f*

charlatan *n* charlatán -na *mf*

charley horse (*fam*) *n* calambre *m*

chart *n* tabla; (*medical record*) expediente *m*; **eye** —— carta de examen visual; **Snellen** —— carta de Snellen

chatter *vi* (*one's teeth*) castañetear

check *vt* revisar, chequear (*Ang*)

checkup *n* chequeo

cheek *n* mejilla; (*fam, buttock*) nalga

cheekbone *n* pómulo

cheerful *adj* alegre

cheese *n* queso

chelated *adj* quelado

chemical *adj* químico; *n* substancia química

chemistry *n* química

chemo *V.* **chemotherapy**.

chemotherapy *n* (*pl* -**pies**) quimioterapia

chest *n* pecho

chew *vt, vi* masticar

chewable *adj* masticable

chewing gum *n* chicle *m*

chicken *n* pollo

chickenpox *n* varicela, viruelas locas (*Mex, CA*)

chickweed *n* (*bot*) pamplina

chigger *n* nigua

child *n* (*pl* **children**) niño -ña *mf*

childbirth *n* parto, alumbramiento

childhood *n* niñez *f*, infancia

childproof *adj* a prueba de niños

children *pl de* **child**

Chilean *adj & n* chileno -na *mf*

chili *n* chile *m*

chill *n* escalofrío

chin *n* barbilla, mentón *m*

chip *n* pedacito, astilla; *vt, vi* astillar(se), quebrar(se)

chiropodist *n* quiropodista *mf*, podíatra *or* podiatra *mf*

chiropractic *n* quiropráctica

chiropractor *n* quiropráctico -ca *mf*

Chlamydia Chlamydia

chloral hydrate *n* hidrato de cloral

chlorambucil *n* clorambucilo
chloramphenicol *n* cloranfenicol *m*
chlordane *n* clordano
chlorhexidine *n* clorhexidina
chloride *n* cloruro
chlorinated *adj* clorado
chlorination *n* cloración *f*
chlorine *n* cloro
chloroform *n* cloroformo
chloroquine *n* cloroquina
chlorpheniramine *n* clorfeniramina
chlorpromazine *n* cloropromacina
chlorpropamide *n* clorpropamida
chocolate *n* chocolate *m*
choke *vt* estrangular; *vi* (*due to fumes, lack of air, etc.*) asfixiarse, sofocarse, ahogarse; **to —— on** (*food, etc.*) atragantarse con
cholangiocarcinoma *n* colangiocarcinoma *m*
cholangiogram *n* colangiograma *m*, colangiografía
cholangiography *n* colangiografía; **percutaneous transhepatic —— (PTC)** colangiografía transhepática percutánea
cholangitis *n* colangitis *f*
cholecystectomy *n* (*pl* -**mies**) colecistectomía
cholecystitis *n* colecistitis *f*
cholelithiasis *n* colelitiasis *f*
cholera *n* cólera *m*
cholesteatoma *n* colesteatoma
cholesterol *n* colesterol *m*
cholestyramine *n* colestiramina
chondrosarcoma *n* condrosarcoma *m*
chorea *n* corea; **Huntington's ——** corea de Huntington
choriocarcinoma *n* coriocarcinoma *m*
chorioretinitis *n* coriorretinitis *f*
chromium *n* cromo
chromomycosis *n* cromomicosis *f*
chromosome *n* cromosoma *m*
chronic *adj* crónico
cigar *n* puro, tabaco (*esp Carib*)
cigarette *n* cigarro, cigarrillo
cimetidine *n* cimetidina
ciprofloxacin *n* ciprofloxacina
circadian *adj* circadiano
circle *n* círculo; (*under one's eye*) ojera
circulate *vi* circular

circulation *n* circulación *f*; **collateral ——** circulación colateral; **fetal ——** circulación fetal; **pulmonary ——** circulación pulmonar; **systemic ——** circulación sistémica *or* mayor
circulatory *adj* circulatorio
circumcise *vt* circuncidar
circumcised *adj* circunciso
circumcision *n* circuncisión *f*
cirrhosis *n* cirrosis *f*
cirrhotic *adj & n* cirrótico -ca *mf*
cisapride *n* cisaprida
cisplatin *n* cisplatin *m*
citrate *n* citrato
citric *adj* cítrico
citrus fruit *n* (*pl* **fruit** *o* **fruits**) fruta cítrica
clammy *adj* pegajoso y frío
clamp *n* pinza *or* pinzas; *vt* pinzar
clap *n* (*vulg*) gonorrea
clarithromycin *n* claritromicina
class *n* clase *f*
classic *adj* clásico
claudication *n* claudicación *f*; **intermittent ——** claudicación intermitente
claustrophobia *n* claustrofobia
clavicle *n* clavícula
claw *n* garra; *vt* arañar
clean *adj* limpio; *vt* limpiar
cleaning *n* (*dent, etc.*) limpieza
cleanliness *n* limpieza
clear *adj* claro, transparente; *vi* **to —— one's throat** aclarar la garganta, garraspear *or* carraspear; **to —— up** (*a rash, illness, etc.*) resolverse
cleft palate *n* paladar hendido
clench *vt* (*teeth, fist*) apretar *or* cerrar fuerte (*los dientes, el puño*)
click *n* (*card*) chasquido; *vi* (*joint*) tronar; **My knee clicks when I bend it.**..Me truena la rodilla al doblarla.
climate *n* clima *m*
climax *n* orgasmo
clindamycin *n* clindamicina
clinic *n* clínica; **urgent care ——** clínica de urgencias
clinical *adj* clínico
clinician *n* médico clínico
clip (*surg*) *n* pinza; *vt* pinzar

clitoris *n* (*pl* -**rides**) clítoris *m*
clofazimine *n* clofazimina
clofibrate *n* clofibrato
clomiphene *n* clomifén *m*
clonazepam *n* clonacepam *m*
clone *n* clona
clonic *adj* clónico
clonidine *n* clonidina
clonus *n* clonus *m*, clono
close *vt* cerrar; **Close your eyes**..Cierre los ojos; *vi* cerrar(se)
Clostridium Clostridium
clot *n* coágulo; *vt, vi* (*pret & pp* **clotted**; *ger* **clotting**) coagular(se)
cloth *n* (*for compress, etc.*) lienzo, paño
clothes *npl* ropa
clothing *n* ropa
clotrimazole *n* clotrimazol *m*
cloud *vi* (*también* to —— up) (*one's vision*) nublarse
cloudy *adj* (*comp* -**ier**; *super* -**iest**) (*vision*) nublado; (*urine*) turbio
clubfoot *n* (*pl* -**feet**) pie deforme congénito
clumsy *adj* torpe
cm. *V.* **centimeter**.
CNS *abbr* **central nervous system**. *V.* **system**.
coagulate *vt, vi* coagular(se)
coagulation *n* coagulación *f*; **disseminated intravascular** —— (**DIC**) coagulación intravascular diseminada
coagulopathy *n* coagulopatía
coal *n* carbón *m*
coal tar *n* alquitrán *m* de hulla
coarctation *n* coartación *f*
coat *n* abrigo; *vt* (*one's stomach, etc.*) cubrir, revestir, recubrir
coated *adj* cubierto, revestido, que tiene capa
coating *n* capa, revestimiento, recubrimiento
cobalt *n* cobalto
coca *n* (*bot*) coca
cocaine *n* cocaína
coccidioidomycosis *n* coccidioidomicosis *f*
coccus *n* (*pl* -**ci**) coco
coccyx *n* (*pl* -**cyges**) cóccix *m*
cochlea *n* (*pl* -**leae**) cóclea
cockroach *n* cucaracha

cocoa *n* cacao; —— **butter** manteca de cacao
coconut *n* coco; —— **oil** aceite *m* de coco
coddle *vt* mimar, consentir
codeine *n* codeína
cod-liver oil *n* aceite *m* de hígado de bacalao
coffee *n* café *m*; —— **grounds** posos del café, café molido
coitus *n* coito; —— **interruptus** coito interrumpido
coke (*vulg*) *n* cocaína, coca (*vulg*)
colchicine *n* colchicina
cold *adj* frío; **to be** *o* **feel** —— tener *or* sentir frío; **Are you cold?**..¿Tiene frío? **to be** —— (*the weather*) hacer frío; *n* frío; (*illness*) resfriado, catarro
cold cream *n* crema limpiadora
cold sore *n* fuego, úlcera en los labios (*debida al herpes*)
cold turkey *adv* (*fam*) bruscamente (*refiriéndose a la suspensión de un hábito o adicción*)
colectomy *n* (*pl* -**mies**) colectomía
colic *adj* (*anat*) cólico; *n* cólico
colitis *n* colitis *f*; **pseudomembranous** —— colitis seudomembranosa; **ulcerative** —— colitis ulcerosa
collagen *n* colágeno, colágena
collapse *n* colapso; *vi* desplomarse, caerse, sufrir un colapso; (*a lung*) colapsarse
collar *n* cuello; **cervical** —— (*hard, soft*) collarín, collar cervical, (*rígido, blando*)
collateral *adj* colateral
colleague *n* colega *mf*
colloid *n* coloide *m*
colloidal *adj* coloidal
Colombian *adj & n* colombiano -na *mf*
colon *n* colon *m*; **ascending** —— colon ascendente; **descending** —— colon descendente; **sigmoid** —— colon sigmoide; **spastic** —— colon espástico; **transverse** —— colon transverso
colonic *adj* colónico; *n* (*fam*) enema *m&f*
colonization *n* colonización *f*
colonoscope *n* colonoscopio
colonoscopy *n* (*pl* -**pies**) colonoscopia *or* (*esp spoken*) colonoscopía

color *n* color *m*; —— **blindness** daltonismo (*form*), dificultad *f* para diferenciar ciertos colores

color-blind *adj* daltónico (*form*), que no diferencia bien ciertos colores

colostomy *n* colostomía; —— **bag** bolsa para colostomía

colostrum *n* calostro

colposcopy *n* (*pl* -**pies**) colposcopia *or* (*esp spoken*) colposcopía

coltsfoot *n* (*bot*) tusílago

coma *n* coma *m*

comatose *adj* comatoso (*form*), en coma

comb *n* peine *m*; *vt* peinar; **to** —— **one's hair** peinarse

combination *n* combinación *f*

come *vi* **to** —— **and go** ir y venir; **Does the pain come and go?**..¿Le va y le viene el dolor? **to** —— **down** bajar(se); **Your sugar came down**..Se bajó el azúcar; **to** —— **on** (*to begin*) empezar; **When did the pain come on?**..¿Cuándo le empezó el dolor?

comfort *n* comodidad *f*; *vt* consolar

comfortable *adj* cómodo, confortable

comfrey *n* (*bot*) consuelda

comminuted *adj* conminuto

commode *n* inodoro portátil (*para inválidos, etc.*)

common *adj* común

communicable *adj* transmisible

communication *n* comunicación *f*

community *adj* comunitario; *n* comunidad *f*

companion *n* compañero -ra *mf*

compassion *n* compasión *f*

compatible *adj* compatible

compensate *vt, vi* compensar

complain *vi* quejarse

complaint *n* queja

complement *n* complemento

complete *adj* completo

complex *n* complejo; **AIDS-related** —— **(ARC)** complejo relacionado con el SIDA; **Oedipal** —— complejo de Edipo

complexion *n* cutis *m*, tez *f*

complication *n* complicación *f*

component *n* componente *m*

compound *n* compuesto

compress *n* compresa; *vt* comprimir

compression *n* compresión *f*; **chest compressions** masaje cardiaco externo (MCE), compresiones torácicas

compromise *vt* comprometer

compulsion *n* compulsión *f*

compulsive *adj* compulsivo

computer *n* computadora

concave *adj* cóncavo

conceive *vi* concebir

concentrate *n* concentrado; *vt, vi* concentrar(se)

concentrated *adj* concentrado

concentration *n* concentración *f*

conception *n* concepción *f*

concussion *n* concusión *f*, conmoción *f*

condition *n* condición *f*, estado

conditioned *adj* condicionado

conditioner *n* acondicionador *m*

condom *n* condón *m*, preservativo

cone *n* cono

confabulation *n* confabulación *f*

confidence *n* confianza

confidential *adj* confidencial

conflict *n* conflicto

confront *vt* confrontar

confuse *vt* confundir; **to become confused** confundirse

confused *adj* confundido

confusion *n* confusión *f*

congenital *adj* congénito

congested *adj* congestionado

congestion *n* congestión *f*

congestive *adj* congestivo

congratulations *interj* (*obst, etc.*) ¡Felicidades!

conjugated *adj* conjugado; —— **estrogens** estrógenos conjugados

conjunctiva *n* (*pl* -**vae**) conjuntiva

conjunctivitis *n* conjuntivitis *f*

connect *vt* conectar

connection *n* conexión *f*, unión *f*

conscience *n* conciencia; **guilty** —— conciencia culpable

conscious *adj* consciente

consciousness *n* conciencia, conocimiento; **to lose** —— perder el conocimiento *or* la conciencia; **to regain** —— volver en sí

consecutive *adj* consecutivo

consent *n* consentimiento, permiso; *vi* consentir; **to —— to** consentir en

consequence *n* consecuencia

conservative *adj* (*measures, etc.*) conservador

consistency *n* (*pl* **-cies**) consistencia

console *vt* consolar

consommé *n* consomé *m*

constant *adj* constante

constipate *vt* estreñir

constipated *adj* estreñido; **to become ——** estreñirse

constipation *n* estreñimiento

constitution *n* constitución *f*

constrict *vt* apretar

constriction *n* constricción *f*

consult *vt* consultar

consultation *n* consulta

consumption *n* consumo

contact *n* contacto; **—— lens** (*hard, soft*) lente *m&f* de contacto (*duro, blando*)

contagious *adj* contagioso, que se pasa (*fam*); **It's not contagious..**No es contagioso..No se pasa a los demás.

container *n* recipiente *m*

contaminate *vt* contaminar; **to become contaminated** contaminarse

contamination *n* contaminación *f*

content, contents *n, npl* contenido

continual *adj* continuo

contour *n* contorno

contraception *n* anticoncepción *f*, contracepción *f*

contraceptive *adj & n* anticonceptivo

contract *vt, vi* contraer(se)

contraction *n* contracción *f*; (*obst*) contracción, dolor *m* del parto; **premature atrial —— (PAC)** contracción auricular prematura; **premature ventricular —— (PVC)** contracción ventricular prematura

contracture *n* contractura

contraindication *n* contraindicación *f*

contrast medium *n* medio de contraste

control *n* control *m*; **birth —— control** de la natalidad; **out of ——** fuera de control; *vt* (*pret & pp* **-trolled**; *ger* **-trolling**) controlar

contusion *n* contusión *f*

convalesce *vi* convalecerse

convalescence *n* convalecencia

convalescent *adj* convaleciente

conversion *n* conversión *f*; **—— reaction** reacción conversiva

convex *adj* convexo

convulsion *n* convulsión *f*, ataque *m* (*fam*)

coo *vi* (*pret & pp* **cooed**) arrullar(se)

cook *n* cocinero -na *mf*; *vt, vi* cocinar

cookie *n* galleta

cool *adj* fresco

cooperate *vi* cooperar

cooperative *adj* cooperativo

coordination *n* coordinación *f*

COPD *abbr* **chronic obstructive pulmonary disease.** *V.* **disease.**

cope *vi* **to —— with** enfrentarse a, hacer frente a

copper *n* cobre *m*; **—— sulfate** sulfato de cobre

coral *n* coral *m*

cord *n* cordón *m*, cuerda; **spinal ——** médula espinal; **umbilical ——** cordón umbilical; **vocal ——** cuerda vocal

core *n* corazón *m*

corn *n* maíz *m*; (*on the foot*) callo; **—— oil** aceite *m* de maíz

cornea *n* córnea

cornstarch *n* almidón *m* de maíz, maicena

coronary *adj* coronario

coroner *n* médico forense; oficial *m* del gobierno que investiga casos de muerte

corporal *adj* corporal

corpse *n* cadáver *m*, difunto -ta *mf*

corpuscle *n* corpúsculo

correct *adj* correcto; *vt* corregir, ajustar

correction *n* corrección *f*, ajuste *m*

corrective *adj* correctivo

correlation *n* correlación *f*

corrosive *adj* corrosivo

cortex *n* (*pl* **-tices**) corteza

cortical *adj* cortical

corticosteroid *n* corticosteroide *m*

cortisol *n* cortisol *m*

cortisone *n* cortisona

cosmetic *adj & n* cosmético

Costa Rican *adj & n* costarricense *mf*

costochondritis *n* costocondritis *f*

cottage cheese *n* requesón *m*

cotton *n* algodón *m*; —— **ball** bolita de algodón, torunda de algodón (*esp Mex, CA*)

couch *n* (*psych*) diván *m*

cough *n* tos *f*; —— **drop** pastilla para la tos; —— **syrup** jarabe *m* para la tos; **dry** —— tos seca; **hacking** —— tos fuerte; *vt* **to** —— **up** expectorar (*form*), desgarrar; **Are you coughing up phlegm?**..¿Desgarra flema?..¿Cuándo tose, saca flema?.. ¿Tiene flema al toser?...**Try to cough up phlegm from your lungs**..Trate de desgarrar flema de sus pulmones..Trate de toser y sacar flema de sus pulmones; *vi* toser; **Cough hard**..Tosa fuerte.

coumarin *n* cumarina

counseling *n* terapia con un consejero, consejo

counselor *n* consejero -ra *mf*

count *n* recuento; **blood** —— biometría hemática, recuento sanguíneo; **white blood cell** —— recuento de glóbulos blancos; *vt, vi* contar

counteract *vt* contrarrestar

country *n* (*pl* -**tries**) país *m*; (*rural area*) campo

county *n* (*US*) condado

couple *n* pareja; **married** —— matrimonio

course *n* (*of a disease, etc.*) transcurso, curso; (*educational*) curso

cousin *n* primo -ma *mf*

cover *vt* cubrir, tapar; **Cover your right eye**..Tape su ojo derecho.

coverage *n* cobertura

cow *n* vaca

CPR *abbr* **cardiopulmonary resuscitation**. *V.* **resuscitation**.

crab louse *n* ladilla

crack *n* (*bone, teeth*) fisura, (*skin*) grieta; (*cocaine*) crack *m* (*Ang*), roca (*fam*), forma de cocaína que se fuma; *vt* (*one's joints, one's back*) tronar(se) (*los huesos, la espalda*); *vi* agrietarse, partirse

cracked *adj* agrietado, partido

cracker *n* galleta

cradle *n* cuna, moisés *m*

cradle cap *n* inflamación escamosa del cuero cabelludo en infantes

cramp *n* calambre *m*; (*abdominal*) retorcijón *or* retortijón *m*; (*menstrual*) dolor *m* menstrual, cólico menstrual, dolor de regla; (*postpartum*) entuertos; *vi* **My leg is cramping**..Tengo un calambre en la pierna.

cranial *adj* craneal, craneano

craniopharyngioma *n* craneofaringioma *m*

cranium *n* (*pl* -**nia**) cráneo

craving *n* (*obst*) antojo

crawl *vi* (*ped*) gatear

craziness *n* locura

crazy *adj* (*comp* -**ier**; *super* -**iest**) loco; **to drive** (*someone*) —— volver loco (*a alguien*), trastornar; **His mother drove him crazy**..Su madre lo volvió loco; **to go** —— volverse loco, enloquecer(se)

cream *n* crema; **hand** —— crema para las manos

creatinine *n* creatinina

cretin *n* cretino

cretinism *n* cretinismo

crib *n* cuna

cried *pret & pp de* **cry**

cries *pl de* **cry**

cripple *vt* lisiar

crippled *adj* lisiado, cojo (*fam*)

crisis *n* (*pl* -**ses**) crisis *f*; **blast** —— crisis blástica; **identity** —— crisis de identidad; **midlife** —— crisis de la edad madura

critical *adj* crítico

cromolyn sodium *n* cromoglicato de sodio

crooked *adj* torcido, chueco (*Mex*)

crop-dust *vt, vi* fumigar con avioneta

cross-eyed *adj* bizco

crossmatch *n* prueba cruzada; *vt* hacer prueba(s) cruzada(s), cruzar (*la sangre*) (*fam*)

crotch *n* entrepiernas *or* entrepierna

croup *n* crup *m*

crown *n* (*anat, dent*) corona

cruel *adj* cruel

cruelty *n* crueldad *f*

crush *vt* aplastar, (*one's finger, hand, etc.*) machucar; (*a tablet*) triturar (*form*), moler, desbaratar

crushing *adj* (*sensation, pain*) opresivo (*form*), aplastante, apretado

crust *n* costra

crutch *n* muleta

cry *n* (*pl* **cries**) (*with tears*) llanto, lloro, (*yell*) grito; *vi* (*pret & pp* **cried**) llorar, gritar

cryotherapy *n* crioterapia

Cryptococcus Cryptococcus

cryptorchidism *n* criptorquidia

crystal *n* cristal *m*

CSF *abbr* **cerebrospinal fluid**. V. **fluid**.

CT *abbr* **computed tomography**. V. **tomography**.

Cuban *adj & n* cubano -na *mf*

cubic centimeter (cc.) *n* centímetro cúbico (cc.)

cucumber *n* pepino

cuddle *vt* abrazar, acariciar

culdocentesis *n* (*pl* **-ses**) culdocentesis *f*

culdoscope *n* culdoscopio

culdoscopy *n* (*pl* **-pies**) culdoscopia *or* (*esp spoken*) culdoscopía

culture *n* cultura; (*micro*) cultivo; **blood** —— hemocultivo; **stool** —— coprocultivo; **urine** —— urocultivo; *vt* cultivar

cumulative *adj* acumulativo

cunnilingus *n* cunilinguo

cup, cupful *n* (*pl* **-fuls**) taza

curable *adj* curable

curative *adj* curativo

cure *n* cura, remedio, curación *f*; *vt* curar; **to be cured** curarse

curettage *n* curetaje *m*, legrado (*fam*), raspado (*fam*)

curvature *n* curvatura, (*of the spine*) encorvamiento

curve *n* curva; **growth** —— curva de crecimiento; *vt* doblar, encorvar; *vi* encorvarse

cushion *n* cojín *m*, almohada; *vt* (*a blow, etc.*) amortiguar; (*to place cushions*) acojinar, acolchar

cushioning *n* amortiguamiento

cuspid *n* diente canino, colmillo (*fam*)

cut *n* cortada, cortadura, corte *m*; *vt* (*pret & pp* **cut**; *ger* **cutting**) cortar; **Did you cut your finger?**..¿Se cortó el dedo? **to —— down (on)** (*fam*) disminuir; **You have to cut down on salt**..Tiene que tomar menos sal; **to —— off** cortar, amputar; **to —— one's hair** cortarse el pelo; **to —— one's nails** cortarse las uñas; **to —— oneself** cortarse; **Did you cut yourself?**..¿Se cortó?

cutaneous *adj* cutáneo

cutdown *n* venodisección *f*

cuticle *n* cutícula

cyanide *n* cianuro

cyanosis *n* cianosis *f*

cyanotic *adj* cianótico, morado (*fam*), amoratado (*fam*)

cyclamate *n* ciclamato

cycle *n* ciclo; **anovulatory** —— ciclo anovulatorio; **menstrual** —— ciclo menstrual; **ovulatory** —— ciclo ovulatorio; **reproductive** —— ciclo reproductor

cyclic, cyclical *adj* cíclico

cycling *n* ciclismo

cyclophosphamide *n* ciclofosfamida

cyclosporin *n* ciclosporina

cyst *n* quiste *m*; **Baker's** —— quiste de Baker; **Bartholin's** —— quiste de Bartholin; **dermoid** —— quiste dermoide; **hydatid** —— quiste hidátide; **ovarian** —— quiste ovárico; **pilonidal** —— quiste pilonidal; **popliteal** —— quiste poplíteo; **sebaceous** —— quiste sebáceo; **thyroglossal duct** —— quiste del conducto tirogloso

cystectomy *n* (*pl* **-mies**) cistectomía

cysteine *n* cisteína

cystic *adj* quístico; (*duct, artery*) cístico

cysticercosis *n* cisticercosis *f*

cystic fibrosis *n* fibrosis quística

cystinuria *n* cistinuria

cystitis *n* cistitis *f*, infección *f* de la vejiga

cystocele *n* cistocele *m*

cystoscope *n* cistoscopio

cystoscopy *n* (*pl* **-pies**) cistoscopia *or* (*esp spoken*) cistoscopía

cytomegalovirus *n* citomegalovirus *m*

cytotoxic *adj* citotóxico

D

dacryocystitis *n* dacriocistitis *f*
dad *n* papá *m*
daily *adj* diario; *adv* diariamente, a diario, cada día
dairy product *n* producto lácteo, producto de leche
damage *n* daño; *vt* dañar, hacer daño
damiana *n* (*bot*) damiana
damp *adj* húmedo, mojado
dampness *n* humedad *f*
danazol *n* danazol *m*
dandelion *n* (*bot*) diente *m* de león
dandruff *n* caspa
danger *n* peligro
dangerous *adj* peligroso
dangle *vt, vi* colgar; **Sit with your legs dangling**..Siéntese con las piernas colgando.
dapsone *n* dapsona
dark *adj* oscuro; (*complexion*) moreno
dark-skinned *adj* moreno
data *n o npl* datos, información *f*
date *n* fecha; (*fruit*) dátil *m*
daub *vt* untar(se)
daughter *n* hija
daughter-in-law *n* (*pl* **daughters-in-law**) nuera
day *n* día *m*; —— **care** cuidado para niños durante el día (*esp niños de madres que trabajan*); **every** —— todos los días; **every other** —— cada dos días; **the —— after** *o* **the following** —— el día siguiente; **the —— after tomorrow** pasado mañana; **the —— before** el día anterior; **the —— before yesterday** anteayer
daydream *vi* (*pret & pp* **-dreamed** *o* **-dreamt**) soñar despierto
daze *n* aturdimiento, mareo, estado de confusión o desorientación sin agitación; **in a** —— aturdido, atarantado, mareado; *vt* aturdir, atarantar
dazed *adj* aturdido, atarantado, mareado; **to become** —— aturdirse, atarantarse
D&C *V.* **dilation and curettage**.
DDT *V.* **dichlorodiphenyltrichloroethane**.
dead *adj* muerto
deaf *adj* sordo
deaf-and-dumb *adj* (*vulg*) sordomudo
deaf-mute *n* sordomudo -da *mf*
deafmutism *n* sordomudez *f*
deafness *n* sordera
death *n* muerte *f*, —— **certificate** certificado de defunción; **brain** —— muerte cerebral
debilitated *adj* debilitado
debilitating *adj* debilitante
debilitation *n* debilitación *f*
debridement *n* desbridamiento
decaffeinated *adj* descafeinado
decay *n* **tooth** —— caries *f*
deceased *adj & n* difunto -ta *mf*
decibel *n* decibel *m*
deciliter *n* decilitro
decision *n* decisión *f*
decongestant *adj* descongestivo, descongestionante; *n* descongestionante *m*, descongestivo
decontaminate *vt* descontaminar, desinfectar
decrease *n* disminución *f*; *vt, vi* disminuir(se)
deep *adj* profundo, hondo
deep-fried *adj* frito con mucho aceite
defecate *vi* defecar
defect *n* defecto; **atrial septal** —— (**ASD**) comunicación *f* interauricular (**CIA**); **birth** —— defecto de nacimiento; **neural tube** —— defecto del tubo neural; **ventricular septal** —— (**VSD**) comunicación *f* inter-

ventricular (CIV)

defense mechanism *n* (*psych*) mecanismo de defensa

defibrillate *vt* desfibrilar

defibrillation *n* desfibrilación *f*

deficiency *n* (*pl* -cies) carencia, deficiencia

deficient *adj* deficiente

deficit *n* déficit *m*

definitive *adj* definitivo

deformed *adj* deforme

deformity *n* (*pl* -ties) deformidad *f*

degenerate *vi* degenerar

degenerative *adj* degenerativo

degree *n* grado

dehumanizing *adj* deshumanizante

dehumidifier *n* deshumidificador *m*

dehumidify *vt* deshumedecer

dehydrated *adj* deshidratado

dehydration *n* deshidratación *f*

delay *n* (*developmental*) retraso, retardo; *vt* retrasar, retardar

delayed *adj* tardío, retardado, retrasado

deletion *n* deleción *f*

delicate *adj* delicado, frágil

delirious *adj* delirante; **to be** —— delirar; **He's delirious**..Está delirante..Está delirando.

delirium *n* delirio; —— **tremens** delirium tremens

deliver (*obst*) *vt* dar a luz; (*action performed by doctor or midwife*) atender (*un parto*); **Mrs. Mata delivered a baby boy at four in the morning**..La señora Mata dio a luz un niño a las cuatro de la mañana...**Dr. Ford delivered Mrs. Mata**..El doctor Ford atendió el parto de la señora Mata..El Dr. Ford atendió a la señora Mata...**Dr. Ford delivered the twins**..El Dr. Ford atendió el parto de los gemelos..El Dr. Ford atendió a los gemelos; *vi* dar a luz, aliviarse (*Mex, fam*)

delivery *n* (*pl* -ries) parto; —— **room** sala de partos

delta *n* delta

deltoid *n* deltoides *m*

delusion *n* falsa creencia patológica

demented *adj* demente

dementia *n* demencia

demonstrate *vt* demostrar

demoralize *vt* desmoralizar; **to become demoralized** desmoralizarse, desalentarse, desanimarse

demyelinating *adj* desmielinizante

dengue *n* dengue *m*, fiebre *f* rompehuesos

denial *n* negación *f*

dense *adj* denso

dental *adj* dental; —— **floss** hilo dental

dentin *n* dentina

dentist *n* dentista *mf*, odontólogo -ga *mf*

dentistry *n* odontología

denture *n* dentadura postiza; **partial** —— dentadura parcial

deodorant *n* desodorante *m*

deoxyribonucleic acid (DNA) *n* ácido desoxirribonucleico (ADN *or* DNA)

department *n* departamento

dependence *n* dependencia, (*on drugs*) farmacodependencia

dependency *n* dependencia, (*on drugs*) farmacodependencia

dependent *adj* dependiente

depersonalization *n* despersonalización *f*

depigmentation *n* despigmentación *f*

depilatory *adj* & *n* depilatorio

deplete *vt* agotar

depletion *n* agotamiento

deposit *n* depósito, sedimento; *vt*, *vi* depositar(se)

depot *adj* (*pharm*) de depósito

depressant *adj* & *n* depresor *m*

depressed *adj* deprimido, decaído; **to get** —— deprimirse

depression *n* depresión *f*

depressive *adj* depresivo

depth *n* profundidad *f*; —— **perception** visión profunda, percepción *f* de la profundidad

deranged *adj* (*mentally*) trastornado, loco

dermatitis *n* dermatitis *f*; **atopic** —— dermatitis atópica; **contact** —— dermatitis por contacto; **seborrheic** —— dermatitis seborreica; **stasis** —— dermatitis por estasis

dermatologist *n* dermatólogo -ga *mf*

dermatology *n* dermatología

dermatomyositis *n* dermatomiositis *f*

DES *V.* **diethylstilbestrol.**

descendant *n* descendiente *mf*

descending *adj* descendente

describe *vt* describir

desensitization *n* desensibilización *f*

desensitize *vt* desensibilizar

desiccant *adj & n* desecante *m*, desecativo

desiccated *adj* desecado

desire *n* deseo; *vt* desear

desperate *adj* desesperado; **to become ——** desesperarse

despondent *adj* abatido, deprimido, desalentado, desanimado

dessert *n* postre *m*

destroy *vt* destruir

destructive *adj* destructivo

detect *vt* detectar

detectable *adj* perceptible

detection *n* detección *f*

detergent *adj & n* detergente *m*

deteriorate *vi* (*condition of patient*) empeorar(se), deteriorarse; (*substance*) deteriorarse

deterioration *n* deterioro

detoxification *n* desintoxicación *f*

develop *vt, vi* desarrollar(se)

development *n* desarrollo

device *n* aparato, dispositivo

dexamethasone *n* dexametasona

dextromethorphan *n* dextrometorfano

diabetes *n* diabetes *f*; **—— insipidus** diabetes insípida; **—— mellitus** diabetes mellitus

diabetic *adj & n* diabético -ca *mf*

diagnose *vt* diagnosticar

diagnosis *n* (*pl* **-ses**) diagnóstico, diagnosis *f*

diagnostic *adj* diagnóstico

diagram *n* diagrama *m*

dialysis *n* diálisis *f*; **peritoneal ——** diálisis peritoneal

diameter *n* diámetro

diaper *n* pañal *m*; **—— rash** dermatitis *f* por pañal, salpullido *or* sarpullido

diaphragm *n* (*anat, gyn*) diafragma *m*

diarrhea *n* diarrea; **traveler's ——** diarrea del viajero

diastolic *adj* diastólico

diazepam *n* diacepam *m*

DIC *abbr* **disseminated intravascular coagulation.** *V.* **coagulation.**

dichlorodiphenyltrichloroethane (DDT) *n* diclorodifeniltricloroetano (DDT)

diclofenac *n* diclofenaco

dicloxacillin *n* dicloxacilina

die *vi* (*pret & pp* **died**; *ger* **dying**) morir(se), fallecer

dieldrin *n* dieldrín *m*

diet *n* dieta, régimen *m*; **high-fiber ——** dieta con alto contenido de fibra; *vi* (*también* **to be on a ——**) estar a dieta

dietary *adj* dietético, de dieta

diethylstilbestrol (DES) *n* dietilestilbestrol *m* (DES)

dietician *n* dietista *mf*

diffusion *n* difusión *f*

digest *vt* digerir

digestible *adj* digerible

digestion *n* digestión *f*

digestive *adj* digestivo

digital *adj* digital

digitalis *n* (*pharm*) digital *f*

digoxin *n* digoxina

dilate *vt, vi* dilatar(se)

dilation *n* dilatación *f*; **—— and curettage (D&C)** dilatación y legrado

dilator *n* dilatador *m*

dildo *n* (*pl* **-dos**) consolador *m* (*fam*)

diltiazem *n* diltiazem *m*

dilute *adj* diluido; *vt* diluir

dim *adj* (*comp* **dimmer**; *super* **dimmest**) oscuro, indistinto

dimension *n* dimensión *f*

dimethyl sulfoxide (DMSO) *n* dimetilsulfóxido

dimethyltryptamine (DMT) *n* dimetiltriptamina (DMT)

diminish *vt, vi* disminuir(se)

dimple *n* hoyuelo

dinner *n* cena

dioxide *n* bióxido *or* dióxido

diphenhydramine *n* difenhidramina

diphtheria *n* difteria

diplococcus *n* (*pl* **-ci**) diplococo

dipstick *n* (*for urine, etc.*) tira reactiva

direction *n* dirección *f*, instrucción *f*

dirt *n* suciedad *f*

dirty *adj* (*comp* -ier; *super* -iest) sucio; **to get** —— ensuciar(se)

disability *n* (*pl* -ties) incapacidad *f*

disabled *adj* inválido, incapacitado, inhabilitado; —— **person** inválido -da *mf*

disadvantage *n* desventaja

disappear *vi* desaparecerse

discharge *n* secreción *f*; *vt* (*from the hospital*) dar de alta; **We are going to discharge you the day after tomorrow**..Le vamos a dar de alta pasado mañana.

discipline *n* disciplina; *vt* disciplinar

discomfort *n* molestia; **You're going to feel a little discomfort**..Va a sentir un poco de molestia.

discontinue *vt* descontinuar, (*a medication*) dejar de tomar

discouraged *adj* desalentado, desanimado; **to get** —— desalentarse, desanimarse

disease *n* enfermedad *f*, mal *m*; **Addison's** —— enfermedad de Addison; **Alzheimer's** —— enfermedad de Alzheimer; **benign breast** —— enfermedad mamaria benigna; **cat-scratch** —— enfermedad por arañazo de gato; **celiac** —— enfermedad celiaca; **Chagas'** —— enfermedad de Chagas; **chronic obstructive pulmonary** —— **(COPD)** enfermedad pulmonar obstructiva crónica (EPOC); **collagen-vascular** —— enfermedad colágeno-vascular *or* del colágeno; **connective tissue** —— enfermedad del tejido conectivo *or* conjuntivo; **Crohn's** —— enfermedad de Crohn; **Cushing's** —— enfermedad de Cushing; **degenerative joint** —— enfermedad articular degenerativa; **fibrocystic** —— enfermedad fibroquística; **fifth** —— quinta enfermedad; **Gaucher's** —— enfermedad de Gaucher; **Gilbert's** —— enfermedad de Gilbert; **glycogen storage** —— enfermedad de almacenamiento de glucógeno; **graft-versus-host** —— enfermedad *or* reacción *f* del injerto contra el huésped; **Graves'** —— enfermedad de Graves; **hand-foot-and-mouth** —— enfermedad de mano, pie y boca; **Hansen's** —— enfermedad de Hansen; **Hirschsprung's** —— enfermedad de Hirschsprung; **Hodgkin's** —— enfermedad de Hodgkin; **Huntington's** —— enfermedad de Huntington; **hyaline membrane** —— enfermedad de membrana hialina; **interstitial lung** —— enfermedad intersticial pulmonar; **Kawasaki's** —— enfermedad de Kawasaki; **Legionnaire's** —— enfermedad de los legionarios; **Lyme** —— enfermedad de Lyme; **minimal change** —— enfermedad de lesiones mínimas; **Paget's** —— enfermedad de Paget; **Parkinson's** —— enfermedad de Parkinson; **pelvic inflammatory** —— **(PID)** enfermedad inflamatoria pélvica, infección pélvica; **peripheral vascular** —— enfermedad vascular periférica; **Pott's** —— enfermedad de Pott; **rheumatic heart** —— cardiopatía reumática; **sexually transmitted** —— **(STD)** enfermedad de transmisión sexual (*form*), enfermedad venérea; **sickle cell** —— enfermedad de células falciformes, drepanocitemia; **venereal** —— **(VD)** (*ant*) enfermedad venérea; **von Willebrand's** —— enfermedad de von Willebrand; **Whipple's** —— enfermedad de Whipple; **Wilson's** —— enfermedad de Wilson

disinfect *vt* desinfectar

disinfectant *adj* & *n* desinfectante *m*

disk *n* disco; **herniated** —— disco herniado; **slipped** —— disco desplazado

dislocate *vt* dislocar(se), zafar(se) (*fam*); **Did you dislocate your ankle?**..¿Se dislocó el tobillo?

dislocation *n* dislocación *f*, zafada (*fam*)

disopyramide *n* disopiramida

disorder *n* trastorno, desorden *m*; **bipolar** —— trastorno bipolar; **personality** —— trastorno de la personalidad; **post-traumatic stress** —— trastorno del estrés postraumático; **sleep** —— trastorno del sueño

disoriented *adj* desorientado

dispense *vt* (*pharm*) dispensar

disposable *adj* desechable

dissection *n* disección *f*

disseminate *vt, vi* diseminar(se)

disseminated *adj* diseminado

dissociation *n* (*psych*) disociación *f*

dissolve *vt, vi* disolver(se)

distend *vt* distender; *vi* distender(se)

distention, distension *n* distensión *f*

distilled *adj* destilado

distinguish *vt* distinguir

distress *n* aflicción *f*

disturbance *n* trastorno, alteración *f*; **sleep —** trastorno del sueño

disulfiram *n* disulfiramo

diuresis *n* diuresis *f*

diuretic *adj & n* diurético

diverticulitis *n* diverticulitis *f*

diverticulosis *n* diverticulosis *f*

diverticulum *n* (*pl* **-la**) divertículo

divorce *n* divorcio; *vt, vi* divorciar(se)

dizziness *n* mareo

dizzy *adj* (*comp* **-zier**; *super* **-ziest**) mareado; **to make —** dar mareo

DMSO *V.* **dimethyl sulfoxide.**

DMT *V.* **dimethlytryptamine.**

DNA *V.* **deoxyribonucleic acid.**

doctor *n* médico, doctor -ra *mf*; **family —** médico de cabecera *or* de la familia; **private —** médico privado

Doctor of Medicine (M.D.) *n* médico

dog *n* perro

dominant *adj* dominante

Dominican *adj & n* dominicano -na *mf*

donate *vt* donar

donor *adj* donado; *n* donante *mf*, donador -ra *mf*

dopamine *n* dopamina

dope (*vulg*) *n* narcótico(s)

Doppler *n* Doppler *m*

dorsal *adj* dorsal

dosage *n* dosificación *f*

dose *n* dosis *f*

double *adj & adv* doble; **— chin** papada; **— vision** visión *f or* vista doble; *vt* doblar

double-jointed *adj* hiperextensible

douche *n* ducha; *vi* ducharse

doxycycline *n* doxiciclina

doze *vi* dormitar

drain *n* dren *m*, drenaje *m*; *vt* drenar, vaciar; *vi* drenarse, salir; **Is it draining pus?**..¿Le sale pus?

drainage *n* drenaje *m*, (*from a wound, etc.*) secreción *f*, flujo

drank *pret de* **drink**

draw *vt* **to — blood** sacar sangre

dream *n* sueño; *vt, vi* (*pret & pp* **dreamed** *o* **dreamt**) soñar; **to — of** *o* **about** soñar con

dress *n* vestido; *vt* vestir; (*a wound*) vendar; *vi* vestirse

dressing *n* venda, apósito

dried (*pret & pp de* **dry**) *adj* seco, desecado; **— fruit** fruta seca

drill (*dent*) *n* taladro; *vt* taladrar

drink *n* bebida; *vt, vi* (*pret* **drank**; *pp* **drunk**) tomar, beber; **Do you drink alcohol?**..¿Acostumbra Ud. tomar bebidas alcohólicas?

drinker *n* bebedor -ra *mf*

drinking fountain *n* fuente *f* para beber, bebedero

drip *n* goteo; **postnasal —** secreción *f or* descarga posterior nasal, goteo postnasal

drip *vi* gotear

drive *n* (*sex, hunger, etc.*) instinto; *vt, vi* (*pret* **drove**; *pp* **driven**) (*a vehicle*) manejar, conducir

drool *n* baba; *vi* babear

droop *vi* (*eyelids, etc.*) caerse

drop *n* gota; (*in level of something being measured*) baja; *vi* bajar(se); **Your sugar dropped**..Su azúcar bajó.

dropper *n* gotero

drove *pret de* **drive**

drown *vt, vi* ahogar(se)

drowsy *adj* (*comp* **-sier**; *super* **-siest**) soñoliento, somnoliento, adormilado

drug *n* droga, medicamento; *vt* drogar

druggist *n* farmacéutico -ca *mf*, boticario -ria *mf*

drugstore *n* farmacia, botica

drunk (*pp de* **drink**) *adj* borracho; **to get — emborracharse**; *n* (*person*) borracho -cha *mf*; (*binge*) borrachera

dry *adj* seco, reseco; **— heaves** (*fam*) vomitar sin nada que expulsar; **— mouth** resequedad *f or* sequedad *f* de boca; *vt* (*pret & pp* **dried**) secar; *vi*

(*también* **to get** —— o **to** —— **out**)
secarse, resecarse

drying *adj* secante

dryness *n* resequedad *f*, sequedad *f*

d.t.'s, the *npl* alucinaciones (*debidas a la suspensión del alcohol*), visiones *fpl* (*fam*), delirios; **Have you ever had the d.t.'s?**..¿Ha tenido alucinaciones alguna vez (*al dejar de tomar alcohol*)?

duct *n* conducto

ductus arteriosus *n* conducto arterioso; **patent** —— —— **(PDA)** conducto arterioso persistente

due *adj* —— **to** debido a; **to be** —— (*obst*) esperar aliviarse; **When are you due?**..¿Cuándo espera aliviarse?

dull *adj* (*pain*) sordo; *vt* (*pain*) calmar

duodenal *adj* duodenal

duodenitis *n* duodenitis *f*

duodenum *n* duodeno

durable *adj* duradero

duration *n* duración *f*

dust *n* polvo

dwarf *n* enano -na *mf*

dwarfism *n* enanismo

dye *n* colorante *m*

dying *ger de* **die**

dyscrasia *n* discrasia; **blood** —— discrasia sanguínea

dysentery *n* disentería

dysfunction *n* disfunción *f*

dyslexia *n* dislexia

dysphasia *n* disfasia

dysplasia *n* displasia

E

ear *n* oreja, (*organ of hearing*) oído; ——, **nose, and throat (ENT)** oídos, nariz, y garganta; **external** —— oído externo; **inner** —— oído interno; **middle** —— oído medio

earache *n* dolor *m* de oído

eardrum *n* tímpano

earlobe *n* lóbulo (*del oído*), pulpejo (*del oído*)

earplug *n* tapón *m* para el oído

earring *n* arete *m*

earthquake *n* temblor *m*, sismo, (*severe*) terremoto

earwax *n* cerilla

eat *vt, vi* (*pret* ate; *pp* eaten) comer

EBV *abbr* **Epstein-Barr virus.** V. **virus.**

ECG V. **electrocardiogram.**

echinococcosis *n* equinococosis *f*

Echinococcus Echinococcus

echocardiogram *n* ecocardiograma *m*, ecocardiografía

eclampsia *n* eclampsia

ECT *abbr* **electroconvulsive therapy.** V. **therapy.**

ectopic *adj* ectópico; —— **pregnancy** embarazo ectópico

Ecuadoran *adj & n* ecuatoriano -na *mf*

eczema *n* eccema *m&f*

edema *n* edema *m*; **pulmonary** —— edema pulmonar

edge *n* borde *m*, margen *m*

educate *vt* educar

education *n* educación *f*; **health** —— educación para la salud

EEG V. **electroencephalogram.**

effect *n* efecto; **adverse** —— efecto adverso; **side** —— efecto colateral *or* secundario; **to take** —— hacer efecto

effective *adj* eficaz, efectivo

effeminate *adj* afeminado

efficient *adj* eficiente

effort *n* esfuerzo

effusion *n* derrame *m*; **pericardial** —— derrame pericardiaco; **pleural** —— derrame pleural

egg *n* huevo; (*small, e.g., of a parasite*) huevecillo; (*fam, ovum*) óvulo, huevo (*fam*); —— **yolk** yema de huevo

eggplant *n* berenjena

ego *n* (*pl* **egos**) ego *m*, (el) yo

egocentric *adj* egocéntrico

egoism *n* egoísmo

egoist *n* egoísta *mf*

egoistic *adj* egoísta

egotism *n* egotismo

egotist *n* egotista *mf*

egotistic *adj* egotista

ejaculate *vi* eyacular

ejaculation *n* eyaculación *f*; **premature** —— eyaculación precoz

EKG *V.* **electrocardiogram.**

elastic *adj & n* elástico

elbow *n* codo

elderly *adj* anciano

electric, electrical *adj* eléctrico

electrocardiogram (ECG *o* **EKG)** *n* electrocardiograma *m* (ECG), electrocardiografía

electrocute *vt* electrocutar

electrode *n* electrodo

electroencephalogram (EEG) *n* electroencefalograma *m* (EEG)

electrolyte *adj* electrolítico; *n* electrólito *or* (*esp spoken*) electrolito

electromyography (EMG) *n* electromiografía (EMG)

electrophoresis *n* electroforesis *f*

element *n* elemento; **trace** —— oligoelemento

elephantiasis *n* elefantiasis *f*

elevate *vt* elevar

elevation *n* elevación *f*

eligible *adj* elegible

eliminate *vt* eliminar

elixir *n* elíxir *or* elixir *m*

emaciated *adj* severamente enflaquecido, demacrado

emasculate *vt* emascular

embarrass *vt* Don't feel embarrassed..No le dé vergüenza.

embarrassment *n* vergüenza

embolectomy *n* (*pl* **-mies**) embolectomía

embolism *n* embolia; **pulmonary** —— embolia pulmonar

embolus *n* (*pl* **-li**) émbolo

embrace *n* abrazo; *vt* abrazar

embryo *n* (*pl* **-os**) embrión *m*

embryology *n* embriología

emergency *n* (*pl* **-cies**) emergencia; —— **room (ER)** sala de emergencia *or* urgencias

emery board *n* lima para uñas

emesis basin *n* riñón *m*, riñonera, escupidera

emetic *adj & n* emético

EMG *V.* **electromyography.**

emotion *n* emoción *f*

emotional *adj* emocional; (*person*) emotivo

empathy *n* empatía

emphysema *n* enfisema *m*

employer *n* empleador -ra *mf*, patrón -na *mf*, jefe -fa *mf*

employment *n* empleo

empty *adj* vacío; *vt* vaciar; **You need to empty your bladder.**.Necesita vaciar su vejiga.

empyema *n* empiema *m*

enalapril *n* enalapril *m*

enamel *n* esmalte *m*

encephalitis *n* encefalitis *f*

encephalomyelitis *n* encefalomielitis *f*

encephalopathy *n* encefalopatía; **Wernicke's** —— encefalopatía de Wernicke

end *n* fin *m*

endarterectomy *n* endarterectomía

endemic *adj* endémico

endocarditis *n* endocarditis *f*

endocardium *n* endocardio

endocrine *adj* endocrino

endocrinologist *n* endocrinólogo -ga *mf*

endocrinology *n* endocrinología

endometriosis *n* endometriosis *f*

endometritis *n* endometritis *f*

endometrium *n* endometrio

endorphin *n* endorfina

endoscope *n* endoscopio

endoscopic *adj* endoscópico; —— **retrograde cholangiopancreatography (ERCP)** *n* colangiopancreatografía retrógrada endoscópica

endoscopy *n* (*pl* -**pies**) endoscopia *or* (*esp spoken*) endoscopía

endotracheal *adj* endotraqueal

endure *vt* aguantar, soportar

enema *n* enema *m&f*, lavativa (*fam*); **barium** —— enema de bario

energetic *adj* enérgico

energy *n* energía

engineering *n* ingeniería; **genetic** —— ingeniería genética

enlarge *vt* agrandar, aumentar

enriched *adj* enriquecido

ENT *abbr* **ear, nose, and throat.** *V.* **ear.**

enteric *adj* entérico; **enteric-coated** con capa entérica

enteritis *n* enteritis *f*; **regional** —— enteritis regional

enterococcus *n* (*pl* -**ci**) enterococo

enterocolitis *n* enterocolitis *f*

enteropathy *n* enteropatía; **protein-losing** —— enteropatía con pérdida de proteínas

enterotoxin *n* enterotoxina

entrails *npl* entrañas

entrance *n* entrada

entrapment *n* compresión *f*; **peripheral nerve** —— compresión de un nervio periférico

environment *n* medio ambiente; (*surroundings*) ambiente *m*

environmental *adj* ambiental

enzyme *n* enzima

eosinophil *n* eosinófilo

ephedra *n* (*bot* belcho, canadillo

ephedrine *n* efedrina

epidemic *adj* epidémico; *n* epidemia

epidemiology *n* epidemiología

epididymis *n* (*pl* -**mides**) epidídimo

epididymitis *n* epididimitis *f*

epidural *adj* epidural

epiglottis *n* epiglotis *f*

epiglottitis *n* epiglotitis *f*

epilepsy *n* epilepsia

epinephrine *n* epinefrina

episiotomy *n* (*pl* -**mies**) episiotomía

episode *n* episodio

epispadias *n* epispadias *m*

epulis *n* épulis *m*

equilibrium *n* equilibrio

equivalent *adj* & *n* equivalente *m*

eradicate *vt* erradicar

ERCP *V.* **endoscopic retrograde cholangiopancreatography.**

erect *adj* erecto

erectile *adj* eréctil

erection *n* erección *f*

ergocalciferol *n* ergocalciferol *m*

ergotamine *n* ergotamina

erode *vt, vi* erosionar(se)

erogenous *adj* erógeno

erosion *n* erosión *f*

erotic *adj* erótico

error *n* error *m*

eruption *n* erupción *f*

erysipelas *n* erisipela

erythema *n* eritema *m*; —— **infectiosum** eritema infeccioso; —— **multiforme** eritema multiforme; —— **nodosum** eritema nodoso

erythrocyte *n* eritrocito

erythromycin *n* eritromicina

Escherichia coli Escherichia coli

esophagitis *n* esofagitis *f*; **reflux** —— esofagitis por reflujo

esophagus *n* (*pl* -**gi**) esófago

essential *adj* esencial

estradiol *n* estradiol *m*

estriol *n* estriol *m*

estrogen *n* estrógeno

ethambutol *n* etambutol *m*

ethanol *n* etanol *m*

ether *n* éter *m*

ethical *adj* ético

ethionamide *n* etionamida

ethnic *adj* étnico

ethosuximide *n* etosuximida

ethyl alcohol *n* alcohol etílico

ethylene glycol *n* etilenglicol *m*

etodolac *n* etodolaco

eucalyptus *n* (*bot*) eucalipto

eunuch *n* eunuco

euphoria *n* euforia

Eustachian tube *n* trompa de Eustaquio

euthanasia *n* eutanasia

evacuate *vt* evacuar

evaluate *vt* evaluar, valorar

evaluation *n* evaluación *f*, valoración *f*

evaporate *vi* evaporarse

evaporation *n* evaporación *f*

even *adj* liso, parejo, plano

evening *adj* vespertino (*form*), (*early*) de la tarde, (*after dark*) de noche; *n* tarde *f*, noche *f*

eventually *adv* con el tiempo

evil eye *n* mal *m* de ojo

evolution *n* evolución *f*

exact *adj* exacto

exam *V.* examination.

examination *n* examen *m*, revisión *f*; **breast** —— examen de los senos; **eye** —— examen visual; **pelvic** —— examen ginecológico, revisión *f* de (*sus*) partes (*fam*); **physical** —— examen físico; **rectal** —— tacto rectal

examine *vt* examinar, revisar; **May I examine your leg?**..¿Puedo examinarle la pierna?

exanthem subitum *n* exantema súbito

excess *n* exceso

excessive *adj* excesivo

excessively *adv* en exceso

excite *vt* excitar

excuse *n* excusa; **work** —— certificado para no trabajar, incapacidad *f* de trabajo (*Mex*)

exercise *n* ejercicio; *vt* hacer ejercicio con; **You need to exercise your arm**..Tiene que hacer ejercicio con su brazo; *vi* hacer ejercicio

exert *vt* **to** —— **oneself** esforzarse

exertion *n* esfuerzo, actividad *f* fuerte

exhale *vt, vi* exhalar

exhausted *adj* exhausto, agotado; **to become** —— agotarse

exhaustion *n* agotamiento

exit *n* salida

expect *vt* esperar

expectorant *adj* & *n* expectorante *m*

expel *vt* expeler, expulsar

experiment *n* experimento; *vi* experimentar

experimental *adj* experimental

expert *adj* & *n* experto -ta *mf*

expiration date *n* fecha de caducidad

expire *vt, vi* (*to breathe out*) espirar; (*to die*) fallecer, expirar

exploratory *adj* (*surg*) explorador, exploratorio

explore *vt* (*surg*) explorar

expose *vt* exponer; **Have you been exposed to tuberculosis?**..¿Ha estado expuesto a la tuberculosis?..¿Ha estado en contacto con algún enfermo de tuberculosis?

exposure *n* exposición *f*

expulsion *n* expulsión *f*

extend *vt, vi* extender(se)

extension *n* extensión *f*, prolongación *f*

extensive *adj* extenso

exterior *adj* & *n* exterior *m*

external *adj* externo

extra *adj* extra

extract *n* (*pharm*) extracto; *vt* (*to remove, take out*) extraer, sacar

extraction *n* extracción *f*

extreme unction *n* santos óleos

extremity *n* extremidad *f*

extrovert *n* extrovertido -da *mf*

extroverted *adj* extrovertido

eye *n* ojo; —— **chart** carta de examen visual; **angle** *o* **corner of the** —— ángulo del ojo

eyeball *n* globo ocular (*form*), globo del ojo

eyebright *n* (*bot*) eufrasia

eyebrow *n* ceja; **Raise your eyebrows**..Levante las cejas.

eyedropper *n* gotero

eyeglasses *npl* lentes *mpl*, anteojos

eyeground *n* fondo de ojo

eyelash *n* pestaña

eyelid *n* párpado

eyesight *n* vista, visión *f*

eyestrain *n* vista cansada, cansancio visual

eyewash *n* colirio

eyewear *n* lentes *mpl*; **protective** —— lentes protectores

F

face *n* cara
facedown *adj* boca abajo
face-lift *n* cirugía plástica *or* estética (*para eliminar las arrugas de la cara*)
face mask *n* máscara, mascarilla; (*shield*) careta
faceup *adj* boca arriba
facial *adj* facial; *n* tratamiento *or* masaje *m* facial
factor *n* factor *m*; **intrinsic** —— factor intrínseco; **Rh** —— factor Rh; **risk** —— factor de riesgo; **solar protection** —— **(SPF)** factor de protección solar (FPS)
faculty *n* (*pl* **-ties**) facultad *f*; *npl* facultades *fpl*
Fahrenheit *adj* Fahrenheit
fail *vi* fracasar, fallar
failure *n* (*treatment*) fracaso; (*organ*) insuficiencia, falla; **heart** ——, **kidney** ——, **respiratory** ——, etc. insuficiencia cardiaca, renal, respiratoria, etc.
faint *adj* mareado, débil, que tiene sensación de desmayo; **Do you feel faint?**..¿Se siente mareado?..¿Tiene sensación de desmayo? *n* desmayo; *vi* desmayarse, desvanecerse
fair *adj* (*complexion*) blanco, güero (*Mex*)
faith healer *n* curandero -ra *mf*
faith healing *n* curanderismo
fall *n* caída; (*in level of something being measured*) baja; (*season*) otoño; *vi* (*pret* **fell**; *pp* **fallen**) caerse; bajar(se)
false *adj* falso, (*tooth, eye, etc.*) postizo; —— **teeth** dientes postizos, dentaduras postizas
familial *adj* familiar
family *adj* familiar; —— **member** familiar *m*; —— **planning** planificación *f* familiar; —— **practice** medicina familiar; *n* (*pl*

-**lies**) familia
famotidine *n* famotidina
fan *n* abanico, (*electric*) ventilador *m*
fang *n* colmillo
fantasy *n* (*pl* **-sies**) fantasía
farmer's lung *n* enfermedad *f* pulmonar de los granjeros
farsighted *adj* hipermétrope (*form*), que tiene dificultad para ver los objetos cercanos
farsightedness *n* hipermetropía, dificultad *f* para ver los objetos cercanos
fascia *n* (*pl* **-ciae**) fascia
fasciitis *n* fascitis *f*
fascioliasis *n* fascioliasis *f*
fasciotomy *n* (*pl* **-mies**) fasciotomía
fast *n* ayuno; *vi* ayunar
fasting *adj* en ayunas; —— **glucose** glucosa en ayunas *or* en ayuno; *n* ayuno, (el) ayunar
fat *adj* (*comp* **fatter**; *super* **fattest**) gordo; **to get** —— engordar; *n* grasa, (*lard*) manteca
fatal *adj* fatal, mortal
father *n* padre *m*
father-in-law *n* (*pl* **fathers-in-law**) suegro
fatigue *n* fatiga, cansancio
fatiguing *adj* fatigoso, agotador
fatty *adj* (*comp* **-tier**; *super* **-tiest**) grasoso; —— **acid** ácido graso
fear *n* miedo, temor *m*
features *npl* facciones *fpl*, rasgos
febrile *adj* febril
feces *npl* heces *fpl* fecales, heces
fed *pret* & *pp de* **feed**
fee *n* honorarios
feeble *adj* débil
feed *vt* (*pret* & *pp* **fed**) alimentar (*form*), dar de comer
feedback *n* retroalimentación *f*

feeding *n* alimentación *f*
feel *vt* (*pret & pp* **felt**) (*touch, pinprick, etc.*) sentir; **Can you feel the cotton?**..¿Puede sentir el algodón? *vi* (*sick, tired, well, etc.*) sentirse; **How do you feel?**..¿Cómo se siente?...**Do you feel sick?**..¿Se siente enfermo?
feeling *n* (*sensation*) sensación *f*; (*emotion*) sentimiento, emoción *f*
feet *pl de* **foot**
fell *pret de* **fall**
fellatio *n* felación *f*, coito bucal *or* oral
felon *n* panadizo
felt *pret & pp de* **feel**
female *adj & n* hembra
feminization *n* feminización *f*
femoral *adj* femoral
femur *n* fémur *m*
fentanyl *n* fentanil *m*
ferric *adj* férrico
ferrous sulfate *n* sulfato ferroso
fertile *adj* fértil
fertilization *n* fecundación *f*, fertilización *f*
fertilize *vt* fecundar
fester *vi* enconarse
fetal *adj* fetal
fetish *n* fetiche *m*
fetishism *n* fetichismo
fetus *n* feto
fever *n* fiebre *f*, calentura; **breakbone** —— fiebre rompehuesos; **dengue** —— dengue *m*; **hay** —— fiebre del heno, alergia al polen; **paratyphoid** —— fiebre paratifoidea; **Q** —— fiebre Q; **relapsing** —— fiebre recurrente; **rheumatic** —— fiebre reumática; **Rocky Mountain spotted** —— fiebre manchada de las Montañas Rocosas; **scarlet** —— fiebre escarlatina; **trench** —— fiebre de las trincheras; **typhoid** —— fiebre tifoidea; **yellow** —— fiebre amarilla
fever blister *n* fuego, ampolla en los labios (*debida al herpes*)
feverfew *n* (*bot*) matricaria
feverish *adj* con fiebre *or* calentura, acalenturado
few *adj* pocos; **just a few times**..unas pocas veces

fiancé *n* novio
fiancée *n* novia
fiber *n* fibra; **muscle** —— fibra muscular; **nerve** —— fibra nerviosa
fiberoptic *adj* de fibra óptica
fibrillation *n* fibrilación *f*; **atrial** —— fibrilación auricular; **ventricular** —— fibrilación ventricular
fibrinogen *n* fibrinógeno
fibroadenoma *n* fibroadenoma *m*
fibrocystic *adj* fibroquístico
fibroid *n* (*of the uterus*) mioma *or* fibromioma uterino (*form*), tumor (*benigno*) del útero, bolita del útero (*fam*)
fibroma *n* fibroma *m*
fibromyalgia *V.* **fibrositis.**
fibrosis *n* fibrosis *f*
fibrositis *n* fibrositis *f*
fibrotic *adj* fibrótico
fibula *n* fíbula, peroné *m*
field *n* campo; **visual** —— campo visual
fig *n* higo
figure *n* (*of a person*) figura
filariasis *n* filariasis *f*
file *n* (*for nails*) lima; (*patient chart*) expediente *m*; *vt* limar
fill *vt* llenar; (*a prescription*) surtir; (*a tooth*) obturar (*form*), rellenar, tapar
filling *n* (*dent*) empaste *m*, relleno
film *n* capa, tela; (*X-ray*) placa
filter *n* filtro; *vt, vi* filtrar(se)
filtration *n* filtración *f*
final *adj* final
finding *n* hallazgo
finger *n* dedo (*de la mano*); —— **cot** dedo de hule; —— **pad** yema del dedo; **index** —— dedo índice; **little** —— dedo meñique; **middle** —— dedo medio; **ring** —— dedo anular
fingernail *n* uña (*de un dedo de la mano*)
finger pad *n* pulpejo (*del dedo*)
fingerstick *n* punción *f* digital (*form*), pinchazo del dedo, piquete *m* del dedo (*esp Mex*)
fingertip *n* punta del dedo
fire *n* fuego, incendio; —— **department** cuerpo de bomberos; —— **extinguisher** extinguidor *m*

firearm *n* arma de fuego
fireman *n* (*pl* -**men**) bombero
firm *adj* firme
firmness *n* firmeza
first *adj* primero; —— **aid** primeros auxilios; **first-aid kit** botiquín *m* de primeros auxilios
fish *n* (*pl* **fish** *o* **fishes**) pez *m*; (*after being caught, as a food*) pescado
fish bone *n* espina
fisherman *n* (*pl* -**men**) pescador *m*
fishhook *n* anzuelo
fissure *n* fisura
fist *n* puño; **to make a** —— apretar el puño, cerrar la mano
fistula *n* (*pl* -**lae** *o* -**las**) fístula
fit *adj* (*comp* **fitter**; *super* **fittest**) en forma; *n* (*attack*) ataque *m*, acceso; *vt* (*glasses, etc.*) ajustar
fitting *n* ajuste *m*
fix *vt* arreglar, reparar
fixation *n* fijación *f*
flabby *adj* (*comp* -**bier**; *super* -**biest**) fláccido, flojo
flaccid *adj* fláccido *or* flácido
flake (*skin*) *n* escama; *vi* descamarse (*form*), caerse en escamas
flaky *adj* (*comp* -**ier**; *super* -**iest**) escamoso
flammable *adj* inflamable
flank *n* flanco
flap *n* colgajo
flare *vi* **to** —— **up** recrudecer (*form*), agravar(se), volver(se) a agravar
flask *n* frasco, pomo
flat *adj* (*comp* **flatter**; *super* **flattest**) plano
flatfoot *n* (*pl* -**feet**) pie plano
flatulence *n* flatulencia
flatulent *adj* flatulento
flatworm *n* platelminto, gusano plano
flavor *n* sabor *m*, gusto; **cherry-flavored, banana-flavored, etc.** sabor a cereza, sabor a plátano, etc.
flea *n* pulga
fleeting *adj* (*pain, etc.*) pasajero, momentáneo, fugaz
flesh *n* carne *f*; **raw** —— carne viva
fleshy *adj* carnoso
flex *vt, vi* flexionar(se) (*form*), doblar(se)

flexible *adj* flexible
flies *pl de* **fly**
floater *n* (*in the eye*) estrellita, lucecita
flood *n* inundación *f*, diluvio
flora *n* (*pl* -**ras** *o* -**rae**) flora
floss *n* hilo dental; *vt, vi* limpiar (*los dientes*) con hilo dental
flour *n* harina
flow *n* flujo; **blood** —— flujo sanguíneo (*form*), circulación *f*; **menstrual** —— flujo *or* sangrado menstrual; *vi* fluir
flu *n* gripe *f*, influenza; **Asian** —— gripe asiática; **swine** —— gripe porcina
fluconazole *n* fluconazol *m*
fluctuate *vi* fluctuar, variar
fluid *n* líquido, fluido; **amniotic** —— líquido amniótico; **cerebrospinal** —— (**CSF**) líquido cefalorraquídeo (**LCR**); **pleural** —— líquido pleural; **seminal** —— líquido seminal; **synovial** —— líquido sinovial
fluke *n* duela
fluorescent *adj* fluorescente
fluoridation *n* fluorización *f*
fluoride *n* fluoruro
fluoroscopy *n* (*pl* -**pies**) fluoroscopia *or* (*esp spoken*) fluoroscopía
fluorouracil *n* fluorouracilo
fluoxetine *n* fluoxetina
fluphenazine *n* flufenacina
flurazepam *n* fluracepam *m*
flush (*physio*) *n* rubor *m*, sonrojamiento, bochorno; *vi* ruborizarse, sonrojarse
flushing *n* sonrojamiento
flutter *n* aleteo; **atrial** —— aleteo auricular
fly *n* (*pl* **flies**) mosca; (*of trousers*) bragueta
foam *n* espuma; (*at the mouth*) espumarajo
foamy *adj* (*comp* -**ier**; *super* -**iest**) espumoso
focal *adj* focal
focus *n* (*pl* **foci** *o* **focuses**) foco; *vt* (*pret & pp* **focused** *o* **focussed**; *ger* **focusing** *o* **focussing**) enfocar
fold *n* pliegue *m*; **skin** —— pliegue cutáneo; *vt* **to** —— **one's arms** cruzar los brazos
folic acid *n* ácido fólico
follicle *n* folículo; **hair** —— folículo piloso; **ovarian** —— folículo ovárico
folliculitis *n* foliculitis *f*

follow-up *n* seguimiento, atención médica subsecuente, vigilancia

follow *vt* (*to take care of*) atender; **Who follows you for your diabetes?**..¿Quién le atiende su diabetes?

fondle *vt* acariciar, molestar

fontanel, fontanelle *n* fontanela, mollera

food *n* comida, alimento(s); —— **poisoning** intoxicación alimenticia *or* alimentaria; **baby** —— comida para niños; **canned** —— alimentos enlatados; **fast** —— comida rápida, comida preparada en un restaurant de servicio rápido; **processed** —— alimentos procesados

food-borne *adj* transmitido por los alimentos

foot *n* (*pl* **feet**) pie *m*; —— **drop** pie péndulo

football *n* fútbol *m*

footpad *n* (*fam*) plantilla

footstool *n* banquito para los pies

footwear *n* calzado (*zapatos, botas*)

force *n* fuerza

forceps *n* (*pl* **-ceps** *o* **-cipes**) (*obst*) fórceps *m*; (*surg*) pinzas de disección, pinzas

forearm *n* antebrazo

forehead *n* frente *f*

foreign body *n* cuerpo extraño

forensic *adj* forense

foreplay *n* caricias eróticas que anteceden al acto sexual

foreskin *n* prepucio

forget *vt, vi* (*pret* **-got**; *pp* **-gotten**; *ger* **-getting**) olvidar

forgetful *adj* olvidadizo

form *n* forma; (*paper to fill out*) formulario; *vt, vi* formar(se)

formaldehyde *n* formaldehido

formation *n* formación *f*

formula *n* fórmula

formulary *n* formulario

fortify *vt* fortificar, fortalecer

forward *adv* adelante, hacia adelante

fossa *n* fosa

foster care *n* (*US*) crianza de huérfanos por alguien que no es padre adoptivo y que recibe remuneración del gobierno

fox *n* zorro

fracture *n* fractura; **closed** —— fractura

cerrada; **comminuted** —— fractura conminuta; **compound** —— fractura expuesta *or* abierta; **compression** —— fractura por compresión; **cranial** —— fractura del cráneo; **hairline** —— fisura; **open** —— fractura expuesta *or* abierta; **skull** —— fractura del cráneo; **spiral** —— fractura en espiral *or* espiroidea; **stress** —— fractura por esfuerzo; *vt, vi* fracturar(se), quebrar(se) (*fam*); **You fractured your neck?**..¿Se fracturó el cuello?

fragile *adj* frágil, quebradizo

fragment *n* fragmento

frail *adj* frágil, débil

frambesia *n* frambesia

frames *npl* (*for eyeglasses*) armazón *m*

fraternal *adj* fraterno

freckle *n* peca

freckled *adj* pecoso

free *adj* (*loose, unattached*) suelto, libre; *vt* soltar

freebase *n* (*cocaine*) base *f* libre de cocaína, coca en pasta

freeze *vt, vi* (*pret* **froze**; *pp* **frozen**) congelar(se)

frequency *n* (*pl* **-cies**) frecuencia

fresh *adj* (*food, air*) fresco

friction *n* fricción *f*

fried *adj* frito

friend *n* amigo **-ga** *mf*

friendly *adj* amable, simpático, amistoso

friendship *n* amistad *f*

fright *n* susto

frigid *adj* (*ant*) frígido, que no responde sexualmente

frigidity *n* (*ant*) frigidez *f*, incapacidad *f* para responder sexualmente

front *adj* de enfrente; *n* **the** —— **of**..la parte de enfrente de

frontal *adj* frontal

frostbite *n* congelación *f*

froth *n* (*at the mouth*) espumarajo

frothy *adj* (*comp* **-ier**; *super* **-iest**) espumoso

frown *vi* fruncir el entrecejo *or* el ceño

froze *pret de* **freeze**

frozen *pp de* **freeze**

fructose *n* fructosa

fruit *n* (*pl* **fruit** *o* **fruits**) fruta(s); **You can**

eat fruit..Puede comer frutas.
fry *vt* freír
FSH *abbr* **follicle-stimulating hormone**. *V.*
  hormone.
fuel *n* combustible *m*
full *adj* lleno; **I feel full**..Me siento lleno.
fullness *n* plenitud *f* (*form*), llenura
fumes *npl* humo, vapor *m*, gas *m*
fumigate *vt* fumigar

function *n* función *f*; *vi* funcionar
funeral home *n* funeraria
fungal *adj* relativo a los hongos
fungus *n* (*pl* **-guses** *o* **-gi**) hongo
funny bone *n* (*fam*) codo
furosemide *n* furosemida
furuncle *n* furúnculo
fuse *vt* (*ortho*) fusionar; *vi* fusionarse, soldar
fusion *n* fusión *f*; **spinal** —— fusión espinal

G

gag *vt* (*pret* & *pp* **gagged**; *ger* **gagging**)
  (*también* **to make** ——) provocar
  náusea(s); *vi* sentir náusea(s)
gain *n* ganancia, aumento; *vt* **to** —— **weight**
  aumentar de peso
gait *n* marcha (*form*), forma de andar
galactose *n* galactosa
galactosemia *n* galactosemia
gallbladder *n* vesícula biliar, vesícula (*fam*)
gallium *n* galio
gallop *n* (*card*) galope *m*
gallstone *n* cálculo biliar
gamma *n* gamma
gancyclovir *n* ganciclovir *m*
ganglion *n* (*pl* **-glia** *o* **-glions**) ganglio
ganglioneuroma *n* ganglioneuroma *m*
gangrene *n* gangrena; **dry** —— gangrena
  seca; **gas** —— gangrena gaseosa
gap *n* espacio
gardener *n* jardinero -ra *mf*
Gardnerella vaginalis Gardnerella vaginalis
gargle *vi* hacer gárgaras
garlic *n* ajo
gas *n* gas *m*; (*fam*) gasolina; **arterial blood**
  —— gasometría, gases arteriales; **natural**
  —— gas natural; **tear** —— gas lacrimógeno; **to have** —— tener gas; **to pass**
  —— tirar gases *or* vientos, pasar gas
gash *n* tajo, cuchillada
gasoline *n* gasolina

gasp *vi* hacer esfuerzos para respirar, jalar
  aire
gastrectomy *n* (*pl* **-mies**) gastrectomía
gastric *adj* gástrico
gastrin *n* gastrina
gastrinoma *n* gastrinoma *m*
gastritis *n* gastritis *f*
gastrocnemius *n* gastrocnemio
gastroenteritis *n* gastroenteritis *f*
gastroenterologist *n* gastroenterólogo -ga *mf*
gastroenterology *n* gastroenterología
gastrointestinal (GI) *adj* gastrointestinal
gauze *n* gasa
gave *pret de* **give**
gay *adj* & *n* homosexual *mf*
gaze *n* mirada, el acto de mantener fija la
  vista en una dirección determinada
gel *n* gel *m*
gelatin *n* gelatina
gemfibrozil *n* gemfibrosilo
gender *n* género
gene *n* gen *m*
generic *adj* genérico
genetic *adj* genético; —— **engineering**
  ingeniería genética
genetics *n* genética
genital *adj* genital; *n* **genitals** genitales *mpl*
genius *n* genio
gentamicin *n* gentamicina
gentle *adj* suave, ligero

geriatric *adj* geriátrico
geriatrician *n* geriatra *mf*
geriatrics *n* geriatría
germ *n* germen *m*
German measles *n* sarampión *m* alemán, rubeola *or* rubéola
germinoma *n* germinoma *m*
gerontologist *n* gerontólogo -ga *mf*
gerontology *n* gerontología
gestation *n* gestación *f*
gestational *adj* gestacional
get *vt* (*pret* **got**; *pp* **gotten**; *ger* **getting**) (*a disease*) darle (*a uno*), pegarle (*a uno*); **I got the flu**..Me dio la gripe; **to —— over** (*an illness, etc.*) recobrarse, recuperarse; **to —— up** levantarse
GH *abbr* **growth hormone**. *V*. **hormone**.
GI *V*. **gastrointestinal**.
Giardia Giardia
giardiasis *n* giardiasis *f*
giddy *adj* (*comp* **-dier**; *super* **-diest**) mareado
gigantism *n* gigantismo
Gila monster *n* monstruo de Gila
ginger *n* (*bot*) jengibre *m*
gingiva *n* (*pl* **-vae**) gingiva, encía
gingivitis *n* gingivitis *f*; **acute necrotizing ulcerative ——** gingivitis ulcerosa necrosante aguda
girdle *n* faja, corsé *m*
girl *n* niña, muchacha
girlfriend *n* novia, amiga íntima, amiga
give *vt* (*pret* **gave**; *pp* **given**) (*a disease*) contagiar, pegar; **Don't give me your cold!**..¡No me pegue su resfriado! **to —— up** (*smoking, etc.*) dejar de; **You have to give up smoking**..Tiene que dejar de fumar; **to —— up on** (*diet, treatment, etc.*) abandonar
gland *n* glándula; **adrenal ——** glándula suprarrenal; **endocrine ——** glándula endocrina; **parathyroid ——** glándula paratiroides; **parotid ——** glándula parótida; **pineal ——** glándula pineal; **pituitary ——** glándula pituitaria; **salivary ——** glándula salival; **thyroid ——** glándula tiroides
glans *n* (*pl* **glandes**) glande *m*

glass *n* (*material*) vidrio; (*tumbler*) vaso; **a glass of milk**..un vaso con leche
glasses *npl* lentes *mpl*, anteojos
glaucoma *n* glaucoma *m*
glioblastoma *n* glioblastoma *m*
glioma *n* glioma *m*
glipizide *n* glipizida
globulin *n* globulina; **gamma —— globulina** gamma; **immune —— globulina** inmune
glomerulonephritis *n* glomerulonefritis *f*
glossitis *n* glositis *f*
glottis *n* glotis *f*
glove *n* guante *m*
glucagon *n* glucagón *m*
glucagonoma *n* glucagonoma *m*
glucometer *n* glucómetro, aparato para medir la glucosa
gluconate *n* gluconato
glucose *n* glucosa
glutamic acid *n* ácido glutámico
glutamine *n* glutamina
gluteal *adj* glúteo
gluten *n* gluten *m*
glyburide *n* gliburida
glycerin *n* glicerina, glicerol *m*
glycerol *n* glicerina, glicerol *m*
glycine *n* glicina
gnash *vt* (*one's teeth*) rechinar (*los dientes*)
gnat *n* jején *m*, mosquito
GnRH *abbr* **gonadotropin-releasing hormone**. *V*. **hormone**.
go *vi* **to —— away** (*pain, etc.*) quitarse; **The pain went away**..El dolor se me quitó; **to —— down** (*temperature, blood glucose, etc.*) bajar(se); **to —— up** subir(se)
goal *n* meta
goat *n* cabra
goggles *npl* lentes protectores
goiter *n* bocio
gold *n* oro
golf *n* golf *m*
gonad *n* gónada
gonadorelin *n* gonadorelina
gonadotropin *n* gonadotropina; **human chorionic ——** (**HCG**) gonadotropina coriónica humana
gonococcus *n* (*pl* **-ci**) gonococo
gonorrhea *n* gonorrea

good adj (comp **better**; super **best**) bueno; n bien m; **for your own ——** por su propio bien
good-looking adj bien parecido, guapo
goose pimples npl piel f de gallina
got pret de **get**
gotten pp de **get**
gout n gota
gouty adj gotoso
gown n bata
grade n (degree) grado
gradually adv poco a poco
graft n injerto; **skin ——** injerto cutáneo; vt injertar
grain n (pharm) grano; (cereal) grano, cereal m; **whole-grain** de grano entero, integral; **whole-grain bread** pan integral
gram n gramo
Gram-negative adj gramnegativo
Gram-positive adj grampositivo
grandchild n (pl **-children**) nieto -ta mf
granddaughter n nieta
grandfather n abuelo
grandiose adj grandioso, pomposo
grandmother n abuela
grandparent n abuelo -la mf
grandson n nieto
granulation n granulación f
granulocyte n granulocito
granuloma n granuloma m
granulomatosis n granulomatosis f; **Wegener's ——** granulomatosis de Wegener
grape n uva
grapefruit n toronja
graph n gráfica or gráfico
grasp n prensión f; vt agarrar, coger
grass n hierba; (fam) marihuana or marijuana
gratification n gratificación f
grave adj grave
gray adj gris; **—— hair** cana(s); **—— matter** substancia gris
grayish adj grisáceo
graze n rozón m; vt rozar(se)
grease n grasa, manteca
greasy adj (comp **-ier**; super **-iest**) grasoso, grasiento
great-grandchild n (pl **-children**) bisnieto

or biznieto -ta mf
great-granddaughter n bisnieta or biznieta
great-grandfather n bisabuelo
great-grandmother n bisabuela
great-grandparent n bisabuelo -la mf
great-grandson n bisnieto or biznieto
green adj verde; (fruit) verde, inmaduro
greenish adj verdoso
greens npl verduras
grew pret de **grow**
grief n pesar m, aflicción f, pena
grieve vi afligirse
grill vt asar a la parrilla
grind vt (a pill, etc.) moler, triturar; (one's teeth) rechinar
grip n prensión f; vt agarrar, coger
griseofulvin n griseofulvina
grit vt (one's teeth) rechinar (los dientes)
groan n gemido; vi gemir
groin n ingle f
group n grupo; **support ——** grupo de apoyo
grow vi (pret **grew**; pp **grown**) crecer; **to —— old** envejecer(se); **to —— out of** (a habit) quitarse (a uno), perder; **They will outgrow it**..Se les quitará; **to —— up** crecer, volverse adulto
growl vi (one's stomach) gruñir, sonar, tronar; **My stomach is growling**..Me gruñen las tripas.
growth n crecimiento; (on the skin) tumor m, tumorcito
grunt n gruñido; vi gruñir
guaifenesin n guaifenesina
guard n protector m
guardian n (legal) tutor -ra mf
Guatemalan adj & n guatemalteco -ca mf
guide n guía; **—— dog** perro guía
guideline n pauta
guilt n culpa; **—— feelings** sentimientos de culpa
guinea pig n cobayo, (esp fig) conejillo de Indias
gum n goma; (anat) encía; **chewing ——** chicle m
gumma n goma m
gun n pistola; (rifle) fusil m
gurgle n gorgoteo; vi gorgotear

gut *n* intestino; *npl* (*fam*) tripas, vísceras
gymnasium *n* gimnasio
gymnastics *n* gimnasia

gynecologic, gynecological *adj* ginecológico
gynecologist *n* ginecólogo -ga *mf*
gynecology *n* ginecología

H

habit *n* hábito, costumbre *f*; **bad —— mal** hábito
habit-forming *adj* que crea hábito
habituation *n* habituación *f*
Haemophilus Haemophilus
hair *n* pelo, cabello; **body —— vello**
haircut *n* corte *m* de pelo; **to get a ——** cortarse el pelo
haircutter *n* peluquero -ra *mf*
half *adj* medio; **—— asleep** medio dormido; **—— brother** medio hermano; **—— sister** media hermana; **—— the** la mitad de; **Take half the medicine now**..Tome la mitad de la medicina ahora; **a —— o —— a** medio; **Take a half pill every morning**..Tome media pastilla todas las mañanas.
half-life *n* vida media
halfway house *n* (*US*) casa de rehabilitación (*esp para farmacodependientes y alcohólicos después de tratamiento y antes de volver a la sociedad*)
halitosis *n* halitosis *f*, mal aliento
hall, hallway *n* corredor *m*, pasillo
hallucination *n* alucinación *f*
hallux valgus *n* hallus *or* hallux valgus *m*
hallux varus *n* hallus *or* hallux varus *m*
haloperidol *n* haloperidol *m*
halothane *n* halotano
ham *n* jamón *m*; (*muscle*) corva
hamartoma *n* hamartoma *m*
hammer *n* martillo
hamstring *n* tendón *m* de la corva
hand *n* mano *f*
hand-held *adj* manual
handkerchief *n* pañuelo

hand lens *n* lupa, lente *m* de aumento
handwriting *n* escritura, letra
hang *vt* (*pret & pp* **hanged** *o* **hung**) (*by the neck*) ahorcar; **to —— oneself** ahorcarse; *vi* colgar
hangnail *n* padrastro
hangover *n* resaca, cruda (*Mex*), goma (*CA*); **to have a —— tener una resaca, tener una** cruda (*Mex*), estar crudo (*Mex*), estar de goma (*CA*)
happiness *n* felicidad *f*
happy *adj* feliz, contento
hard *adj* duro; **—— of hearing** que no oye bien, medio sordo
harden *vt, vi* endurecer(se)
hardened *adj* endurecido
hardening *n* endurecimiento
harm *n* daño; *vt* dañar, hacer daño
harmful *adj* nocivo, dañino, perjudicial
harmless *adj* inofensivo, no dañino, que no hace daño
harsh *adj* áspero
harvest mite *n* nigua
hashish *n* hachís *m*
hat *n* sombrero
hate *n* odio; *vt* odiar
hatred *n* odio
hawthorn *n* (*bot*) espino
hay *n* heno
hazard *n* peligro
hazardous *adj* peligroso
HCG *abbr* **human chorionic gonadotropin.** V. **gonadotropin.**
HDL *abbr* **high density lipoprotein.** V. **lipoprotein.**
head *n* cabeza; (*of an abscess*) centro; (*of a*

bed) cabecera; **to come to a** —— (*abscess*) madurar

headache *n* cefalea (*form*), dolor *m* de cabeza; **cluster** —— cefalea en grupos; **migraine** —— migraña, jaqueca; **tension** —— cefalea por tensión *or* tensional; **vascular** —— cefalea vascular

heal *vt, vi* curar(se), sanar

healing *n* curación *f*, (el) curar; **Steroids can retard healing.**.Los esteroides pueden retardar la curación...**the art of healing.**.el arte de curar

health *n* salud *f*, salubridad *f*; **mental** —— salud mental; **public** —— salud pública

healthcare *n* atención médica, servicios médicos

health club *n* gimnasio

Health Department *n* departamento de salud

health food *n* comida saludable, comida que se cree que es buena para la salud porque no contiene preservativos, sabores artificiales, ni pesticidas

healthy *adj* (*comp* -ier; *super* -iest) sano, saludable

hear *vt, vi* (*pret & pp* **heard**) oír

hearing *n* (*sense*) oído, audición *f* (*form*); **How's your hearing?**..¿Cómo escucha?.. ¿Cómo oye? —— **aid** audífono

heart *n* corazón *m*; —— **attack** ataque cardiaco *or* al corazón; —— **disease** enfermedad *f* del corazón; —— **murmur** soplo cardiaco; **congestive** —— **failure** insuficiencia cardiaca congestiva

heartbeat *n* latido del corazón

heartburn *n* agruras, acidez *f* (*estomacal*), acedía

heat *n* calor *m*; *vt* (*también* **to** —— **up**) calentar

heater *n* calentador *m*

heating *n* calefacción *f*

heating pad *n* cojín eléctrico

heatstroke *n* insolación *f*, golpe *m* de calor

heaviness *n* pesadez *f*

heavy *adj* (*comp* -ier; *super* -iest) pesado

heavyset *adj* robusto, fornido

heel *n* talón *m*; (*of a shoe*) tacón *m*

height *n* altura

helium *n* helio

helmet *n* casco

help *interj* ¡Auxilio!, ¡Socorro!; *n* ayuda, auxilio, socorro; *vt, vi* ayudar

hemangioma *n* hemangioma *m*; **cavernous** —— hemangioma cavernoso

hematocele *n* hematocele *m*

hematocrit *n* hematócrito

hematologist *n* hematólogo -ga *mf*

hematology *n* hematología

hematoma *n* hematoma *m*; **subdural** —— hematoma subdural

hemiplegia *n* hemiplejía

hemisphere *n* hemisferio

hemlock *n* (*bot*) cicuta

hemochromatosis *n* hemocromatosis *f*

hemodialysis *n* hemodiálisis *f*

hemoglobin *n* hemoglobina

hemolysis *n* hemólisis *f*

hemolytic *adj* hemolítico

hemophilia *n* hemofilia

hemophiliac *n* hemofílico -ca *mf*

hemorrhage *n* hemorragia; **subarachnoid** —— hemorragia subaracnoidea

hemorrhagic *adj* hemorrágico

hemorrhoid *n* hemorroide *f*, almorrana

hemorrhoidectomy *n* (*pl* -**mies**) hemorroidectomía

hemosiderosis *n* hemosiderosis *f*

heparin *n* heparina

hepatic *adj* hepático; —— **insufficiency** insuficiencia hepática

hepatitis *n* hepatitis *f*; —— **A; B; non-A, non-B; etc.** hepatitis A, B, no A no B, etc.

hepatoma *n* hepatoma *m*

hepatorenal *adj* hepatorrenal

herb *n* hierba; —— **shop** herbolario, botanica *or* botánica, hierbería

herbal *adj* herbario

herbalist *n* herbolario -ria, hierbero -ra *mf*

herbicide *n* herbicida *m*

hereditary *adj* hereditario

heredity *n* herencia

hermaphrodite *adj & n* hermafrodita *mf*

hermaphroditism *n* hermafroditismo

hernia *n* hernia; **femoral** —— hernia femoral; **incarcerated** —— hernia incarcerada; **incisional** —— hernia incisional; **inguinal** —— hernia inguinal; **hiatal** —— hernia hiatal; **reducible** —— hernia reducible; **strangulated** —— hernia estrangulada; **umbilical** —— hernia umbilical

heroin *n* heroína

herpangina *n* herpangina

herpes *n* herpes *m*; —— **simplex** herpes simple; —— **zoster** herpes zoster, zona

herpetic *adj* herpético

heterosexual *adj & n* heterosexual *mf*

hiccup *n* hipo; *vi* (*pret & pp* -**cuped** *o* -**cupped**; *ger* -**cuping** *o* -**cupping**) (*también* **to have the hiccups**) tener hipo

hickey *n* chupete *m*, chupón *m*, marca roja en la piel debida a un beso fuerte

hidradenitis suppurativa *n* hidradenitis supurativa

high *adj* alto; (*fam*) intoxicado por drogas, drogado

high-heeled *adj* de tacón alto

high-pitched *adj* de tono alto, agudo

hike *n* caminata

hip *n* cadera

hip-joint *n* articulación *f* de la cadera

hipbone *n* hueso de la cadera

hiplength *adj* de largo hasta el muslo

Hippocratic Oath *n* juramento hipocrático

histamine *n* histamina

histidine *n* histidina

histiocytosis X *n* histiocitosis *f* X

histology *n* histología

histoplasmosis *n* histoplasmosis *f*

history *n* (*pl* -**ries**) (*medical*) historia clínica; **past medical** —— historia clínica previa

histrionic *adj* histriónico

hit *vt* (*pret & pp* **hit**; *ger* **hitting**) pegar, golpear; **It hit me here**..Me pegó aquí... **Did you hit your head?**..¿Se golpeó la cabeza?

HIV *abbr* **human immunodeficiency virus**. *V*. **virus**.

hives *npl* ronchas

hoarse *adj* ronco

hoarseness *n* ronquera

hobby *n* (*pl* -**bies**) pasatiempo

hold *vt* **to** —— **one's breath** detener or aguantar la respiración; **to** —— **one's nose** taparse la nariz

hole *n* hoyo, agujero

hollow *adj & n* hueco; —— **of the hand** hueco de la mano

home *n* casa, hogar, domicilio; —— **remedy** remedio casero; **at** —— en casa

homeless *adj* sin hogar

homemade *adj* casero

homemaker *n* ama de casa

homeopath *n* homeópata *mf*

homeopathic *adj* homeopático

homeopathy *n* homeopatía

homesick *adj* **to be** —— sentir nostalgia (*a la tierra de uno*)

homesickness *n* nostalgia (*a la tierra de uno*)

homophobia *n* homofobia

homophobic *adj* homofóbico

homosexual *adj & n* homosexual *mf*

Honduran *adj & n* hondureño -ña *mf*

honey *n* miel *f* (*de abeja*)

hooked *adj* (*on drugs*) prendido (*esp Mex*), adicto

hookworm *n* uncinaria

hop *n* brinco, salto; *vi* (*pret & pp* **hopped**; *ger* **hopping**) brincar, saltar; **Hop on one foot**..Brinque en un pie.

hope *n* esperanza; **to lose** —— perder la esperanza, desesperarse; *vi* esperar; **to** —— **for** esperar

hopeless *adj* desesperado, sin esperanza

hops *n* (*bot*) lúpulo

hormonal *adj* hormonal

hormone *n* hormona; **adrenocorticotropic** —— (**ACTH**) hormona adrenocorticotrópica; **follicle-stimulating** —— (**FSH**) hormona estimulante del folículo; **gonadotropin-releasing** —— (**GnRH**) hormona liberadora de gonadotropinas; **growth** —— (**GH**) hormona del crecimiento; **luteinizing** —— (**LH**) hormona luteinizante; **parathyroid** —— (**PTH**) hormona paratiroidea; **thyroid** —— hormona tiroidea; **thyroid-stimulating** —— (**TSH**) hormona estimulante del tiroides

hornet *n* avispón *m*

horsefly n (pl -**flies**) tábano
horsetail n (bot) cola de caballo
hose n (tube) manguera
hose n (pl hose) (stocking) media
hospice n asilo para pacientes con enfermedades terminales
hospital n hospital m; —— **administration** administración f del hospital; **community** —— hospital de la comunidad; **county** —— (US) hospital del condado; **general** —— hospital general; **mental** —— hospital psiquiátrico; **private** —— hospital privado; **public** —— hospital público; **Veteran's Administration (VA)** —— hospital para veteranos
hospitalize vt hospitalizar, internar; **Have you ever been hospitalized before?**..¿Ha estado hospitalizado alguna vez antes?
hostile adj hostil
hostility n hostilidad f
hot adj (comp **hotter**; super **hottest**) caliente; (to the taste) picante; **to be** o **feel** —— tener or sentir calor; **Do you feel hot all the time?**..¿Se siente con calor todo el tiempo? —— **flash** calor m, bochorno, sensación repentina de calor (esp durante la menopausia)
hot sauce n salsa picante
hot springs npl aguas termales
hot-water bottle o **bag** n bolsa de agua caliente
hour n hora; **office hours** horas de oficina or de consulta; **visiting hours** horas de visita
housecleaner n sirviente -ta mf, limpiador -ra mf de casas
housefly n (pl -**flies**) mosca doméstica
housewife n (pl -**wives**) ama de casa
hug n abrazo; vt (pret & pp **hugged**; ger **hugging**) abrazar
hum n (buzzing or ringing) zumbido; vt (pret & pp **hummed**; ger **humming**) (a note) canturrear; vi zumbar, canturrear
human adj humano; —— **being** ser humano; n humano
humanitarian adj humanitario
humerus n húmero
humid adj húmedo

humidifier n humidificador m, aparato que produce vapor
humidify vt (pret & pp -**fied**) humedecer
humidity n humedad f
humor n (anat) humor m; **aqueous** —— humor acuoso; **vitreous** —— humor vítreo
hump n (on the back) joroba
humpback n jorobado -da mf
humpbacked adj jorobado
hung pret & pp de **hang**
hunger n hambre f
hungover adj crudo (Mex); **to be** —— tener una resaca, tener una cruda (Mex), estar crudo (Mex), estar de goma (CA)
hungry adj **to be** —— tener hambre; **Are you hungry?**..¿Tiene hambre?
hurricane n huracán m
hurt vt (pret & pp **hurt**) (to cause pain) doler, causar dolor; (to injure) lastimar, herir; (to harm) hacer daño; **This won't hurt you**..Esto no le va a doler...**I'm not going to hurt you**..No voy a causarle dolor...**Did you hurt your finger?**..¿Se lastimó el dedo?...**Eating oranges won't hurt you**..Comer naranjas no le hará daño; **to** —— **oneself** o **to get** —— lastimarse; **Did you hurt yourself?**..¿Se lastimó? vi doler, sentir dolor; **Where does it hurt?**..¿Dónde le duele?...**Do you hurt all over?**..¿Le duele todo?...**Tell me if it hurts**..Dígame si siente dolor.
husband n esposo, marido
hydatid adj hidátide, hidatídico
hydatidiform adj hidatiforme, hidatidiforme
hydralazine n hidralacina
hydrangea n (bot) hortensia
hydrate vt hidratar
hydrocarbon n hidrocarburo
hydrocele n hidrocele m
hydrocephalus n hidrocéfalo
hydrocephaly n hidrocefalia
hydrochloric acid n ácido clorhídrico
hydrochlorothiazide n hidroclorotiazida
hydrocortisone n hidrocortisona
hydrogenated adj hidrogenado
hydrogen peroxide n peróxido de hidrógeno (form), agua oxigenada

hydronephrosis *n* hidronefrosis *f*
hydrophobia *n* hidrofobia
hydroquinone *n* hidroquinona
hydrotherapy *n* hidroterapia
hygiene *n* higiene *f*, aseo; **oral** —— aseo oral *or* bucal
hygienic *adj* higiénico
hygienist *n* higienista *mf*
hymen *n* himen *m*
hyoid bone *n* hioides *m*
hyperactive *adj* hiperactivo
hyperactivity *n* hiperactividad *f*
hyperalimentation *n* hiperalimentación *f*
hyperbaric *adj* hiperbárico; —— **chamber** cámara hiperbárica
hypercalcemia *n* hipercalcemia
hyperglycemia *n* hiperglucemia
hyperlipidemia *n* hiperlipemia *or* hiperlipidemia
hyperlipoproteinemia *n* hiperlipoproteinemia
hyperosmolar *adj* hiperosmolar
hyperparathyroid *adj* hiperparatiroideo
hyperparathyroidism *n* hiperparatiroidismo
hyperpigmentation *n* hiperpigmentación *f*
hyperplasia *n* hiperplasia
hypersensitive *adj* hipersensible
hypersensitivity *n* hipersensibilidad *f*
hypertension *n* hipertensión *f*, alta presión (*fam*); **malignant** —— hipertensión maligna; **portal** —— hipertensión portal; **pulmonary** —— hipertensión pulmonar
hyperthermia *n* hipertermia

hyperthyroid *adj* hipertiroideo
hyperthyroidism *n* hipertiroidismo
hypertrophy *n* hipertrofia; **benign prostatic** —— hipertrofia prostática benigna
hyperventilate *vi* respirar demasiado rápido
hyperventilation *n* hiperventilación *f*
hyphema *n* hipema *f*
hypnosis *n* hipnosis *f*
hypnotic *adj & n* hipnótico
hypnotism *n* hipnotismo
hypnotist *n* hipnotizador -ra *mf*
hypnotize *vt* hipnotizar
hypoallergenic *adj* hipoalergénico
hypochondriac *adj & n* hipocondríaco *or* (*esp spoken*) hipocondriaco
hypodermic *adj* hipodérmico
hypoglycemia *n* hipoglucemia
hypoglycemic *adj* hipoglucémico; **oral** —— **agent** hipoglucemiante *m* oral
hypoparathyroid *adj* hipoparatiroideo
hypoparathyroidism *n* hipoparatiroidismo
hypopituitarism *n* hipopituitarismo
hypospadias *n* hipospadias *m*
hypotension *n* hipotensión *f*
hypothalamus *n* hipotálamo
hypothermia *n* hipotermia
hypothyroid *adj* hipotiroideo
hypothyroidism *n* hipotiroidismo
hysterectomy *n* (*pl* **-mies**) histerectomía; **abdominal** —— histerectomía abdominal; **vaginal** —— histerectomía vaginal
hysteria *n* histeria
hysterical *adj* histérico

I

ibuprofen *n* ibuprofén *m*, ibuprofeno
ice *n* hielo; —— **chips** pedacitos de hielo; —— **pack** bolsa con hielo
ice cream *n* helado
I&D *V.* **incision and drainage**.
id *n* (*psych*) id *m*

ideal *adj* ideal
identification *n* identificación *f*; —— **bracelet** brazalete *m* para identificación
identify *vt* identificar; *vi* **to** —— **with** (*psych*) identificarse con
identity *n* (*pl* **-ties**) identidad *f*; —— **crisis**

crisis *f* de identidad
idiopathic *adj* idiopático
ileostomy *n* (*pl* **-mies**) ileostomía
ileum *n* íleon *m*
ileus *n* íleo
iliac *adj* iliaco
ilium *n* hueso iliaco
ill *adj* enfermo, malo
illegal *adj* ilegal
illiteracy *n* analfabetismo
illiterate *adj* analfabeto
illness *n* enfermedad *f*, mal *m*; **mental —** enfermedad mental; **occupational —** enfermedad ocupacional
illusion *n* ilusión *f*
IM *V.* **intramuscular**.
image *n* imagen *f*
imbalance *n* desequilibrio
imipenem *n* imipenem *m*
imipramine *n* imipramina
immature *adj* inmaduro
immediate *adj* inmediato
immediately *adv* inmediatamente
immersion *n* inmersión *f*
immobile *adj* inmóvil
immobilization *n* inmovilización *f*
immobilize *vt* inmovilizar
immobilizer *n* inmovilizador *m*
immune *adj* (*person*) inmune; (*system, reaction, etc.*) inmunitario
immunity *n* inmunidad *f*
immunization *n* inmunización *f*
immunize *vt* inmunizar
immunocompetent *adj* inmunocompetente
immunocompromised *adj* inmunocomprometido
immunodeficiency *n* inmunodeficiencia
immunodepressed *adj* inmunodeprimido
immunodepression *n* inmunodepresión *f*
immunoglobulin *n* inmunoglobulina
immunological, immunologic *adj* inmunológico
immunologist *n* inmunólogo -ga *mf*
immunology *n* inmunología
immunosuppressant *n* inmunosupresor *m*
immunosuppressive *adj* inmunosupresor
immunotherapy *n* inmunoterapia
impact *n* impacto; **low —** bajo impacto

impacted *adj* impactado
impaction *n* impactación *f*
impair *vt* dañar, perjudicar
impaired *adj* dañado; **hearing —** que tiene dificultad para oír
imperforate *adj* imperforado
impetigo *n* impétigo
implant *n* implante *m*; *vt* implantar; **to become implanted** implantarse
implantation *n* implantación *f*
impotence *n* impotencia
impotent *adj* impotente
impregnate *vt* impregnar
improper *adj* indebido
improve *vt, vi* mejorar(se)
improvement *n* mejoría
impulse *n* impulso
impulsive *adj* impulsivo
impure *adj* impuro
impurity *n* impureza
inactive *adj* inactivo
inactivity *n* inactividad *f*
inappropriate *adj* indebido, inapropiado (*Ang*)
incapable *adj* incapaz
incapacitating *adj* incapacitante
incest *n* incesto
incestuous *adj* incestuoso
inch *n* pulgada
incidence *n* incidencia
incision *n* incisión *f*, corte *m*, herida
incisor *n* diente incisivo
incoherent *adj* incoherente
incompatible *adj* incompatible
incompetent *adj* incompetente
incomplete *adj* incompleto
incontinence *n* incontinencia, incapacidad *f* para retener la orina o el excremento; **stress —** incontinencia de esfuerzo
incontinent *adj* (*of urine or stool*) incontinente, incapaz de retener la orina o el excremento
increase *n* aumento; *vt, vi* aumentar
incubator *n* incubadora
incurable *adj* incurable
independent *adj* independiente
index *adj & n* (*pl* **indexes** *o* **indices**) índice *m*; **— finger** dedo índice

indication *n* indicación *f*
indifference *n* indiferencia
indigestion *n* indigestión *f*
indisposition *n* indisposición *f*
indistinct *adj* indistinto
individual *n* individuo (*invariant with respect to gender*)
indomethacin *n* indometacina
induce *vt* inducir
ineffective *adj* ineficaz
ineligible *adj* inelegible
inert *adj* inerte
infancy *n* infancia
infant *n* infante *m*, criatura
infantile *adj* infantil
infarct *n* infarto
infarction *n* infarto, acción *f* y efecto de un infarto; **myocardial** —— infarto de miocardio
infect *vt, vi* infectar(se)
infection *n* infección *f*; **urinary tract** —— **(UTI)** infección del tracto urinario, mal *m* de orín (*fam*)
infectious *adj* infeccioso
inferior *adj* (*anat*) inferior
infertile *adj* estéril
infertility *n* infertilidad *f*, esterilidad *f*
infest *vt* infestar
infestation *n* infestación *f*
infiltrate *vt, vi* infiltrar(se)
infiltration *n* infiltración *f*
infirmary *n* enfermería
inflamed *adj* inflamado; **to become** —— inflamarse
inflammable *adj* inflamable
inflammation *n* inflamación *f*
inflammatory *adj* inflamatorio
influenza *n* influenza, gripe *f*
information *n* información *f*
infrared *adj* infrarrojo
infuse *vt* infundir
infusion *n* infusión *f*
ingest *vt* ingerir
ingredient *n* ingrediente *m*
ingrown nail *n* uña enterrada *or* encarnada, uñero
inguinal *adj* inguinal
INH *V.* isoniazid.

inhalant *adj* inhalador; *n* inhalante *m* (*form*), medicamento para inhalación
inhalation *n* inhalación *f*
inhale *vt, vi* inhalar
inhaler *n* aerosol *m*, inhalador *m*, espray *m* (*Ang*); **metered dose** —— aerosol dosificador; **nasal** —— aerosol *or* inhalador nasal
inherit *vt* heredar
inherited *adj* heredado
inhibit *vt* inhibir
inhibited *adj* inhibido, cohibido
inhibition *n* inhibición *f*, cohibición *f*
initial *adj* inicial; *n* inicial *f*
inject *vt* inyectar
injectable *adj* inyectable
injection *n* inyección *f*; **The nurse will give you an injection..**La enfermera lo va a inyectar..La enfermera le va a poner una inyección.
injure *vt* herir, lastimar
injury *n* (*pl* **-ries**) herida, lesión *f*
inlay *n* (*dent*) incrustación *f*
innards *npl* tripas, entrañas
inner *adj* interno
inoculate *vt* inocular
inoculation *n* inoculación *f*
inoperable *adj* inoperable
inorganic *adj* inorgánico
inquest *n* pesquisa
insane *adj* loco
insanity *n* locura
insect *n* insecto
insecticide *n* insecticida *m*
insecure *adj* inseguro
insecurity *n* inseguridad *f*
inseminate *vt* inseminar
insemination *n* inseminación *f*; **artificial** —— inseminación artificial
insert *n* **package** —— instructivo; *vt* introducir, meter
inside *adj* interior, interno; *adv* dentro, adentro; *n* interior *m*; *prep* dentro de; **inside your body..**dentro de su cuerpo
insole *n* plantilla
insomnia *n* insomnio
inspire *vt, vi* inspirar
instep *n* empeine *m* (*del pie*)

instinct *n* instinto
instruction *n* instrucción *f*
instrument *n* instrumento
insufficiency *n* insuficiencia; **aortic** ——, **renal** ——, **venous** ——, etc. insuficiencia aórtica, renal, venosa, etc.
insulin *n* insulina; **lente** —— insulina lenta; **NPH** —— insulina NPH *or* de acción intermedia; **regular** —— insulina de acción rápida; **semilente** —— insulina semilenta; **ultralente** —— insulina ultralenta
insurance *n* seguro (*frec pl*)
intact *adj* intacto
intellect *n* intelecto
intellectual *adj* intelectual
intellectualize *vi* intelectualizar
intelligence *n* inteligencia; —— **quotient (IQ)** cociente *m* de inteligencia (CI)
intense *adj* intenso
intensify *vt* (*pret & pp* **-fied**) intensificar
intensity *n* (*pl* **-ties**) intensidad *f*
intensive *adj* intensivo
interact *vi* interactuar
interaction *n* interacción *f*
intercourse *n* relación *f* (*sexual*), acto sexual; **When was the last time you had intercourse?**..¿Cuándo fue la última vez que tuvo relaciones?
interferon *n* interferón *m*; **alpha** —— interferón alfa; **beta** —— interferón beta; **gamma** —— interferón gamma
interior *adj & n* interior *m*
intermediate *adj* intermedio
intermittent *adj* intermitente
intern *n* médico interno, interno -na *mf*
internal *adj* interno
internist *n* internista *mf*
interpersonal *adj* interpersonal
interpret *vt, vi* interpretar
interpreter *n* intérprete *mf*
interstitial *adj* intersticial
interval *n* intervalo
intervention *n* intervención *f*
interventricular *adj* interventricular
intestinal *adj* intestinal
intestine *n* intestino, tripa (*frec pl*); **large** —— intestino grueso; **small** ——

intestino delgado
intimacy *n* intimidad *f*
intolerable *adj* intolerable
intolerance *n* intolerancia
intolerant *adj* intolerante
intoxication *n* intoxicación *f*
intraarticular *adj* intraarticular
intracranial *adj* intracraneal
intradermal *adj* intradérmico, intracutáneo
intramuscular (IM) *adj* intramuscular (IM)
intraocular *adj* intraocular
intrauterine device (IUD) *n* dispositivo intrauterino (DIU), aparato (*fam*)
intravenous (IV) *adj* intravenoso (IV), endovenoso
intrinsic factor *n* factor intrínseco
introvert *n* introvertido -da *mf*
introverted *adj* introvertido
intubate *vt* intubar
intubation *n* intubación *f*
intussusception *n* intususcepción *f*
invalid *n* (*ant*, **disabled person** *es preferido*) inválido -da *mf*
invasive *adj* invasor
investigational *adj* (*medication, etc.*) en investigación
invigorate *vt* vigorizar; **to become invigorated** vigorizarse
invisible *adj* invisible
involuntary *adj* involuntario
iodine *n* yodo
iodized *adj* yodado
iontophoresis *n* iontoforesis *f*
ipecac *n* ipecacuana
ipratropium bromide *n* bromuro de ipratropio
IQ *V.* **intelligence quotient.**
iris *n* (*pl* **irides**) iris *m*
iritis *n* iritis *f*
iron *n* hierro
irradiate *vt* irradiar, tratar con radiación
irradiation *n* irradiación *f*, tratamiento con radiación
irregular *adj* irregular
irreversible *adj* irreversible
irrigate *vt* irrigar
irrigation *n* irrigación *f*
irritability *n* irritabilidad *f*

irritable *adj* irritable
irritant *n* irritante *m*
irritate *vt* irritar; **to become irritated** irritarse
irritating *adj* irritante, molesto
irritation *n* irritación *f*
ischemia *n* isquemia
ischemic *adj* isquémico
isolate *vt* aislar
isolation *n* aislamiento
isoleucine *n* isoleucina
isometric *adj* isométrico
isoniazid (INH) *n* isoniacida
isosorbide dinitrate *n* dinitrato de isosorbide
isotope *n* isótopo

isotretinoin *n* isotretinoína
isradipine *n* isradipina
itch *n* picazón *f*, comezón *f*; *vi* picar, tener picazón *or* comezón; **Where does it itch?** ..¿Dónde le pica?...**Does your arm itch?**.. ¿Le pica el brazo?...**Do you itch?**..¿Tiene picazón?
itching, itchiness *n* picazón *f*, comezón *f*
ITP *abbr* **idiopathic thrombocytopenic purpura. V. purpura.**
itraconazole *n* itraconazol *m*
IUD *V.* **intrauterine device.**
IV *V.* **intravenous.**
IVP *abbr* **intravenous pyelogram.** *V.* **pyelogram.**

J

jabbing *adj* punzante
jacket *n* chaqueta, chamarra (*Mex*); (*dent*) corona
jail *n* cárcel *f*
jaundice *n* ictericia (*form*), coloración amarilla de la piel, piel amarilla (*fam*)
jaw *n* mandíbula, quijada (*fam*); **lower —— maxilar** *m* inferior, mandíbula, quijada; **upper —— maxilar** *m* superior
jawbone *n* mandíbula, quijada
Jehovah's Witnesses *npl* Testigos de Jehová
jejunal *adj* yeyunal
jejunum *n* yeyuno
jelly *n* (*pl* -lies) jalea
jellyfish *n* (*pl* -fish *o* -fishes) medusa, aguamala

jigger *n* nigua
job *n* trabajo, empleo
jock itch *n* (*fam*) tiña inguinal
jockstrap *n* (*fam*) suspensorio
jog *vi* (*pret & pp* **jogged;** *ger* **jogging**) trotar
join *vt* (*two objects*) ligar, juntar; *vi* unirse, juntarse
joint *n* articulación *f*, coyuntura
judo *n* judo
jugular *adj* yugular
juice *n* jugo, zumo; **fruit —— jugo de fruta; orange —— jugo de naranja
junk *n* (*vulg*) heroína
junkie *n* (*vulg*) persona que se inyecta heroína
juvenile *adj* juvenil

K

karate *n* karate *m*
keloid *n* queloide *m*
keratin *n* queratina
keratotomy *n* queratotomía; **radial ——** queratotomía radiada
ketoacidosis *n* cetoacidosis *f*
ketoconazole *n* ketoconazol *m*
ketone *n* cetona
ketorolac *n* ketorolaco
ketotic *adj* cetónico
kick *n* patada; *vt* dar una patada; *vi* dar patadas
kid *n* (*fam, child*) niño -ña *mf*
kidney *n* riñón *m*; **—— disease** enfermedad *f* de los riñones; **—— failure** insuficiencia renal; **polycystic ——** riñón poliquístico
kidney belt *n* (*fam*) faja, cinturón *m* (*para prevenir hernias*)
kill *vt* matar
kilogram *n* kilogramo
kind *adj* amable, amistoso

kiss *n* beso; *vt* besar
kissing bug *n* chinche besucona (*vector de la enfermedad de Chagas*)
kit *n* botiquín *m*; **first-aid ——** botiquín de primeros auxilios
Klebsiella Klebsiella
knee *n* rodilla; **—— jerk** reflejo patelar *or* rotuliano; **back of the ——** corva
kneecap *n* rótula
kneelength *adj* de largo hasta la rodilla
kneepad *n* rodillera
knife-like *adj* (*pain*) punzante
knife *n* (*pl* **knives**) cuchillo
knit *vi* (*ortho*) soldar
knock-kneed *adj* con las rodillas hacia adentro, patizambo
knuckle *n* nudillo
kwashiorkor *n* kwashiorkor *or* cuasiorcor *m*
kyphoscoliosis *n* cifoscoliosis *f*
kyphosis *n* cifosis *f*

L

lab *V.* **laboratory.**
label *n* etiqueta
labetolol *n* labetolol *m*
labial *adj* labial
labium *n* (*pl* **labia**) labio (*genital*)
labor *n* trabajo de parto; **—— pain** dolor *m* del parto; **to be in ——** estar en trabajo de parto
laboratory *n* (*pl* **-ries**) laboratorio

labyrinth *n* laberinto
labyrinthitis *n* laberintitis *f*
lacerate *vt* lacerar
laceration *n* laceración *f*
lack *n* deficiencia, falta; *vt* carecer de, faltarle (*a uno*)
lacrimal, lachrymal *adj* lacrimal *or* lagrimal
lactase *n* lactasa
lactate *vi* lactar, salirle leche (*fam*)

lactation *n* lactancia
lactic acid *n* ácido láctico
lactic dehydrogenase *n* deshidrogenasa láctica
Lactobacillus Lactobacillus
lactose *n* lactosa; —— **intolerance** intolerancia a la lactosa
lactulose *n* lactulosa
lag *n* retraso; *vi* (*pret & pp* **lagged**; *ger* **lagging**) retrasarse
lain *pp de* **lie**
lamb *n* (*meat*) carne *f* de cordero, cordero
lame *adj* cojo
laminectomy *n* (*pl* -**mies**) laminectomía
lamp *n* lámpara
lance *vt* abrir con bisturí (*un absceso*)
lancet *n* lanceta
language *n* (*referring to structure and development*) lenguaje *m*
lanolin *n* lanolina
lanugo *n* lanugo
lap *n* (*of a person*) regazo
laparoscope *n* laparoscopio
laparoscopic *adj* laparoscópico
laparoscopy *n* (*pl* -**pies**) laparoscopia *or* (*esp spoken*) laparoscopía
laparotomy *n* (*pl* -**mies**) laparotomía
lapse *n* lapso
lard *n* manteca
large *adj* grande
larva *n* (*pl* -**vae**) larva
larva migrans *n* larva migrans
laryngeal *adj* laríngeo
laryngectomy *n* (*pl* -**mies**) laringectomía
laryngitis *n* laringitis *f*
laryngoscope *n* laringoscopio
laryngoscopy *n* (*pl* -**pies**) laringoscopia *or* (*esp spoken*) laringoscopía
larynx *n* (*pl* -**inges**) laringe *f*
laser *n* rayo láser, láser *m*
last *adj* último; **your last period**..su última regla; *vi* durar; **How long did the pain last?**..¿Cuánto tiempo le duró el dolor?
last rites *npl* santos óleos
late *adj* (*development, etc.*) tardío
latent *adj* latente
lateral *adj* lateral
latex *n* látex *m*

latrine *n* letrina
laugh *n* risa; *vi* reír(se)
laughing gas *n* gas *m* hilarante
lavage *n* lavado; **bronchoalveolar** —— lavado broncoalveolar; **gastric** —— lavado gástrico; **peritoneal** —— lavado peritoneal
lavatory *n* (*pl* -**ries**) lavatorio
lawsuit *n* demanda (*legal*)
laxative *adj & n* laxante *m*; **bulk** —— laxante que aumenta el bolo fecal
lay *adj* lego, popular, no profesional; —— **opinion** opinión popular *or* no profesional
lay *pret de* **lie**
layer *n* capa
lb. *V.* **pound**.
LDL *abbr* **low density lipoprotein.** *V.* **lipoprotein.**
lead *n* plomo
lean *adj* (*person*) flaco; (*meat*) magro; *vi* inclinarse; **Lean forward**..Inclínese hacia adelante.
learning *n* aprendizaje *m*; —— **disability** dificultad *f* del aprendizaje
leathery *adj* correoso
lecithin *n* lecitina
leech *n* sanguijuela
left *adj* izquierdo; *n* (*left-hand side*) izquierda
left-handed *adj* zurdo
leg *n* pierna
legume *n* legumbre *f*
leiomyofibroma *n* leiomiofibroma *m*
leiomyoma *n* leiomioma *or* liomioma *m*
leiomyosarcoma *n* leiomiosarcoma *or* liomiosarcoma *m*
leishmaniasis *n* leishmaniasis *f*; **American** *o* **mucocutaneous** —— leishmaniasis mucocutánea americana
lemon *n* limón *m*
length *n* longitud *f*, largo
lengthen *vt* alargar, hacer más largo
lens *n* lente *m&f*; (*of the eye*) cristalino; **contact** —— (*hard, soft*) lente de contacto (*duro, blando*)
leprosy *n* lepra
leptospirosis *n* leptospirosis *f*
lesbian *n* lesbiana

lesion *n* lesión *f*
lethal *adj* letal
lethargic *adj* letárgico
lethargy *n* letargo
leucine *n* leucina
leukemia *n* leucemia; **acute lymphocytic** —— leucemia linfocítica aguda; **chronic myelogenous** —— leucemia mielógena crónica; **granulocytic** —— leucemia granulocítica; **lymphoblastic** —— leucemia linfoblástica; **myeloid** —— leucemia mieloide
leukocyte *n* leucocito
level *n* nivel *m*
LGV *V.* **lymphogranuloma venereum.**
LH *abbr* **luteinizing hormone.** *V.* **hormone.**
libido *n* libido *f*, deseo sexual
lice *pl de* **louse**
lichen planus *n* liquen plano
lick *vt* lamer
licorice *n* (*bot*) regaliz *m*
lidocaine *n* lidocaína
lie *vi* (*pret* **lay;** *pp* **lain;** *ger* **lying**) **to** —— **down** acostarse
life *n* vida; —— **expectancy** expectativa *or* esperanza de vida
lifestyle *n* estilo de vida
life-support *adj* se refiere a equipos y métodos para sostener funciones vitales como respirar, eliminar desechos, etc.
life-threatening *adj* que amenaza la vida
lifetime *n* vida, curso de vida, toda una vida
lift *vt* levantar; **to** —— **weights** levantar pesas
ligament *n* ligamento
ligation *n* ligadura; **tubal** —— ligadura de las trompas, amarre *m* de las trompas (*fam*)
light *adj* (*case of disease*) leve; (*touch*) ligero; (*weight*) liviano; *n* luz *f*
lightheaded *adj* mareado, que tiene sensación de desmayo; **to feel** —— tener mareo, estar mareado, tener sensación de desmayo
lightheadedness *n* mareo, sensación *f* de desmayo
lightning *n* relámpago
limb *n* (*arm or leg*) miembro

limber *adj* flexible, ágil
lime *n* (*fruit*) lima
limit *n* límite *m*; **lower** —— **of normal** límite inferior normal **upper** —— **of normal** límite superior normal; *vt* limitar
limp *adj* flojo; *vi* cojear, renquear
lindane *n* lindano
line *n* línea; *vt* (*the intestine, etc.*) revestir; **to** —— **up** alinear; *vi* **to** —— **up** alinearse
liniment *n* linimento
lining *n* (*of the stomach, etc.*) revestimiento, recubrimiento
linoleic acid *n* ácido linoleico
lip *n* labio; (*genital*) labio; **lower** —— labio inferior; **upper** —— labio superior
lipase *n* lipasa
lipid *n* lípido
lipoma *n* lipoma *m*
lipoprotein *n* lipoproteína; **high density** —— **(HDL)** lipoproteína de alta densidad (LAD); **low density** —— **(LDL)** lipoproteína de baja densidad (LBD); **very low density** —— **(VLDL)** lipoproteína de muy baja densidad (LMBD)
liposarcoma *n* liposarcoma *m*
liposuction *n* liposucción *f*
lipread *vi* (*pret & pp* -**read**) leer los labios
liquid *adj & n* líquido
liquor *n* licor *m*, alcohol *m*
lisinopril *n* lisinopril *m*
lisp *n* ceceo; *vi* cecear
listen *vi* escuchar; **I'm going to listen to your lungs.**..Voy a escucharle los pulmones.
listeriosis *n* listeriosis *f*
listless *adj* decaído, letárgico
liter *n* litro
lithium *n* litio
lithotripsy *n* litotripsia
litter *n* camilla
little *adj* pequeño, chico; poco; **a little tumor**..un tumor pequeño...**a little milk**..un poco de leche...**little time**..poco tiempo; *n* poco; —— **by** —— poco a poco
live *adj* (*virus, vaccine*) vivo; *vi* vivir
liver *n* hígado; —— **disease** enfermedad *f*

del hígado; —— **failure** insuficiencia hepática

lives *pl de* **life**

lobar *adj* lobar

lobe *n* lóbulo

lobectomy *n* (*pl* -**mies**) lobectomía

lobelia *n* (*bot*) lobelia

lobotomy *n* (*pl* -**mies**) lobotomía

local *adj* local

lockjaw *n* (*fam*) trismo

lodge *vi* alojarse

loin *n* lomo

long *adj* largo; *adv* **How long have you had diabetes?**..¿Desde cuándo tiene diabetes? ..¿Hace cuánto que tiene diabetes?...**How long were you unconscious?**..¿Por cuánto tiempo estuvo inconsciente?

long-acting *adj* de acción prolongada

longevity *n* longevidad *f*

long-term *adj* a largo plazo

look *vi* mirar; **Look upward**..Mire hacia arriba.

loop *n* lazo

loose *adj* flojo, suelto

loosen *vt* aflojar, soltar, (*clothing*) desabrochar(se); **Loosen your pants**..Desabroche su pantalón.

loperamide *n* loperamida

loracarbef *n* loracarbef *m*

loratidine *n* loratidina

lorazepam *n* lorazepam *m*

lordosis *n* lordosis *f*

lordotic *adj* lordótico

lose *vt* (*pret & pp* **lost**) perder; **to —— consciousness** perder el conocimiento *or* la conciencia; **to —— one's voice** estar afónico; **to —— weight** perder peso, bajar de peso

loss *n* pérdida; **hair ——** caída del pelo; **hearing ——** pérdida de la audición

lot *n* (*pharm*) lote *m*; **a ——** mucho; **Do you sleep a lot?**..¿Duerme mucho? **a ——** (*fam*) mucho(s); **a lot of milk**..mucha leche...**a lot of pimples**..muchos granos

lotion *n* loción *f*, crema; **hand ——** crema para las manos; **suntan ——** loción bronceadora, crema para el sol

louse *n* (*pl* **lice**) piojo

lovastatin *n* lovastatina

love *n* amor *m*; *vt*, *vi* amar, querer

loved one *n* ser amado

loving *adj* cariñoso, afectuoso

low *adj* bajo; —— **in calories** bajo en calorías; **Your potassium is low**..Su potasio está bajo; **to be —— on** faltarle (*a uno*); **You are low on iron**..Le falta hierro.

lower *adj* (*anat*) inferior (*form*), bajo, de abajo; —— **back** parte baja de la espalda; *vt* reducir, bajar; **You need a cholesterol-lowering diet**..Necesita una dieta para reducir el colesterol...**Lower your arm**..Baje el brazo.

low-pitched *adj* grave

lozenge *n* trocisco, pastilla para chupar

LSD *V.* **lysergic acid diethylamide**.

lubricant *adj & n* lubricante *m*

lubricate *vt* lubricar

lubrication *n* lubricación *f*

lukewarm *adj* tibio

lumbar *adj* lumbar

lump *n* bola, bolita, pelota, (*due to trauma, esp about the head*) chichón *m*

lumpectomy *n* lumpectomía (*Ang*)

lumpy *adj* (*comp* -**ier**; *super* -**iest**) que tiene bolitas

lunch *n* comida al mediodía, almuerzo, lonche *m* (*Ang*), comida (*Mex*); **to have —— ** comer al mediodía, almorzar, comer (*Mex*)

lung *n* pulmón *m*

lupus *n* lupus *m*; **systemic —— erythematosus (SLE)** lupus eritematoso generalizado *or* sistémico

luteal *adj* luteínico

lye *n* lejía

lying *ger de* **lie**

lymph *n* linfa; —— **node** ganglio linfático

lymphadenitis *n* linfadenitis *f*

lymphangitis *n* linfangitis *f*

lymphatic *adj* linfático

lymphocyte *n* linfocito; **B ——** linfocito B; **helper T ——** linfocito T ayudante; **suppressor T ——** linfocito T supresor

lymphogranuloma venereum (LGV) *n* linfogranuloma venéreo *or* inguinal

lymphoid *adj* linfoide
lymphoma *n* linfoma *m*; **lymphocytic** *o*
   non-Hodgkin's —— linfoma linfocítico,
   linfoma no Hodgkin

lyophilized *adj* liofilizado
lysergic acid diethylamide (LSD) *n*
   dietilamida del ácido lisérgico (LSD)
lysine *n* lisina

M

macerate *vt* macerar
macrobiotic *adj* macrobiótico
mad *adj* (*comp* **madder**; *super* **maddest**)
   enojado; (*crazy*) loco; **to get** ——
   enojarse
maggot *n* cresa, gusano
magnesium *n* magnesio; —— **sulfate** sulfato de magnesio
magnetic resonance imaging (MRI) *n*
   imágenes *fpl* por resonancia magnética
magnifying glass *n* lupa, lente *m* de aumento
maintain *vt* mantener
maintenance *n* mantenimiento
major *adj* mayor
make-up *n* (*cosmetics*) maquillaje *m*
malabsorption *n* malabsorción *f*
malady *n* (*pl* **-dies**) enfermedad *f*, mal *m*
malaise *n* malestar *m*
malaria *n* paludismo, malaria
malathion *n* malatión *m*
mal del pinto *n* mal *m* del pinto, pinta
male *adj* masculino; *n* varón *m*
malformation *n* malformación *f*
malignancy *n* malignidad *f*
malignant *adj* maligno
malinger *vi* fingirse enfermo
malnourished *adj* desnutrido
malnutrition *n* desnutrición *f*
malpractice *n* negligencia médica
mammary *adj* mamario
mammogram *n* mamografía, mamograma *m*
mammography *n* mamografía
mammoplasty *n* (*pl* **-ties**) mamoplastia *or*

(*esp spoken*) mamoplastía
man *n* (*pl* **men**) hombre
manage *vt* manejar
management *n* manejo
mandible *n* mandíbula
maneuver *n* maniobra; **Heimlich** ——
   maniobra de Heimlich; *vt, vi* maniobrar
mania *n* manía
manic *adj* maniaco *or* maníaco
manic-depressive *adj* maniacodepresivo
manicure *n* manicura
manifestation *n* manifestación *f*
manipulate *vt* manipular
manometry *n* manometría
manual *adj* manual; *n* (*booklet*) manual *m*
manubrium *n* manubrio
many *adj* muchos; **many times**..muchas
   veces
margarine *n* margarina
margin *n* margen *m*
marijuana *n* marihuana *or* marijuana
marital *adj* marital
mark *n* marca
marrow *n* médula; **bone** —— médula ósea
marshmallow *n* (*bot*) malvavisco
masculine *adj* masculino
mash *n* (*crushing injury*) machucón *m*,
   machucadura; *vt* machucar, apachurrar
mask *n* (*for oxygen, etc.*) máscara, mascarilla; (*surg*) cubreboca *m*; (*of pregnancy*)
   paño; *vt* (*signs, symptoms*) enmascarar
masochism *n* masoquismo
masochist *n* masoquista *mf*
masochistic *adj* masoquista

mass *n* masa; **muscle** —— masa muscular

massage *n* masaje *m*; *vt* masajear, dar masaje, sobar (*fam*)

masseur *n* masajista *m*

masseuse *n* masajista *f*

massive *adj* masivo

MAST *V.* **military anti-shock trousers.**

mastectomy *n* (*pl* -**mies**) mastectomía; **modified radical** —— mastectomía radical modificada

mastitis *n* mastitis *f*

mastoid *adj* mastoideo; —— **process** apófisis *f* mastoides

masturbate *vi* masturbarse

match *vt* (*blood, tissue*) ser compatible con (*sangre, tejido*); **We need to find out if your sister's tissue type matches your own..**Tenemos que averiguar si el tejido de su hermana es compatible con el suyo.

material *n* material *m*

maternal *adj* materno; (*motherly*) maternal

maternity *n* maternidad *f*

matter *n* **gray** —— substancia gris; **white** —— substancia blanca

mattress *n* colchón *m*

mature *adj* maduro; *vi* madurar

maturity *n* madurez *f*

maxilla *n* (*pl* -**lae**) maxilar *m* superior

maxillary *adj* maxilar

maxillofacial *adj* maxilofacial

maximum *adj* & *n* (*pl* -**ma** *o* -**mums**) máximo

mayonnaise *n* mayonesa

M.D. *V.* **Doctor of Medicine.**

meal *n* comida; **balanced** —— comida balanceada

measles *n* sarampión *m*; **German** —— *o* **three-day** —— sarampión alemán, rubeola *or* rubéola (*form*)

measure *n* medida; *vt* medir

measurement *n* medida

measuring tape *n* cinta métrica

meat *n* carne *f*; **organ meats** vísceras; **red** —— carne roja

meatus *n* (*pl* **meatus**) meato

mebendazole *n* mebendazol *m*

mechanism *n* mecanismo; **defense** —— (*psych*) mecanismo de defensa

meconium *n* meconio

medial *adj* (*anat*) interno

median *adj* (*anat*) mediano

mediastinum *n* mediastino

medical *adj* médico

medicate *vt* medicar

medication *n* medicamento

medicinal *adj* medicinal

medicine *n* medicina, medicamento; —— **chest** *o* **cabinet** botiquín *m*; —— **dropper** gotero, cuentagotas *m*; **alternative** —— medicina alternativa; **family** —— medicina familiar; **folk** —— curanderismo; **internal** —— medicina interna; **nuclear** —— medicina nuclear; **occupational** —— medicina ocupacional; **podiatric** —— medicina podiátrica; **preventive** —— medicina preventiva; **socialized** —— medicina socializada; **sports** —— medicina deportiva; **veterinary** —— veterinaria

medicolegal *adj* medicolegal

meditate *vi* meditar

medium *adj* mediano; *n* medio; **contrast** —— medio de contraste

medroxyprogesterone *n* medroxiprogesterona

medulla *n* (*pl* -**lae**) bulbo raquídeo; (*of the adrenal gland*) médula

megacolon *n* megacolon *m*

megadose *n* megadosis *f*

melancholy *adj* melancólico; *n* melancolía

melanin *n* melanina

melanoma *n* melanoma *m*

melatonin *n* melatonina

member *n* miembro

membrane *n* membrana; **mucous** —— membrana mucosa; **tympanic** —— membrana timpánica

memory *n* memoria; **long-term** —— memoria remota; **short-term** —— memoria reciente

men *pl de* **man**

meninges *pl de* **meninx**

meningioma *n* meningioma *m*

meningitis *n* meningitis *f*

meningocele *n* meningocele *m*

meningococcus *n* (*pl* -**ci**) meningococo

meninx *n* (*pl* **meninges**) meninge *f*
meniscus *n* (*pl* **menisci** *o* **meniscuses**) menisco
menopause *n* menopausia, cambio de vida
men's room *n* baño para hombres
menstrual *adj* menstrual
menstruate *vi* menstruar, reglar
menstruation *n* menstruación *f*
mental *adj* mental
menthol *n* mentol *m*
meperedine *n* meperedina
mercury *n* mercurio
mercy killing *n* eutanasia, muerte piadosa
mescal *n* mezcal *m*
mescaline *n* mescalina *or* mezcalina
mesenteric *adj* mesentérico
mesentery *n* mesenterio
mesh *n* malla
mesothelioma *n* mesotelioma *m*
metabolic *adj* metabólico
metabolism *n* metabolismo
metacarpal *adj* & *n* metacarpiano
metal *n* metal *m*; **heavy** —— metal pesado
metallic *adj* metálico
metaproterenol *n* metaproterenol *m*, orciprenalina
metastasis *n* (*pl* **-ses**) metástasis *f*
metastasize *vi* metastatizar
metastatic *adj* metastásico
metatarsal *adj* & *n* metatarsiano
meter *n* metro; (*measuring device*) medidor *m*; —— **squared** *o* **square** —— metro cuadrado
methadone *n* metadona
methamphetamine *n* metanfetamina
methane *n* metano
methanol *n* metanol *m*
methaqualone *n* metaqualona
methicillin *n* meticilina
methionine *n* metionina
method *n* método
methotrexate *n* metotrexato
methyl alcohol *n* alcohol metílico
methylcellulose *n* metilcelulosa
methyldopa *n* metildopa
methylphenidate *n* metilfenidato
methylprednisolone *n* metilprednisolona
metoclopramide *n* metoclopramida

metoprolol *n* metoprolol *m*
metric system *n* sistema métrico
metronidazole *n* metronidazol *m*
Mexican *adj* & *n* mexicano -na *mf*
mice *pl de* **mouse**
miconazole *n* miconazol *m*
microbe *n* microbio
microbial *adj* microbiano
microbiology *n* microbiología
microgram *n* microgramo
microorganism *n* microorganismo
microscope *n* microscopio; **electron** —— microscopio electrónico
microscopic *adj* microscópico
microsurgery *n* microcirugía
microwave *n* microonda
midbrain *n* mesencéfalo, cerebro medio
middle *adj* medio; *n* mitad *f*, medio
midget *n* enano -na *mf*
midwife *n* (*pl* **-wives**) partera, (*esp untrained*) comadrona
migraine *n* migraña, jaqueca
mild *adj* (*soap, etc.*) suave; (*illness, injury*) leve
mildew *n* moho
miliary *adj* miliar
military antishock trousers (MAST) *n* pantalones *mpl* antichoque
milk *n* leche *f*; —— **product** producto lácteo *or* de leche; **breast** —— leche materna; **condensed** —— leche condensada; **cow's** —— leche de vaca; **evaporated** —— leche evaporizada; **goat's** —— leche de cabra; **low-fat** —— leche baja en grasa; **pasteurized** —— leche pasteurizada; **powdered** —— leche en polvo; **raw** —— leche sin procesar, leche bronca (*Mex*); **skim** —— leche descremada *or* desnatada; **whole** —— leche entera
milk of magnesia *n* leche *f* de magnesia
milligram *n* miligramo
milliliter *n* mililitro
millimeter *n* milímetro
mind *n* mente *f*; **to lose one's** —— perder la razón, volverse loco
miner *n* minero
mineral *adj* & *n* mineral *m*; —— **oil** aceite *m* mineral; —— **water** agua mineral

minimum *adj* & *n* (*pl* -ma *o* -mums) mínimo

minor *adj* menor; *n* menor *m* (*de edad*)

minoxidil *n* minoxidil *m*

mint *n* (*bot*) menta

minute *n* minuto

miracle *n* milagro

mirror *n* espejo

miscarriage *n* aborto espontáneo *or* natural,
malparto

miscarry *vi* abortar (*sin intención*)

mischievous *adj* travieso

miss *vt* (*work*) faltar a; (*an appointment*)
faltar a, perder; (*dose of medication*) dejar
de tomar, no tomar; (*a loved one, etc.*)
extrañar, echar de menos; **Try not to miss
this appointment..**Procure no faltar a esta
cita...**Don't miss a single dose of this
medicine..**No deje de tomar una sola dosis
de esta medicina...**Do you miss your
husband?..**¿Extraña a su esposo?

missing *adj* ausente; **to be** —— faltarle; **She
is missing two fingers..**Le faltan dos
dedos.

mite *n* ácaro

mitral *adj* mitral

mix *vt* mezclar

mixture *n* mezcla

moan *n* gemido; *vi* gemir

mobile *adj* móvil

mobility *n* movilidad *f*

mobilize *vt* movilizar

moderate *adj* moderado

moderation *n* moderación *f*

modification *n* modificación *f*

modify *vt* (*pret* & *pp* -fied) modificar

moist *adj* húmedo

moisten *vt* humedecer, mojar un poco

moisture *n* humedad *f*

moisturize *vt* humedecer

moisturizing *adj* hidratante, humectante

molar *adj* molar; *n* muela, molar *m* (*form*)

molasses *n* melaza

mold *n* (*dent*) molde *m*; (*fungus*) moho; *vt*
moldear

mole *n* lunar *m*; (*obst*) mola; **hidatidiform**
—— mola hidatiforme

molecule *n* molécula

molluscum contagiosum *n* molusco contagioso

mom *n* mamá

momentary *adj* momentáneo

mometasone *n* furoato de mometasona

monitor *n* monitor *m*; **cardiac** —— monitor
cardiaco; **fetal heart** —— monitor cardiaco fetal, monitor cardiotocográfico;
Holter —— monitor Holter, monitor
cardiaco ambulatorio; *vt* monitorizar

monitoring *n* monitoreo, monitorización *f*,
vigilancia

monoclonal *adj* monoclonal

monogamous *adj* monógamo

monogamy *n* monogamia

mononucleosis *n* mononucleosis *f*

monosodium glutamate (MSG) *n* glutamato
monosódico

monounsaturated *adj* monoinsaturado

monster *n* monstruo

month *n* mes *m*

mood *n* estado de ánimo, humor *m*; ——
swing cambio repentino del estado de
ánimo; **to be in a good (bad)** —— estar
de buen (mal) humor

morbid *adj* (*path*) morboso

morbidity *n* morbilidad *f*

morgue *n* morgue *f*

morning *adj* matutino (*form*), de la mañana;
—— **sickness** náuseas *or* vómitos del
embarazo; *n* mañana

morphine *n* morfina

morphology *n* morfología

mortal *adj* mortal, fatal

mortality *n* mortalidad *f*

mortuary n funeraria

mosquito *n* (*pl* -toes *o* -tos) mosquito

mother *n* madre *f*

mother-in-law *n* (*pl* mothers-in-law) suegra

motion sickness *n* mareo (*producido por el
movimiento*)

motivation *n* motivación *f*

motor *adj* motor

motorcycle *n* motocicleta, moto *f* (*fam*)

mountain sickness *n* mal *m* de montaña,
soroche *m* (*SA*)

mourn *vt*, *vi* lamentar(se)

mouse *n* (*pl* **mice**) ratón *m*

moustache *n* bigote *m*

mouth *n* boca; **by** —— por vía bucal, por la boca; **roof of the** —— paladar *m*

mouthful *n* (*pl* -**fuls**) bocado

mouthpiece *n* boquilla

mouthwash *n* enjuage *m* bucal

move *vt* mover, (*a patient*) trasladar, cambiar; **We have to move you to another room**..Tenemos que trasladarlo a otro cuarto; *vi* moverse; **Don't move**..No se mueva.

movement *n* movimiento; **bowel** —— (**BM**) defecación *f* (*form*), evacuación *f*, deposición *f* (*SA*); **rapid eye movements** (**REM**) movimientos oculares rápidos (**MOR**), movimientos rápidos de los ojos

MRI *V*. **magnetic resonance imaging**.

MSG *V*. **monosodium glutamate**.

much *adj* & *adv* mucho

mucinous *adj* mucinoso

mucocele *n* mucocele *m*

mucocutaneous *adj* mucocutáneo

mucolytic *adj* & *n* mucolítico

mucous *adj* mucoso; —— **membrane** membrana mucosa

mucus *n* mucosidad *f*, moco

mullein *n* (*bot*) gordolobo

multiple *adj* múltiple; —— **myeloma** mieloma *m* múltiple; —— **sclerosis** esclerosis *f* múltiple

multiply *vi* (*pret* & *pp* -**plied**) multiplicarse

multivitamin *adj* multivitamínico; *n* multivitamina

mumps *n* paperas

mupirocin *n* mupirocin *m*

murmur *n* (*card*) soplo

muscle *n* músculo; —— **pull** estiramiento (*form*), desgarro leve (*muscular*)

muscular *adj* muscular; (*person*) musculoso; —— **dystrophe** distrofia muscular progresiva

mushroom *n* hongo

musician *n* músico -ca *mf*

mutant *adj* & *n* mutante *m*

mutation *n* mutación *f*

mute *adj* & *n* mudo -da *mf*

mutilate *vt* mutilar

mutism *n* mudez *f*, (*esp elective*) mutismo

myalgia *n* mialgia

myasthenia gravis *n* miastenia grave *or* gravis

Mycoplasma Mycoplasma

myelin *n* mielina

myelogram *n* mielograma *m*

myelomeningocele *n* mielomeningocele *m*

myocardial *adj* miocárdico

myocarditis *n* miocarditis *f*

myocardium *n* miocardio

myoglobin *n* mioglobina

myoma *n* mioma *m*

myopathy *n* miopatía

myopia *n* miopía

myopic *adj* miope

myositis *n* miositis *f*

myxedema *n* mixedema *m*

myxoma *n* mixoma *m*

N

nabumetone *n* nabumetone *m*

nail *n* (*anat*) uña; (*carpentry*) clavo; —— **file** lima para las uñas; —— **polish** esmalte *m* para las uñas; **ingrown** —— uña enterrada *or* encarnada, uñero

naked *adj* desnudo

nalidixic acid *n* ácido nalidíxico

naloxone *n* naloxona

name *n* nombre *m*; **first** —— nombre; **last** —— apellido

nap *n* siesta; **to take a ——** tomar una siesta
napalm *n* napalm *m*
naproxen *n* naproxén *m*
narcissism *n* narcisismo
narcissist *n* narcisista *mf*
narcissistic *adj* narcisista
narcolepsy *n* narcolepsia
narcotic *adj* & *n* narcótico
narrow *adj* estrecho
narrowing *n* estrechez *f*
nasal *adj* nasal; (*sound of voice*) gangoso; **—— passage** conducto nasal
nasogastric *adj* nasogástrico
nasopharynx *n* nasofaringe *f*
natural *adj* natural
nature *n* (la) naturaleza
naturopath *n* naturópata *mf*, naturista *mf*
naturopathic *adj* naturopático, naturista
naturopathy *n* naturopatía, naturismo
nausea *n* náusea (*frec pl*)
nauseated *adj* **to be ——** tener náusea(s); **to make ——** dar náusea(s)
nauseating *adj* que produce náusea(s)
nauseous *adj* que tiene náusea(s); que produce náusea(s)
navel *n* ombligo
nearsighted *adj* miope, que tiene dificultad para ver los objetos lejanos
nebulizer *n* nebulizador *m*
neck *n* cuello; **back of the ——** nuca
necrophilia *n* necrofilia
necrophobia *n* necrofobia
necrosis *n* necrosis *f*
necrotic *adj* necrótico
needle *n* aguja; **hypodermic ——** aguja hipodérmica
negative *adj* negativo
negativism *n* negativismo
neglect *n* negligencia, descuido; *vt* descuidar, desatender
negligent *adj* negligente, descuidado
neighbor *n* vecino -na *mf*
neighborhood *n* vecindad *f*, barrio
Neisseria Neisseria
neomycin *n* neomicina
neonatal *adj* neonatal
neonatologist *n* neonatólogo -ga *mf*

neonatology *n* neonatología
neoplasm *n* neoplasia
neoplastic *adj* neoplásico
neostigmine *n* neostigmina
nephew *n* sobrino
nephrectomy *n* (*pl* -mies) nefrectomía
nephritis *n* nefritis *f*
nephrologist *n* nefrólogo -ga *mf*
nephrology *n* nefrología
nephropathy *n* nefropatía
nephrosis *n* nefrosis *f*
nephrotic *adj* nefrótico
nerve *n* nervio; **—— block** bloqueo nervioso; **—— root** raíz nerviosa; **acoustic ——** nervio auditivo *or* acústico; **cranial ——** nervio craneal; **entrapped ——** nervio comprimido *or* atrapado; **facial ——** nervio facial; **femoral ——** nervio femoral; **median ——** nervio mediano; **motor ——** nervio motor; **optic ——** nervio óptico; **parasympathetic ——** nervio parasimpático; **peroneal ——** nervio peroneo *or* peroneal; **phrenic ——** nervio frénico; **pinched ——** nervio atrapado; **pudendal ——** nervio pudendo; **radial ——** nervio radial; **recurrent laryngeal ——** nervio laríngeo recurrente; **sciatic ——** nervio ciático; **sensory ——** nervio sensitivo; **spinal ——** nervio raquídeo *or* espinal; **sympathetic ——** nervio simpático; **trigeminal ——** nervio trigémino; **ulnar ——** nervio cubital; **vagus ——** nervio vago
nerves *npl* (*fam, anxiety*) nervios (*fam*)
nervous *adj* nervioso; **—— breakdown** choque *or* colapso nervioso, crisis nerviosa
nervousness *n* nerviosismo
nettle *n* (*bot*) ortiga
network *n* red *f*, retículo
neural *adj* neural
neuralgia *n* neuralgia; **postherpetic ——** neuralgia postherpética
neurinoma *n* neurinoma *m*
neuritis *n* neuritis *f*
neuroblastoma *n* neuroblastoma *m*
neurofibroma *n* neurofibroma *m*
neurofibromatosis *n* neurofibromatosis *f*
neurogenic *adj* neurogénico *or* neurógeno

neuroleptic *adj* & *n* neuroléptico
neurological, neurologic *adj* neurológico
neurologist *n* neurólogo -ga *mf*
neurology *n* neurología
neuroma *n* neuroma *m*; **acoustic** —— neuroma del acústico
neuromuscular *adj* neuromuscular
neuropathy *n* neuropatía *f*; **diabetic** —— neuropatía diabética; **peripheral** —— neuropatía periférica
neurosis *n* (*pl* **-ses**) neurosis *f*
neurosurgeon *n* neurocirujano -na *mf*
neurosurgery *n* (*pl* **-ries**) neurocirugía
neurosyphilis *n* neurosífilis *f*
neurotic *adj* & *n* neurótico -ca *mf*
neutral *adj* neutral
neutralize *vt* neutralizar
neutrophil *n* neutrófilo
nevus *n* (*pl* **nevi**) nevo
newborn *n* recién nacido -da *mf*, **premature** —— prematuro -ra *mf*
next *adj* próximo, siguiente
niacin *n* niacina
Nicaraguan *adj* & *n* nicaragüense *mf*
nick *n* cortada pequeña, herida pequeña
nickel *n* níquel *m*
niclosamide *n* niclosamida
nicotine *n* nicotina
nicotinic acid *n* ácido nicotínico
niece *n* sobrina
nifedipine *n* nifedipina
night *n* noche *f*; **last** —— anoche
night-terrors *npl* terrores nocturnos
nightmare *n* pesadilla
nipple *n* (*female*) pezón *m*; (*male*) tetilla; (*of a nursing bottle*) mamila, tetera, mamadera; —— **shield** pezonera
nit *n* liendre *f*
nitrate *n* nitrato
nitrite *n* nitrito
nitrofurantoin *n* nitrofurantoína
nitrogen *n* nitrógeno
nitroglycerin *n* nitroglicerina
nitrous oxide *n* óxido nitroso
nizatidine *n* nizatidina
nocardiosis *n* nocardiosis *f*
nocturnal *adj* nocturno; —— **emission** eyaculación nocturna

node *n* (*card*) nodo; (*lymph*) ganglio; **atrioventricular** —— nodo auriculoventricular; **lymph** —— ganglio linfático; **sinoatrial** —— nodo sinoauricular
nodular *adj* nodular
nodule *n* nódulo
noise *n* ruido
nonabsorbable *adj* no absorbible
nonflammable *adj* no inflamable, que no se quema
noninvasive *adj* no invasor
nonketotic *adj* no cetónico
nonspecific *adj* inespecífico
nonsteroidal antiinflammatory drug (NSAID) *n* antiinflamatorio no esteroide
noon *n* mediodía *m*
norepinephrine *n* norepinefrina
norfloxacin *n* norfloxacina
norm *n* norma
normal *adj* normal
normalize *vt* normalizar
North American *adj* norteamericano -na *mf*
nortriptyline *n* nortriptilina
nose *n* nariz *f*; **to blow one's** —— sonarse la nariz, soplarse la nariz (*Carib*); **to hold one's** —— taparse la nariz; **to pick one's** —— limpiarse la nariz con el dedo, sacarse los mocos con el dedo
nosebleed *n* hemorragia nasal (*form*), sangrado por la nariz; **Have you had any nosebleeds?**..¿Ha sangrado por la nariz?
no-see-um *n* jején *m*
nostril *n* fosa *or* ventana nasal, hoyo de la nariz (*fam*)
notice *vt* notar, fijarse (en); **When did you first notice blood in your stool?**..¿Cuándo fue la primera vez que notó que había sangre en el excremento?
notify *vt* (*pret* & *pp* **-fied**) notificar
nourish *vt* alimentar, nutrir
nourishing *adj* nutritivo
nourishment *n* nutrición *f*, alimentación *f*
novacaine *n* novacaína
NSAID *V.* **nonsteroidal antiinflammatory drug**.
nuclear *adj* nuclear; —— **magnetic resonance** (*ant*) resonancia magnética nuclear (*ant*), imágenes *fpl* por resonancia

magnética; —— **war** guerra nuclear

numb *adj* dormido, adormecido; **to become** —— dormirse, adormecerse; *vt* (*también* **to —— up**) anestesiar, dormir; **I'm going to numb up your finger**..Le voy a anestesiar el dedo.

number one *n* (*fam, urination*) número uno (*fam*), (el) orinar

number two *n* (*fam, defecation*) número dos (*fam*), (el) defecar

numbing *adj* adormecedor

numbness *n* adormecimiento, falta de sensación

nurse *n* enfermera (enfermero *if male*); **charge** —— jefa de turno (jefe *if male*); **head** —— jefa de enfermeras; **home** —— enfermera domiciliaria; *vt* (*to breast-feed*) amamantar (*form*), dar pecho, dar de mamar; (*to care for patients*) cuidar; *vi* (*to suckle*) mamar

nurse-practitioner *n* (*US*) enfermero -ra *mf*

que tiene entrenamiento adicional para diagnosticar y tratar padecimientos sencillos

nursery *n* (*pl* -**ries**) guardería infantil; **newborn** —— sala de cuneros

nursing *n* enfermería; —— **home** asilo de ancianos

nurture *vt* alimentar, nutrir; criar

nut *n* nuez *f*

nutrient *n* alimento nutritivo, substancia nutritiva

nutrition *n* nutrición *f*; **total parenteral** —— (**TPN**) nutrición parenteral total

nutritional *adj* nutricional

nutritionist *n* nutriólogo -ga *mf*, especialista *mf* en nutrición

nutritious *adj* nutritivo

nutritive *adj* nutritivo

nylon *n* nylon *m* (*Ang*), nilón *m*

nystagmus *n* nistagmo

nystatin *n* nistatina

O

oatmeal *n* avena, hojuelas de avena

oats *n* avena

obese *adj* obeso

obesity *n* obesidad *f*

obsession *n* obsesión *f*

obsessive-compulsive *adj* obsesivo-compulsivo

obstetrical, obstetric *adj* obstétrico

obstetrician *n* obstetra *mf*

obstetrics *n* obstetricia

obstruct *vt* obstruir, tapar (*fam*)

obstruction *n* obstrucción *f*

obstructive *adj* obstructivo

occipital *adj* occipital

occlusion *n* oclusión *f*

occlusive *adj* oclusivo

occupation *n* ocupación *f*, trabajo

occupational *adj* ocupacional

octogenarian *n* octogenario -ria *mf*

ocular *adj* ocular

oculist *n* (*ant*) oculista *mf*

odor *n* olor *m*

off *prep* (*drugs, a medication, etc.*) ya no usando, ya no tomando (*drogas, un medicamento, etc.*); **How long have you been off heroin?**..¿Desde cuándo no usa heroína?...**Are you off prednisone?**..¿Ya no toma prednisona?

office *n* oficina, (*of a doctor*) consultorio; —— **hours** horas de consulta

ofloxacin *n* ofloxacina

often *adv* seguido, muchas veces; **How often do you have chest pain?**..¿Qué tan seguido tiene dolor de pecho?

oil *n* aceite *m*
ointment *n* ungüento, pomada
old *adj* viejo; **How old are you?**..¿Cuántos años tiene? —— **man** viejo, anciano; —— **woman** vieja, anciana; **to grow** —— envejecer(se)
old wives' tale *n* creencia sin base médica
olfactory *adj* olfatorio
olive oil *n* aceite *m* de oliva
olive-skinned *adj* trigueño
omeprazole *n* omeprazol *m*
on *prep* (*drugs, a medication, etc.*) usando, tomando, bajo el efecto de; **Are you on lithium?**..¿Está tomando litio?...**Were you on PCP when you kicked the policeman?**..¿Estaba bajo el efecto de la fenciclidina cuando le dio una patada al policía?
onchocerciasis *n* oncocercosis *f*
oncologist *n* oncólogo -ga *mf*
oncology *n* oncología
one-armed *adj* manco
one-eyed *adj* tuerto
one-handed *adj* manco
onion *n* cebolla
onset *n* comienzo, principio
opacity *n* opacidad *f*, (*of the eye*) nube *f*
opaque *adj* opaco
open *vt, vi* abrir(se); **Open your mouth, please**..Abra la boca, por favor.
opening *n* abertura
operable *adj* operable
operate *vi* operar; **We need to operate on your leg**..Tenemos que operarle la pierna.
operating room (OR) *n* quirófano, sala de operaciones
operating table *n* mesa de operaciones
operation *n* operación *f*; **to have an** —— operarse; **You need to have an operation**..Tiene que operarse.
ophthalmic *adj* oftálmico
ophthalmologist *n* oftalmólogo -ga *mf*
ophthalmology *n* oftalmología
ophthalmoscope *n* oftalmoscopio
opiate *adj & n* opiáceo
opinion *n* opinión *f*; **second** —— segunda opinión
opium *n* opio

opportunistic *adj* oportunista
optical, optic *adj* óptico
optician *n* óptico
optics *n* óptica
optometrist *n* optometrista *mf*
OR *V.* **operating room**.
oral *adj* oral, bucal
orange *adj* naranja, de color naranja; *n* (*fruit*) naranja
orbit *n* (*anat*) órbita
orchiectomy, orchidectomy *n* (*pl* -mies) orquiectomía, orquidectomía
orchitis *n* orquitis *f*
order *n* (*for patient in a hospital*) indicación *f*; *vt* indicar (*form*), recetar, ordenar
orderly *n* (*pl* -lies) asistente *m* de enfermera
organ *n* órgano; —— **meats** vísceras
organic *adj* orgánico; sembrado sin uso de substancias químicas
organism *n* organismo
organophosphate *n* organofosforado
orgasm *n* orgasmo
orifice *n* orificio
oropharynx *n* orofaringe *f*
orphan *n* huérfano -na *mf*
orphanage *n* orfanatorio, orfelinato
orthodontia, orthodontics *n* ortodoncia
orthodontist *n* ortodoncista *mf*
orthopedic, orthopaedic *adj* ortopédico
orthopedics, orthopaedics *n* ortopedia
orthopedist *n* ortopedista *mf*
orthosis *n* (*pl* -ses) ortosis *f*
osseous *adj* óseo
ossicle *n* huesecillo, huesillo
osteitis *n* osteítis *f*; —— **fibrosa cystica** osteítis fibroquística
osteoarthritis *n* osteoartritis *f*
osteogenesis imperfecta *n* osteogénesis *or* osteogenia imperfecta
osteoma *n* osteoma *m*
osteomalacia *n* osteomalacia
osteomyelitis *n* osteomielitis *f*
osteopath *n* osteópata *mf*
osteopathy *n* osteopatía
osteophyte *n* osteofito
osteoporosis *n* osteoporosis *f*
osteosarcoma *n* osteosarcoma *m*
otic *adj* ótico

otitis *n* otitis *f*; ——— **externa** otitis externa; ——— **interna** otitis interna; ——— **media** otitis media

otolaryngologist *n* otorrinolaringólogo -ga *mf*

otolaryngology *n* otorrinolaringología

otosclerosis *n* otosclerosis *f*

otoscope *n* otoscopio

ouch *interj* ¡Ay! *or* ¡Ai!

ounce (oz.) *n* onza (onz.)

outbreak *n* brote *m*

outcome *n* resultado

outdated, out of date *adj* (*medication, etc.*) vencido, caducado

outdoors *adv* al aire libre

outer *adj* externo, exterior

outgrow *vt* (*pret* -**grew**; *pp* -**grown**) (*a habit*) perder con la edad; **She will outgrow it**..Lo perderá con la edad..Se le quitará con el tiempo.

outlet *n* (*psych*) desahogo, escape *m*; (*electrical*) tomacorriente *f*, enchufe *m*

outlook *n* perspectiva

outpatient *n* paciente *mf* externo -na *or* ambulatorio -ria

outside *adj* exterior, externo; *n* exterior *m*; *prep* fuera de

ova *pl de* **ovum**

ovarian *adj* ovárico

ovary *n* (*pl* -**ries**) ovario; **polycystic** ——— ovario poliquístico

overactive *adj* demasiado activo

overcome *vt* superar

overcompensate *vi* sobrecompensar

overdevelop *vt, vi* desarrollar demasiado

overdo *vt* (*pret* -**did**; *pp* -**done**) **to** ——— **it** esforzarse demasiado, excederse; **Don't overdo it**..No se esfuerce demasiado..No se exceda.

overdose *n* sobredosis *f*, dosis excesiva

overeat *vi* (*pret* -**ate**; *pp* -**eaten**) comer demasiado

overexcite *vt* excitar demasiado, sobreexcitar

overexert *vt* agotar; **to** ——— **oneself** hacer un esfuerzo excesivo

overexertion *n* agotamiento (*debido a un esfuerzo excesivo*)

overload *vt* sobrecargar

over-the-counter *adj* que no requiere receta médica

overuse *n* uso excesivo

overweight *adj* pasado de peso, que tiene peso excesivo, que tiene sobrepeso

ovulate *vi* ovular

ovulation *n* ovulación *f*

ovum *n* (*pl* **ova**) óvulo, huevo (*fam*)

oxacillin *n* oxacilina

oxalate *n* oxalato

oxazepam *n* oxacepam *m*

oxide *n* óxido

oxycodone *n* oxicodona

oxygen *n* oxígeno; ——— **tank** tanque *m* de oxígeno

oxytocin *n* oxitocina

oz. *V.* **ounce**.

ozone *n* ozono

P

PAC *abbr* **premature atrial contraction**. *V.* **contraction**.

pace *n* paso; *vi* **to** ——— **oneself** no excederse

pacemaker *n* marcapaso *m*

pacifier *n* chupón *m*, chupete *m*, entretenedor *m*

pacing *n* (*card*) uso de marcapaso

pack *n* compresa; **ice** ——— compresa *or* bolsa de hielo

package insert *n* instructivo

packing *n* material como gasa usado para rellenar una cavidad

pad *n* cojín *m*, almohadilla; **alcohol ——** gasita con alcohol; **heating ——** cojín eléctrico; *vt* acojinar, acolchar

padding *n* (*ortho, surg*) huata

page *n* (*overhead*) llamada por vocina; (*by beeper*) llamada por el bíper; *vt* vocear, llamar por vocina; llamar por el bíper

pager *n* bíper *m* (*Ang*)

pain *n* dolor *m*; **to be in ——** tener dolor; **back —— (*in general*)** dolor de espalda; **a —— in the back** un dolor en la espalda

painful *adj* doloroso; (*sore*) adolorido *or* dolorido

painkiller *n* (*fam*) medicamento para quitar el dolor

painless *adj* sin dolor, indoloro

paint *n* pintura

palatable *adj* de sabor aceptable, que no sabe mal

palate *n* paladar *m*; **cleft ——** paladar hendido; **hard ——** paladar duro; **soft ——** paladar blando

pale *adj* pálido

paleness *n* palidez *f*

palliative *adj & n* paliativo

pallor *n* palidez *f*

palm *n* (*anat, bot*) palma; **—— oil** aceite *m* de palma

palmar *adj* palmar

palpate *vt* palpar

palpitate *vi* palpitar

palpitation *n* palpitación *f*, latido rápido o fuerte del corazón

palsy *n* (*pl* -**sies**) parálisis *f*; **Bell's ——** parálisis de Bell

pamper *vt* mimar, consentir

pamphlet *n* folleto

Panamanian *adj & n* panameño -ña *mf*

pancreas *n* (*pl* -**creases** *o* -**creata**) páncreas *m*

pancreatectomy *n* (*pl* -**mies**) pancreatectomía

pancreatic *adj* pancreático

pancreatitis *n* pancreatitis *f*

pang *n* punzada, dolor breve y agudo; **hunger ——** dolor de hambre

panic *n* pánico; **—— attack** ataque *m* de pánico

pant *vi* jadear

panties *npl* calzón *m* (*frec pl*), pantaletas (*Mex*), bloomer *m* (*esp CA*), panties *mpl* (*Carib*)

pantothenic acid *n* ácido pantoténico

pants *npl* pantalones *mpl*

pantyhose *n* (*pl* -**hose**) pantimedias

Papanicolaou smear *n* examen *m* de Papanicolaou, prueba del cáncer (*fam*)

Pap smear *V.* **Papanicolaou smear.**

paper *n* papel *m*

papilla *n* papila

papillary *adj* papilar

papillomavirus *n* papilomavirus *m*

paracoccidioidomycosis *n* paracoccidioidomicosis *f*

paradoxical *adj* paradójico

paragonimiasis *n* paragonimiasis *f*

Paraguayan *adj & n* paraguayo -ya *mf*

paralysis *n* parálisis *f*

paralyze *vt* paralizar

paralyzing *adj* paralizador, paralizante

paramedic *adj* paramédico; *n* paramédico, persona con entrenamiento médico básico encargada de llevar heridos y enfermos al hospital

paranasal *adj* paranasal

paranoia *n* paranoia

paranoid *adj* paranoide, paranoico

paraplegic *adj & n* parapléjico -ca *mf*

paraquat *n* paraquat *m*

parasite *n* parásito

parasitic *adj* parasitario

paraspinal, paraspinous *adj* paraespinal

parathion *n* paratión *m*

parathyroid *adj* paratiroideo

paregoric *n* paregórico

parent *n* padre *m*, madre *f*

parenteral *adj* parenteral

paresis *n* paresia

parietal *adj* parietal

paronychia *n* paroniquia

parotid *adj* parotídeo; *n* parótida

parotiditis, parotitis *n* parotiditis *f*

paroxetine *n* paroxetina

paroxysm *n* paroxismo

paroxysmal *adj* paroxismal, paroxístico

parsley *n* perejil *m*

partial *adj* parcial
particle *n* partícula
partner *n* (*marital, sexual*) pareja; (*professional*) socio -cia *mf*
pass *n* paso; *vt* (*parasites, a stone, etc.*) eliminar, expulsar, botar, arrojar (*esp Mex*), echar; **Have you ever passed a stone?**..¿Ha eliminado alguna vez una piedra (*al orinar*)? **to —— gas** tirar gases *or* vientos, pasar gas; **Are you passing gas yet?**..¿Está tirando gases ya? *vi* **to —— out** desmayarse
passage *n* pasaje *m*; **nasal passages** pasajes nasales
passionflower *n* (*bot*) pasionaria
passive *adj* pasivo
passive-aggressive *adj* pasivo-agresivo
paste *n* pasta
pastime *n* pasatiempo
pat *n* palmada, palmadita, golpecito; *vt* (*pret & pp* **patted**; *ger* **patting**) dar palmadas, dar palmaditas, dar golpecitos
patch *n* parche *m*
patella *n* (*pl* **-lae**) patela, rótula
paternal *adj* paterno
paternity *n* paternidad *f*
pathological, pathologic *adj* patológico
pathologist *n* patólogo -ga *mf*
pathology *n* patología
patient *adj* paciente; *n* paciente *mf*, enfermo -ma *mf*
pattern *n* patrón *m*
paunch *n* panza, barriga
PCP *V.* **phencyclidine.**
PDA *abbr* **patent ductus arteriosus.** *V.* **ductus arteriosus.**
pea *n* guisante *m*
peak *n* punto máximo, pico; *vi* alcanzar el punto máximo, alcanzar el pico
peanut *n* cacahuate *m*; **—— butter** mantequilla de cacahuate; **—— oil** aceite *m* de cacahuate
pear *n* pera
pectoral *adj* pectoral
pediatric *adj* pediátrico
pediatrician *n* pediatra *or* pedíatra *mf*
pediatrics *n* pediatría
pediculosis *n* pediculosis *f*

pedicure *n* pedicure *m*
pee (*esp ped*) *n* pipí *m*; *vi* hacer pipí
peel *vi* (*skin*) descamarse (*form*), pelarse, despellejarse (*fam*); **I'm peeling** *o* **My skin is peeling**..Me estoy pelando.
pellagra *n* pelagra
pelvic *adj* pélvico; *n* (*fam*) examen ginecológico; revisión *f* de (sus) partes (*fam*)
pelvis *n* pelvis *f*
pemphigoid *adj & n* penfigoide *m*
pemphigus *n* pénfigo
pending *adj* pendiente
penetrate *vt* penetrar
penetrating *adj* penetrante
penetration *n* penetración *f*
penicillamine *n* penicilamina
penicillin *n* penicilina
penis *n* (*pl* **penises** *o* **penes**) pene *m*, miembro (*fam*)
pentamidine *n* pentamidina
pentazocine *n* pentazocina
pentoxifylline *n* pentoxifilina
pepsin *n* pepsina
peptic *adj* péptico; **—— ulcer** úlcera péptica
per *prep* por; **beats per minute**..latidos por minuto; **—— day** por día, al día
percent *n* por ciento
percentage *n* porcentaje *m*
perception *n* percepción *f*; **depth ——** visión profunda, percepción de la profundidad
percutaneous *adj* percutáneo
perfectionism *n* perfeccionismo
perfectionist *adj & n* perfeccionista *mf*
perforate *vt* perforar
perforation *n* perforación *f*
perform *vt* practicar; **We need to perform more tests**..Tenemos que practicarle más estudios.
performance *n* rendimiento
perfume *n* perfume *m*
pericardial *adj* pericárdico
pericarditis *n* pericarditis *f*; **constrictive —— ** pericarditis constrictiva
pericardium *n* pericardio
perineal *adj* perineal
period *n* periodo *or* período, regla; **Do you still have periods?**..¿Todavía tiene la

regla?...**When was your last period?**..
¿Cuándo fue su último periodo? **incuba-**
tion —— periodo de incubación
periodontal *adj* periodontal
periodontist *n* periodoncista *mf*
peripheral *adj* periférico
periphery *n* periferia
peristalsis *n* peristalsis *f*
peritoneal *adj* peritoneal
peritoneum *n* peritoneo
peritonitis *n* peritonitis *f*
permanent *adj* permanente
permission *n* permiso
peroxide *n* peróxido
persist *vi* persistir
person *n* persona
personal *adj* personal
personality *n* (*pl* **-ties**) personalidad *f*; ——
  disorder trastorno de personalidad;
  antisocial —— personalidad antisocial;
  borderline —— personalidad limítrofe;
  cyclothymic —— personalidad ciclotímica; **histrionic** —— personalidad
  histriónica; **narcissistic** —— personalidad narcisista; **obsessive-compulsive**
  —— personalidad obsesivo-compulsiva;
  paranoid —— personalidad paranoide;
  passive-aggressive —— personalidad
  pasivo-agresiva; **schizoid** —— personalidad esquizoide
perspiration *n* transpiración *f*, sudor *m*
perspire *vi* transpirar, sudar
pertussis *n* pertussis *f*, tos ferina, coqueluche
  m&f
Peruvian *adj* & *n* peruano -na *mf*
pessary *n* pesario
pessimism *n* pesimismo
pest *n* peste *f*
pesticide *n* pesticida *m*
pestilence *n* pestilencia
pet *n* mascota, animal doméstico; **Do you**
  have pets at home?..¿Tiene animales en
  la casa?
PET *abbr* **positive emission tomography**.
  V. **tomography**.
petroleum *n* petróleo; —— **jelly** vaselina,
  petrolato
peyote *n* peyote *m*

pH *n* pH *m*
phallic *adj* fálico
phallus *n* (*pl* **-li**) falo
pharmaceutical, pharmaceutic *adj*
  farmacéutico
pharmacist *n* farmacéutico -ca *mf*, boticario
  -ria *mf*
pharmacological, pharmacologic *adj*
  farmacológico
pharmacologist *n* farmacólogo -ga *mf*
pharmacology *n* farmacología
pharmacopoeia *n* farmacopea
pharmacy *n* (*pl* **-cies**) farmacia, botica
pharyngitis *n* faringitis *f*
pharynx *n* (*pl* **-inges**) faringe *f*
phase *n* fase *f*
phenacetin *n* fenacetina
phencyclidine (PCP) *n* fenciclidina (PCP)
phenobarbital *n* fenobarbital *m*
phenol *n* fenol *m*
phenomenon *n* fenómeno; **Raynaud's** ——
  fenómeno de Raynaud
phenothiazine *n* fenotiacina
phenotype *n* fenotipo
phenylalanine *n* fenilalanina
phenylbutazone *n* fenilbutazona
phenylephrine *n* fenilefrina
phenylketonuria (PKU) *n* fenilcetonuria
phenylpropanolamine *n* fenilpropanolamina
phenytoin *n* fenitoína
pheochromocytoma *n* feocromocitoma *m*
phlebitis *n* flebitis *f*
phlebotomist *n* persona que extrae sangre
phlebotomy *n* extracción *f* de sangre de una
  vena, flebotomía (*Ang*); (*therapeutic*)
  flebotomía, sangría (*fam*)
phlegm *n* flema
phlegmon *n* flemón *m*
phobia *n* fobia, temor morboso y obsesivo
phosphate *n* fosfato
phosphorus *n* fósforo
photosensitive *adj* fotosensible
phototherapy *n* fototerapia
phrenic *adj* frénico
physiatrist *n* fisiatra *mf*, médico espe-
  cializado en medicina física
physiatry, physiatrics *n* fisiatría, medicina
  física

physical *adj* físico; *n* (*fam*) examen físico
physician *n* médico, doctor -ra *mf*; **attending** —— médico adscrito; **family** —— médico de cabecera *or* de la familia; **private** —— médico privado
physician's assistant *n* (*US*) técnico entrenado para asistir al médico
physiological, physiologic *adj* fisiológico
physiologist *n* fisiólogo -ga *mf*
physiology *n* fisiología
physiotherapist *n* fisioterapista *mf*, fisioterapeuta *mf* (*form*)
physiotherapy *n* fisioterapia
physique *n* físico, complexión *f*
physostigmine *n* fisostigmina
pick *vt* (*a scab, etc.*) rascarse; **to** —— **one's nose** limpiarse la nariz con el dedo, sacarse los mocos con el dedo
PID *abbr* **pelvic inflammatory disease**. *V.* **disease**.
pierce *vt* perforar, atravesar, penetrar
piercing *adj* (*pain*) penetrante, punzante
pigeon-toed *adj* con los pies torcidos hacia dentro
pigment *n* pigmento
pigmentation *n* pigmentación *f*
piles *npl* (*fam*) hemorroides *fpl*, almorranas *fpl*
pill *n* (*capsule*) cápsula; (*solid*) píldora, pastilla, tableta; **birth control** —— píldora anticonceptiva
pillow *n* almohada
pillowcase *n* funda de almohada
pilonidal *adj* pilonidal
pimple *n* (*any cause*) grano, (*due to acne*) barro, espinilla
pin *n* alfiler *m*; (*ortho*) clavo
pinch *vt, vi* (*to bind*) apretar
pindolol *n* pindolol *m*
pineal *adj* pineal
pineapple *n* piña
pink *adj* rosado
pinkeye *n* ojo enrojecido, ojo rojo, conjuntivitis *f* (*form*),
pins and needles *n* (*sensation*) hormigueo
pint *n* pinta
pinta *n* pinta, mal *m* del pinto
pinworm *n* oxiuro
pipe *n* (*for smoking*) pipa

piperacillin *n* piperacilina
piss *vi* (*vulg*) mear (*vulg*), orinar
pitch *n* (*sound*) tono
pitcher *n* jarra
pituitary *adj* pituitario
pityriasis *n* pitiriasis *f*; —— **versicolor** pitiriasis versicolor
PKU *V.* **phenylketonuria**.
placebo *n* (*pl* **-bos** *o* **-boes**) placebo
placenta *n* (*pl* **-tae** *o* **-tas**) placenta; —— **abruptio** desprendimiento prematuro de placenta; —— **previa** placenta previa
plague *n* peste *f*, plaga; **bubonic** —— peste bubónica
planned parenthood *n* planificación *f* familiar
plant *n* (*bot*) planta
plantar *adj* plantar
plaque *n* (*dent*) placa (*bacteriana*)
plasma *n* plasma *m*
plasmapheresis *n* plasmaféresis *f*
plaster *n* (*for a cast*) yeso; (*medicinal*) cataplasma, emplasto
plastic *adj* & *n* plástico
plate *n* (*dent, surg*) placa
platelet *n* plaqueta
platinum *n* platino
pleasure *n* placer *m*
plethysmography *n* pletismografía
pleura *n* (*pl* **-rae**) pleura
pleural *adj* pleural
pleurisy *n* pleuresía
pleuritic *adj* pleurítico
pleuritis *n* pleuritis *f*
plexus *n* (*pl* **-xuses**) plexo
plug *n* tapón *m*
plum *n* ciruela
plunger *n* (*of a syringe*) émbolo
pneumococcus *n* (*pl* **-ci**) neumococo
pneumoconiosis *n* (*pl* **-ses**) neumoconiosis *f*
Pneumocystis carinii Pneumocystis carinii
pneumonia *n* pulmonía, neumonía; **aspiration** —— pulmonía *or* neumonía por aspiración
pneumonitis *n* neumonitis *f*
pneumothorax *n* neumotórax *m*
pockmark *n* cicatriz producida por la viruela; **to have pockmarks** estar cacarizo;

She has pockmarks..Está cacariza.
podiatrist *n* podíatra *or* podiatra *mf*
podiatry *n* podiatría
podophyllin *n* podofilina
point *n* (*anat*) punto
poison *n* veneno; **ant** ——, **rat** ——, etc.
veneno para hormiga, veneno para rata *or*
raticida *m*, etc.; *vt* envenenar
poisoning *n* envenenamiento, intoxicación *f*
poison ivy *n* hiedra venenosa
polio *n* polio *f*
poliomyelitis *n* poliomielitis *f*
polish *vt* (*teeth, etc.*) pulir
pollen *n* polen *m*
pollution *n* contaminación *f*, polución *f*; **air**
—— contaminación atmosférica *or* del
aire
polyarteritis nodosa *n* poliarteritis nudosa
polycystic *adj* poliquístico
polycythemia vera *n* policitemia vera
polymyalgia rheumatica *n* polimialgia reumática
polymyositis *n* polimiositis *f*
polymyxin *n* polimixina
polyp *n* pólipo; **adenomatous** —— pólipo
adenomatoso; **juvenile polyps** pólipos
juveniles; **nasal** —— pólipo nasal
polypectomy *n* (*pl* -**mies**) polipectomía
polyposis *n* poliposis *f*
polyunsaturated *adj* poliinsaturado
pons *n* puente *m*
pool *vi* (*blood*) estancarse (*la sangre*)
poopoo *n* (*ped*) popó *or* pupú *m*, caca (*esp
Carib*)
poorly *adv* mal
popliteal *adj* poplíteo
porcelain *n* porcelana
porcine *adj* porcino
pore *n* poro
pork *n* carne *f* de cerdo *or* puerco
porphyria *n* porfiria
portable *adj* portátil
portal *adj* portal
portion *n* porción *f*
port-wine stain *n* mancha de vino oporto
position *n* posición *f*; *vt* poner en posición
positive *adj* positivo
posterior *adj* posterior

postmortem *adj & adv* post mortem
postnasal *adj* postnasal; —— **drip** secreción
f or descarga nasal posterior, goteo postnasal
postnatal *adj* postnatal
postoperative *adj* postoperatorio
postpartum *adj* postparto (*invariant with
respect to gender*); **the second week
postpartum**.la segunda semana postparto
postpone *vt* aplazar, posponer
postural *adj* postural
posture *n* postura
pot *n* (*fam*) marihuana *or* marijuana
potable *adj* potable
potassium *n* potasio
potato *n* (*pl* -**toes**) papa
potbellied *adj* barrigón, panzón (*fam*)
potbelly *n* panza, barriga
potency *n* (*pl* -**cies**) potencia
potent *adj* potente
potential *adj & n* potencial *m*; **evoked** ——
potencial evocado
potion *n* poción *f*, pócima
potty *n* (*ped*) excusado, excusado pequeño
para niños
pouch *n* bolsa
poultry *n* aves *fpl* de corral
pound (lb.) *n* libra (lb.)
powder *n* polvo
powdered *adj* en polvo
power *n* poder *m*; **durable** —— **of attorney
for health care** (*US*) poder duradero para
la atención médica; —— **of attorney**
poder legal
powerful *adj* (*medication, etc.*) potente,
fuerte
PPD *abbr* **purified protein derivative of
tuberculin.** *V.* **purified.**
practice *n* práctica; *vt, vi* practicar
practitioner *n* médico clínico; **general** ——
médico general
pravastatin *n* pravastatina
praziquantel *n* praziquantel *m*
prazosin *n* prazosina
precaution *n* precaución *f*
precise *adj* preciso
precision *n* precisión *f*
precocious *adj* precoz

precordial thump *n* golpe precordial *or* torácico

predict *vt* predecir, pronosticar

predispose *vt* predisponer

predisposed *adj* predispuesto

predisposition *n* predisposición *f*

prednisone *n* prednisona

preeclampsia *n* preeclampsia

preemie *n* (*fam*) prematuro -ra *mf*

pregnancy *n* (*pl* **-cies**) embarazo; **ectopic** —— embarazo ectópico; **tubal** —— embarazo tubárico

pregnant *adj* embarazada, encinta; **You are three months pregnant.**.Tiene tres meses de embarazo.

preliminary *adj* preliminar

premature *adj* prematuro, precoz

premedication *n* premedicación *f*

premolar *adj* & *n* premolar *m*

prenatal *adj* prenatal

preoperative *adj* preoperatorio

preparation *n* (*pharm*) preparado, preparación *f*

prepare *vt* preparar

presbycusis *n* presbiacusia

presbyopia *n* presbiopía

prescribe *vt* recetar, prescribir

prescription *n* receta (*médica*), prescripción *f*

presentation *n* presentación *f*

preservative *n* preservativo

preserve *vt* preservar

press *vt* (*to apply pressure*) presionar, apretar; **Does it hurt when I press here?** ..¿Le duele cuando presiono aquí?

pressure *n* presión *f*; —— **sore** escara de presión, úlcera por presión, llaga (*debida a permanecer mucho tiempo sin cambiar de posición*); **blood** —— presión arterial (*form*), presión sanguínea, presión (*de la sangre*) (*fam*); **You have high blood pressure.**.Tiene alta presión; **diastolic** —— presión diastólica; **systolic** —— presión sistólica

preterm *adj* pretérmino (*invariant with respect to gender*)

prevalence *n* prevalencia

prevent *vt* (*disease, etc.*) prevenir, evitar; **Brushing your teeth every day helps prevent cavities.**.Cepillarse los dientes todos los días ayuda a prevenir la caries.

preventible *adj* prevenible

prevention *n* prevención *f*

preventive *adj* preventivo

previous *adj* previo, anterior

prick *n* pinchazo, piquete *m* (*esp Mex*), picadura; *vt* pinchar, picar (*esp Mex*)

priest *n* sacerdote *m*, padre *m*, cura *m*

primary *adj* primario, del primer nivel

prison *n* cárcel *f*, prisión *f*

privacy *n* privacidad *f*

private *adj* privado, confidencial; —— **doctor** médico privado; —— **parts** (*fam*) genitales *mpl*, partes privadas *or* íntimas, partes (*fam, esp female*)

probability *n* (*pl* **-ties**) probabilidad *f*

probably *adv* probablemente

probe *n* sonda; *vt* sondear *or* sondar

problem *n* problema *m*

probucol *n* probucol *m*

procainamide *n* procainamida

procaine *n* procaína

procedure *n* procedimiento

process *n* (*anat*) apófisis *f*; **mastoid** —— apófisis mastoides; **xiphoid** —— apófisis xifoides

proctitis *n* proctitis *f*

prodrome *n* pródromo

produce *vt* producir

product *n* producto; **milk** *o* **dairy** —— producto lácteo *or* de leche

professional *adj* profesional

profile *n* perfil *m*

progeria *n* progeria

progesterone *n* progesterona

prognosis *n* (*pl* **-ses**) pronóstico

program *n* programa *m*

progress *n* progreso; *vi* progresar

progression *n* progresión *f*

progressive *adj* progresivo; —— **multifocal leukoencephalopathy** leucoencefalopatía multifocal progresiva; —— **systemic sclerosis** esclerosis sistémica progresiva

projectile *n* proyectil *m*

projection *n* (*psyche, etc.*) proyección *f*

prolactin *n* prolactina

prolactinoma *n* tumor secretor de prolactina, prolactinoma *m*

prolapse *n* prolapso; **mitral-valve** —— prolapso valvular mitral

prolapsed *adj* —— **umbilical cord,** —— **uterus, etc.** prolapso del cordón umbilical, prolapso del útero, etc.

proline *n* prolina

prolong *vt* prolongar

prone *adj* prono, acostado boca abajo

proof *n* prueba

proper *adj* adecuado, apropiado

prophylactic *adj* & *n* profiláctico

prophylaxis *n* profilaxis *f*

proportion *n* proporción *f*

propoxyphene *n* propoxifeno

propranolol *n* propranolol *m*

proprioceptive *adj* propioceptivo

proptosis *n* proptosis *f*

propylthiouracil *n* propiltiouracilo

prostaglandin *n* prostaglandina

prostate *n* próstata

prostatectomy *n* (*pl* **-mies**) prostatectomía

prostatitis *n* prostatitis *f*

prosthesis *n* (*pl* **-ses**) prótesis *f*

prosthetic *adj* protésico *or* protético (*form*), postizo

prostitute *n* prostituto -ta *mf*

prostrate *adj* postrado

protect *vt* proteger; **Protect your skin**..Proteja su piel; **to** —— **oneself** protegerse

protection *n* protección *f*

protective *adj* protector

protein *n* proteína

Proteus Proteus

protocol *n* protocolo

protozoan *adj* & *n* protozoario

protuberance *n* protuberancia

provide *vt* suministrar, proporcionar

provoke *vt* provocar

prune *n* ciruela pasa

pruritis *n* prurito

pseudocyst *n* seudoquiste *m*; **pancreatic** —— seudoquiste pancreático

pseudoephedrine *n* seudoefedrina

pseudogout *n* seudogota

pseudohypoparathyroidism *n* seudohipoparatiroidismo

Pseudomonas Pseudomonas

psilocybin *n* psilocibina

psittacosis *n* psitacosis *f*

psoas *n* psoas *m*

psoriasis *n* psoriasis *f*

psyche *n* psique *f*

psychedelic *adj* psicodélico

psychiatric *adj* psiquiátrico

psychiatrist *n* psiquiatra *mf*

psychiatry *n* psiquiatría

psychoactive *adj* psicoactivo

psychoanalysis *n* psicoanálisis *m*

psychoanalyst *n* psicoanalista *mf*

psychoanalyze *vt* psicoanalizar

psychological *adj* psicológico

psychologist *n* psicólogo -ga *mf*

psychology *n* psicología

psychopath *n* psicópata *mf*

psychosis *n* (*pl* **-ses**) psicosis *f*

psychosomatic *adj* psicosomático

psychotherapist *n* psicoterapista *mf*, psicoterapeuta *mf* (*form*)

psychotherapy *n* psicoterapia

psychotic *adj* & *n* psicótico -ca *mf*

psychotropic *adj* & *n* psicotrópico

PTC *abbr* **percutaneous transhepatic cholangiography.** *V.* **cholangiography.**

pterygium *n* pterigión *m*, carnosidad *f*

ptomaine *n* tomaína

ptosis *n* ptosis *f*

puberty *n* pubertad *f*

pubic *adj* púbico

public *adj* público

pudendal *adj* pudendo

puerperal *adj* puerperal

puerperium *n* puerperio

Puerto Rican *adj* & *n* puertorriqueño -ña *mf*

puffy *adj* (*comp* **-fier**; *super* **-fiest**) hinchado

puke (*vulg*) *n* vómito; *vt*, *vi* arrojar, devolver, deponer (*Mex*), tener basca, vomitar

pull *n* **muscle** —— estiramiento (*form*), desgarro leve (*muscular*); *vt* **to** —— **a muscle** estirarse un músculo, desgarrarse un músculo, sufrir un tirón

pulmonary *adj* pulmonar; —— **edema** edema *m* pulmonar; —— **embolism** embolia pulmonar

pulmonic *adj* pulmonar

pulmonologist *n* neumólogo -ga *mf*
pulmonology *n* neumología
pulsation *n* pulsación *f*
pulse *n* pulso; **I'm going to take your pulse**..Voy a tomarle el pulso.
pumice stone *n* piedra pómez
pump *n* bomba; *vt* (*blood*) bombear, impulsar
puncture *n* punción *f* (*form*), pinchazo, piquete *m* (*esp Mex*), picadura; —— **wound** herida por punción; **lumbar** —— punción lumbar; *vt* puncionar (*form*), hacer una punción, pinchar, picar, penetrar
pupil *n* (*of the eye*) pupila
pure *adj* puro
purée *n* puré *m*
purgative *adj* & *n* purgante *m*
purified *adj* purificado; —— **protein derivative of tuberculin (PPD)** proteína purificada derivada de la tuberculina (PPD)
purifier *n* purificador *m*, depurador *m*
purify *vt* purificar, depurar
purine *n* purina
purple *adj* morado
purpura *n* púrpura; **Henoch-Schönlein** —— púrpura de Henoch-Schönlein; **idiopathic thrombocytopenic** —— **(ITP)** púrpura trombocitopénica idiopática; **thrombotic thrombocytopenic** —— **(TTP)** púrpura trombocitopénica trombótica

purse *vt* (*one's lips*) fruncir (*los labios*)
pus *n* pus *m*
push *vi* (*obst*) pujar; **Take a deep breath and push!**..¡Respire profundo y puje!
push-up *n* lagartija
pustule *n* pústula
put *vt* (*pret & pp* **put**; *ger* **putting**) **to —— on** (*clothing, etc.*) ponerse; (*lipstick*) pintarse (*los labios*); (*makeup*) pintarse (*la cara*); (*nail polish*) pintarse (*las uñas*); **Put on this gown so that it opens over your back**..Póngase esta bata con la abertura atrás.
PVC *abbr* **premature ventricular contraction**. *V.* **contraction**.
pyelogram *n* urograma *m*, pielograma *m*; **intravenous** —— **(IVP)** urograma excretorio, pielograma intravenoso
pyelography *n* urografía, pielografía
pyelonephritis *n* pielonefritis *f*
pyloric *adj* pilórico
pyloroplasty *n* (*pl* -**ties**) piloroplastia
pylorus *n* píloro
pyoderma *n* piodermia *m&f*
pyogenic *adj* piógeno; —— **granuloma** granuloma piógeno
pyorrhea *n* piorrea
pyrazinamide *n* pirazinamida
pyridoxine *n* piridoxina
pyrosis *n* pirosis *f*

Q

quack *n* (*fam*) charlatán -na *mf*; matasanos *m*, medicastro, medicucho, mediquillo
quadrant *n* cuadrante *m*
quadriceps *n* cuádriceps *m*
quadriplegia *n* cuadriplejía
quadriplegic *adj* & *n* cuadripléjico -ca *mf*
quadruplet *n* cuadrillizo -za *mf*, cuadrupleto

-ta *mf*
quality *n* calidad *f*; —— **of life** calidad de vida
quarantine *n* cuarentena; *vt* poner en cuarentena
quart *n* cuarto
queasy *adj* (*comp* -**ier**; *super* -**iest**) con un

poco de náusea, que tiene náusea(s); **I feel queasy** *o* **My stomach is queasy**..Siento un poco de náusea.

questionnaire *n* cuestionario

quickening *n* percepción *f* por la madre de los movimientos fetales

quiet *adj* quieto; *vi* **to —— down** calmarse

quinacrine *n* quinacrina

quinapril *n* quinaprilo

quinidine *n* quinidina

quinine *n* quinina

quintuplet *n* quintillizo -za *mf*

quit *vt* (*pret & pp* **quit**; *ger* **quitting**) dejar de, parar; **You need to quit drinking**.. Tiene que dejar de tomar.

R

rabid *adj* rabioso

rabies *n* rabia

raccoon *n* mapache *m*

race *n* (*of people*) raza; *vi* (*one's heart*) latir rápido

radial *adj* radial

radiate *vi* (*pain, heat*) radiarse

radiation *n* radiación *f*

radical *adj* radical

radiculopathy *n* radiculopatía

radioactive *adj* radiactivo *or* radioactivo

radioactivity *n* radiactividad *or* radioactividad *f*

radiography *n* radiografía

radioisotope *n* radioisótopo

radiologist *n* radiólogo -ga *mf*

radiology *n* radiología

radionuclide *n* radionúclido

radiotherapy *n* radioterapia

radium *n* radio, rádium *m*

radius *n* (*pl* **radii** *o* **radiuses**) radio

radon *n* radón *m*

rage *n* ira, enojo

ragweed *n* (*bot*) ambrosia

raise *vt* levantar, elevar; (*a child*) criar; **Raise your leg**..Levante su pierna...**This medicine may raise your sugar**..Esta medicina le puede elevar el azúcar.

ramipril *n* ramipril *m*

ran *pret de* **run**

range *n* rango; **—— of motion** rango de movimiento; **—— of values** rango de valores

ranitidine *n* ranitidina

rape *n* violación *f*; *vt* violar

rare *adj* (*disease, etc.*) raro; (*meat*) casi crudo, poco asado

rash *n* erupción *f*, rash *m*, (*esp due to heat or chafing*) salpullido *or* sarpullido

raspberry *n* frambuesa

rat *n* rata

rate *n* índice *m*, tasa, frecuencia; **basal metabolic ——** índice *or* tasa de metabolismo basal; **birth ——** índice *or* tasa de natalidad; **death ——** índice *or* tasa de mortalidad; **heart ——** frecuencia cardiaca; **respiratory ——** frecuencia respiratoria

rationalization *n* racionalización *f*

rationalize *vi* racionalizar

rattlesnake *n* serpiente *f* de cascabel

rave *vi* delirar, desvariar

raw *adj* (*food*) crudo; (*skin, mucous membrane*) pelado

ray *n* rayo

Raynaud's phenomenon *n* fenómeno de Raynaud

razor *n* rastrillo; (*electric*) rasuradora, máquina de afeitar; **—— blade** navaja *or* hoja de afeitar *or* rasurar

RDA *V.* **recommended dietary allowance**.

reach *n* alcance *m*; **out of —— of children**

fuera del alcance de los niños; *vt, vi* alcanzar

react *vi* reaccionar

reaction *n* reacción *f*; **adverse** —— reacción adversa; **allergic** —— reacción alérgica; **conversion** —— reacción conversiva; **cross** —— reacción cruzada; **delayed** —— reacción tardía

reactivate *vt* reactivar

reactivation *n* reactivación *f*

reactive *adj* reactivo

read *vt, vi* (*pret & pp* **read**) leer

reading *n* (*of an instrument*) lectura

reality *n* realidad *f*

rebound *n* rebote *m*

recently *adv* últimamente, recientemente

recessive *adj* recesivo

recombinant *adj* recombinante

recommend *vt* recomendar

recommendation *n* recomendación *f*

recommended dietary allowance (RDA) *n* dosis diaria recomendada

reconstruct *vt* reconstruir

record *n* (*patient chart*) expediente *m*; (*of temperatures, etc.*) registro

recourse *n* recurso

recover *vt* recobrar, recuperar; *vi* recuperarse, aliviarse, restablecerse

recovery *n* recuperación *f*, restablecimiento; —— **room** sala de recuperación

recreation *n* recreación *f*, (*esp during school*) recreo

rectal *adj* rectal

rectocele *n* rectocele *m*

rectum *n* (*pl* **-tums** *o* **-ta**) recto

recumbent *adj* recostado

recuperate *vi* recuperarse

recuperation *n* recuperación *f*

recur *vi* (*pret & pp* **recurred**; *ger* **recurring**) volver (*una enfermedad, condición, etc.*)

recurrence *n* recurrencia

red *adj* (*comp* **redder**; *super* **reddest**) rojo, colorado

redbug *n* nigua

Red Cross *n* Cruz Roja

reddening *n* enrojecimiento

reddish *adj* rojizo

redness *n* enrojecimiento

reduce *vt* reducir, disminuir, bajar; (*ortho*) reducir; *vi* (*fam, to lose weight*) rebajar

reducible *adj* reducible

reduction *n* reducción *f*

reevaluate *vt* reevaluar, revalorar

reference *n* referencia

refill *n* surtido nuevo (*de medicamentos*); *vt* surtir de nuevo

refined *adj* refinado

reflex *n* reflejo; **conditioned** —— reflejo condicionado; **gag** —— reflejo nauseoso; **patellar** —— reflejo patelar *or* rotuliano

reflux *n* reflujo; **esophageal** —— reflujo esofágico

refraction *n* refracción *f*

refractive *adj* refractivo

refresh *vt* refrescar; **to get refreshed** refrescarse

refreshing *adj* refrescante

refrigeration *n* refrigeración *f*

refrigerator *n* refrigerador *m*

regain *vt* recuperar; **to** —— **consciousness** volver en sí

regenerate *vi* regenerarse

regeneration *n* regeneración *f*

regimen *n* régimen *m*

register *n* (*of births, etc.*) registro

regression *n* regresión *f*

regular *adj* regular

regulate *vt* regular

regulator *n* regulador *m*

regurgitate *vt* regurgitar

regurgitation *n* regurgitación *f*; **aortic** ——, **mitral** ——, **etc.** regurgitación aórtica, regurgitación mitral, etc.

rehabilitate *vt* rehabilitar

rehabilitation *n* rehabilitación *f*

rehydrate *n* rehidratar

rehydration *n* rehidratación *f*

reinfection *n* reinfección *f*

reinfestation *n* reinfestación *f*

reinforce *vt* reforzar

reinforcement *n* refuerzo

reject *vt* rechazar

rejection *n* rechazo

rejuvenate *vt* rejuvenecer; **to become rejuvenated** rejuvenecerse

relapse *n* recaída; *vi* recaer

relation *n* relación *f*

relative *n* familiar *m*, pariente *mf*; **blood** —— pariente consanguíneo, pariente que tiene la misma sangre (*fam*)

relax *vt, vi* relajar(se), aflojar(se); **Relax..** Relájese...**Relax your leg.**.Afloje la pierna.

relaxant *n* relajante *m*

relaxation *n* relajación *f*, (*rest*) descanso

relaxing *adj* relajante

release *n* liberación *f*; **slow** —— liberación prolongada; **sustained** —— liberación sostenida; **timed** —— difusión regulada; *vt* liberar; **copper-releasing, hormone-releasing, etc.** liberador de cobre, liberador de hormona, etc.

reliable *adj* confiable

relief *n* alivio, (*emotional*) desahogo

relieve *vt* aliviar

REM *abbr* **rapid eye movement.** *V.* **movement.**

remedy *n* (*pl* **-dies**) remedio; **home** —— remedio casero

remember *vt* recordar, acordarse (de)

remission *n* remisión *f*

remorse *n* remordimiento

removable *adj* que se puede sacar

removal *n* extracción *f*, (el) quitar, (el) sacar

remove *vt* extraer (*form*), sacar, quitar

renal *adj* renal; —— **failure** insuficiencia renal

renew *vt* renovar

renovascular *adj* renovascular

repair *n* reparación *f*; *vt* reparar, arreglar

repeat *vt* repetir

repellant *n* repelente *m*; **insect** —— repelente de insectos

repetitive *adj* repetitivo

replace *vt* reemplazar

replacement *n* reemplazo; **total hip** —— reemplazo total de cadera

replenish *vt* reponer

report *vt* reportar; **The law requires me to report your condition to the public health department.**.La ley requiere que yo reporte su condición al departamento de salud pública.

reportable *adj* reportable

repress *vt* reprimir

repression *n* represión *f*

reproduce *vt, vi* reproducir(se)

reproduction *n* reproducción *f*

reproductive *adj* reproductor, reproductivo

rescue *n* rescate *m*, salvamento; *vt* rescatar, salvar

rescuer *n* socorrista *mf*

research *n* investigación *f*

resection *n* resección *f*

reserpine *n* reserpina

reserve *n* reserva

reservoir *n* reservorio

resident *n* (*physician*) residente *mf*

residue *n* residuo

resin *n* resina

resist *vt, vi* resistir(se)

resistance *n* resistencia

resistant *adj* resistente

resolve *vi* resolverse

resorb *vt, vi* reabsorber, resorber

respect *n* respeto

respiration *n* respiración *f*

respirator *n* mascarilla (*para filtrar el aire*), respirador *m*; aparato para suministrar respiración artificial, respirador *m*

respiratory *adj* respiratorio; —— **failure** insuficiencia respiratoria

respire *vt, vi* respirar

respond *vi* responder

response *n* respuesta; **immune** —— respuesta inmune

rest *n* descanso, reposo; **at** —— en reposo; *vt, vi* descansar

restless *adj* inquieto, intranquilo

restoration *n* restauración *f*

restore *vt* reponer, restablecer

restrain *vt* sujetar

restraints *npl* sujetadores *mpl*

restrict *vt* restringir

restriction *n* restricción *f*

rest room *n* baño

result *n* resultado

resuscitate *vt* resucitar

resuscitation *n* resucitación *f*, reanimación *f*; **cardiopulmonary** —— **(CPR)** resucitación *or* reanimación cardiopulmonar (RCP); **mouth-to-mouth** —— resucitación *or* respiración *f* boca-a-boca

retain *vt* retener; **to —— water** retener agua

retainer *n* (*orthodontia*) arco de Hawley

retardation *n* retardo, retraso; **mental ——** retardo *or* retraso mental

retarded *adj* retardado, retrasado; **mentally —— retardado** *or* retrasado mental

retch *vi* vomitar sin tener nada que expulsar

retention *n* retención *f*

reticulocyte *n* reticulocito

retina *n* (*pl* -nas *o* -nae) retina; **detached —— retina** desprendida

retinopathy *n* retinopatía

retrograde *adj* retrógrado

reusable *adj* reusable, para uso repetido

revaccination *n* revacunación *f*

reversible *adj* reversible

revitalize *vt* revitalizar

revitalizing *adj* revitalizador

revive *vt, vi* reanimar(se), revivir

rhabdomyolysis *n* rabdomiólisis *f*

rhabdomyoma *n* rabdomioma *m*

rhabdomyosarcoma *n* rabdomiosarcoma *m*

rhabdosarcoma *n* rabdosarcoma *m*

rheumatic *adj* reumático

rheumatoid *adj* reumatoide

rheumatologist *n* reumatólogo -ga *mf*

rheumatology *n* reumatología

Rh factor *n* factor *m* Rh

rhinitis *n* rinitis *f*; **allergic ——** rinitis alérgica

rhinoplasty *n* (*pl* -ties) rinoplastia

rhubarb *n* ruibarbo

rhythm *n* ritmo; **—— method** método del ritmo

rhythmic *adj* rítmico

rib *n* costilla; **—— cage** caja torácica

ribavarin *n* ribavarina

riboflavin *n* riboflavina

ribonucleic acid *n* ácido ribonucleico

rice *n* arroz *m*

rich *adj* (*food, etc.*) rico

rickets *n* raquitismo

Rickettsia Rickettsia

rid *vt* **to get —— of** deshacerse de

rifampin *n* rifampicina

right *adj* derecho; *n* (*right-hand side*) derecha; (*legal, moral*) derecho

right-handed *adj* que usa la mano derecha; **Are you right-handed or left-handed?..** ¿Ud. escribe con la derecha o la izquierda?

rigid *adj* rígido

rigor mortis *n* rigor mortis *m*

ring *n* anillo; *vi* (*in one's ears*) zumbar

ringing *n* (*in one's ears*) zumbido

ringworm *n* tiña del cuerpo

rinse *n* enjuague *m*; *vt* enjuagar

ripe *adj* (*abscess, fruit*) maduro

rise *n* aumento, elevación *f*, subida; *vi* (*pret* **rose**; *pp* **risen**) subir(se), elevar(se); (*to get up*) levantarse; **Your sugar rose..Su** azúcar subió.

risk *n* riesgo; **—— factor** factor *m* de riesgo; **high ——** alto riesgo; **to run the —— of** correr el riesgo de; **to take a —— arriesgarse**; *vt* arriesgar

ritual *n* ritual *m*

roast *vt* asar

rod *n* (*bacteria*) bacilo; (*of the eye*) bastón *m*

rodent *adj & n* roedor *m*

role *n* papel *m*; **—— model** modelo (*a seguir*)

roll *vi* **to —— over** voltearse, darse vuelta; **Roll over facing the wall..**Voltéese viendo hacia la pared.

room *n* cuarto, sala; **delivery ——** sala de partos; **emergency —— (ER)** sala de emergencia *or* urgencias; **operating —— (OR)** quirófano, sala de operaciones; **recovery ——** sala de recuperación; **waiting ——** sala de espera

root *n* raíz *f*

root canal *n* endodoncia (*form*), tratamiento de nervio (*fam*), curación *f* de nervio (*fam*)

rose *pret de* **rise**

roseola infantum *n* roséola *or* roseola infantil

rot *vt, vi* (*pret & pp* **rotted**; *ger* **rotting**) pudrir(se)

rotten *adj* podrido

rough *adj* áspero

roughness *n* aspereza

round *adj* redondo

rounds *npl* visitas, rondas (*Ang*); **to make**

—— pasar visita, hacer rondas

roundworm *n* ascáride *m* (*form*), gusano redondo, lombriz *f* (*fam*)

routine *adj* rutinario; *n* rutina; **daily** —— rutina cotidiana

rub *vt* (*pret* & *pp* **rubbed**; *ger* **rubbing**) (*to massage*) sobar; (*to chafe*) rozar; *vi* rozar

rubber *n* hule *m*, goma; (*fam*) condón *m*, preservativo

rubbing *n* fricción *f*

rubdown *n* masaje *m*

rubella *n* rubeola *or* rubéola, sarampión *m* alemán (*fam*)

rubeola *n* (*form*) sarampión *m*

rule *vt* **to** —— **out** descartar; **Cancer was ruled out**..Se descartó el cáncer.

rum *n* ron *m*

run *n* **to have the runs** (*fam*) tener diarrea; *vt* (*pret* **ran**; *pp* **run**; *ger* **running**) **to** —— **over** atropellar; *vi* correr; (*to flow*) fluir, correr, chorrear; **to** —— **in one's family** venir de familia; **to** —— **out** acabarse; **When did your medicine run out?**..¿Cuándo se le acabó la medicina?

runaway *n* niño -ña *mf* que ha abandonado el hogar

run-down *adj* agotado, exhausto, debilitado, decaído

runny *adj* (*comp* **-nier**; *super* **-niest**) líquido, de consistencia líquida; **to have a** —— **nose** tener secreciones por la nariz, fluirle la nariz, tener mocosidad, tener moquera (*fam*)

rupture *n* ruptura; **premature** —— **of membranes** ruptura prematura de membranas; *vt, vi* reventar(se)

rural *adj* rural, del campo

rusty *adj* oxidado; —— **nail** clavo oxidado

S

S-A *V.* **sinoatrial**.

saccharin *n* sacarina

sacral *adj* sacro

sacroiliac *adj* sacroiliaco

sacrum *n* (*pl* **-cra**) sacro

sad *adj* (*comp* **sadder**; *super* **saddest**) triste

sadism *n* sadismo

sadist *n* sádico -ca *mf*

sadistic *adj* sádico

safe *adj* seguro, sin peligro

safety *n* seguridad *f*; —— **cap** tapa de seguridad; —— **pin** imperdible *m*, alfiler *m* de seguridad, seguro (*Mex*), gancho

safflower oil *n* aceite *m* de cártamo

sag *vi* (*pret* & *pp* **sagged**; *ger* **sagging**) caerse

salad *n* ensalada

salbutamol *n* salbutamol *m*

salicylate *n* salicilato

salicylic acid *n* ácido salicílico

saline *adj* salino; **normal** —— **solution** solución salina isotónica

saliva *n* saliva

salivary *adj* salival

salivation *n* salivación *f*

Salmonella Salmonella

salmonellosis *n* salmonelosis *f*

salpingitis *n* salpingitis *f*

salt *n* sal *f*; —— **substitute** substituto de sal; **Epsom** —— sal de Epsom; **smelling salts** sales aromáticas

salted *adj* salado, que tiene sal

saltine *n* galleta salada

salty *adj* salado

Salvadoran, Salvadorian *adj* & *n* salvadoreño -ña *mf*

salvage *vt* salvar

salve *n* ungüento, pomada

sample *n* muestra

sanatorium *n* sanatorio

sandfly *n* (*pl* -**flies**) jején *m*, mosquito, mosquito simúlido

sane *adj* cuerdo

sanitarium *n* centro de recreo para la salud; sanatorio

sanitary *adj* sanitario; —— **napkin** toalla sanitaria, toalla femenina (*esp Mex*)

sanitation *n* saneamiento (*ambiental*), medidas sanitarias

sanity *n* cordura

saphenous *adj* safeno

sarcoidosis *n* sarcoidosis *f*

sarcoma *n* sarcoma *m*; **Ewing's** —— sarcoma de Ewing; **Kaposi's** —— sarcoma de Kaposi

sarsaparilla *n* (*bot*) zarzaparrilla

sassafras *n* (*bot*) sasafrás *m*

sat *pret* & *pp de* **sit**

satellite *adj* (*lesion, clinic*) satélite

saturated *adj* saturado

sauce *n* salsa; **hot** —— salsa picante

sauna *n* sauna *m*

sausage *n* chorizo

save *vt* salvar; **We want to save your leg** ..Queremos salvarle la pierna.

saw *n* sierra

saw *pret de* **see**

scab *n* costra

scabies *n* sarna

scald *n* escaldadura; *vt* escaldar

scale *n* (*for weighing*) báscula, balanza; (*piece of skin*) escama; (*of measurement*) escala; **sliding** —— escala flexible *or* móvil

scalp *n* cuero cabelludo

scalpel *n* escalpelo, bisturí *m*

scaly *adj* (*comp* -**ier**; *super* -**iest**) escamoso

scan *n* escán *m* (*Ang*), imagen diagnóstica, (*nuclear*) gammagrama *m*, gammagrafía; **bone** —— serie ósea; **CAT** —— tomografía axial computarizada, TAC *m* (*fam*), tomografía (*fam*); **CT** —— tomografía computada, tomografía (*fam*); **gallium** —— gammagrama de galio; **thallium** —— gammagrama de talio

scapula *n* (*pl* -**lae** *o* -**las**) escápula (*form*), omóplato, paleta (*fam*)

scar *n* cicatriz *f*

scarce *adj* escaso

scare *n* susto; *vt* **to be scared** tener miedo; **Don't be scared**..No tenga miedo.

schedule *n* horario; (*of vaccinations*) esquema

schistosomiasis *n* esquistosomiasis *f*

schizoid *adj* esquizoide

schizophrenia *n* esquizofrenia

schizophrenic *adj* & *n* esquizofrénico -ca *mf*

school *n* escuela

sciatic *adj* ciático

sciatica *n* ciática

scientific *adj* científico

scientist *n* científico -ca *mf*

scissors *npl* tijeras

sclera *n* (*pl* -**rae**) esclerótica, esclera

scleritis *n* escleritis *f*

scleroderma *n* esclerodermia

sclerosis *n* esclerosis *f*

sclerotherapy *n* escleroterapia

scoliosis *n* escoliosis *f*

scopolamine *n* escopolamina

scored *adj* (*tablet*) ranurado

scorpion *n* escorpión *m*, alacrán *m*

scrape *n* raspón *m*, raspadura; *vt* raspar(se)

scratch *n* rasguño, raspado, (*with claws*) arañazo; *vt* rasguñar(se), raspar(se), arañar(se); (*an itch, etc.*) rascar(se); **How did you scratch yourself?**..¿Cómo se rasguñó?...**You have to quit scratching (yourself)**..Tiene que dejar de rascarse.

screen *n* examen *m* de detección; *vt, vi* practicar exámenes de detección

screening *n* detección *f*, práctica de exámenes de detección; —— **for cancer, glaucoma, etc.** detección del cáncer, glaucoma, etc.

scrofula *n* escrófula

scrotum *n* escroto

scurvy *n* escorbuto

seafood *n* marisco(s); **Are you allergic to seafood?**..¿Es alérgico a los mariscos?

seasickness *n* mareo (*en un barco*)

season *n* (*winter, spring, etc.*) estación *f*; (*for a disease, rain, etc.*) temporada

seat belt *n* cinturón *m* de seguridad

sea urchin *n* erizo de mar

sebaceous *adj* sebáceo

seborrhea *n* seborrea
sebum *n* sebo
second *adj* segundo; *n* segundo
secondary *adj* secundario
secretary *n* (*pl* -**ries**) secretario -ria *mf*
secrete *vt* secretar
secretion *n* secreción *f*
secretory *adj* secretorio
section *n* sección *f*; **frozen** —— corte *m* por congelación
sedate *vt* sedar, dar un sedante
sedative *adj* & *n* sedante *m*, calmante *m*
sedentary *adj* sedentario
sediment *n* sedimento
see *vt, vi* (*pret* **saw**; *pp* **seen**) ver; **When was the last time you saw an eye doctor?**..¿Cuándo fue la última vez que vio a un médico de los ojos?
Seeing Eye dog *n* perro guía
seize *vi* tener una convulsión
seizure *n* crisis convulsiva *or* epiléptica (*form*), convulsión *f* (*form*), ataque *m*; **Did you have a seizure?**..¿Tuvo una convulsión?..¿Le dio un ataque?; **absence** —— crisis de ausencia; **complex partial** —— crisis parcial compleja; **focal** —— crisis focal; **generalized** —— crisis generalizada; **gran mal** —— crisis gran mal; **Jacksonian** —— crisis jacksoniana; **partial** —— crisis parcial; **petit mal** —— crisis pequeño mal; **psychomotor** —— crisis psicomotora; **temporal lobe** —— crisis del lóbulo temporal; **tonic-clonic** —— crisis tonicoclónica
selenium *n* selenio
self-absorbed *adj* ensimismado
self-centered *adj* egocéntrico
self-confidence *n* confianza en sí mismo
self-conscious *adj* consciente de sí mismo
self-control *n* dominio de sí mismo
self-destructive *adj* autodestructivo
self-discipline *n* autodisciplina
self-esteem *n* autoestima (*form*), amor propio
self-examination *n* autoevaluación *f*, autoexamen *m*
self-help *n* autoayuda
self-limited *adj* autolimitado
self-prescribe *vt* autorrecetarse, autoprescribirse
self-respect *n* respeto de sí mismo, autorrespeto
self-treatment *n* autotratamiento
semen *n* semen *m*
semicircular canal *n* conducto semicircular
seminoma *n* seminoma *m*
senile *adj* senil
senior citizen *n* (*US*) persona anciana, persona que recibe ciertos derechos debido a su edad mayor
senna *n* (*bot*) sen *m*
sensation *n* sensación *f*
sense *n* sentido; —— **of hearing** sentido del oído; —— **of sight** sentido de la vista; —— **of smell** sentido del olfato; —— **of taste** sentido del gusto; —— **of touch** sentido del tacto
sensitive *adj* sensible
sensitivity *n* (*pl* -**ties**) sensibilidad *f*
sensitize *vt* sensibilizar; **to become sensitized** sensibilizarse
sensory *adj* (*nerve*) sensitivo; (*perception*) sensorio
sepsis *n* sepsis *f*
septic *adj* séptico
septum *n* (*pl* -**ta**) tabique *m*; **deviated** —— tabique desviado; **interventricular** —— tabique interventricular; **nasal** —— tabique nasal
sera *pl de* serum
serial *adj* seriado
series *n* (*pl* **series**) serie *f*
serine *n* serina
serious *adj* serio, grave
seroconversion *n* seroconversión *f*
serology *n* (*pl* -**gies**) serología
seronegative *adj* seronegativo
seropositive *adj* seropositivo
sertraline *n* sertralina
serum *n* sérico; *n* (*pl* **sera** *o* **serums**) suero; —— **sickness** enfermedad *f* del suero
service *n* servicio
set *vt* (*a bone*) reducir (*form*), acomodar
severe *adj* severo
severity *n* gravedad *f*
sew *vt* (*fam, to suture*) suturar, coser (*fam*)

sewage *n* aguas negras

sewer *n* drenaje *m*

sex *n* sexo; —— **change** cambio de sexo; —— **life** vida sexual; **oral** —— sexo oral; **safe** —— sexo sin riesgo de infección, sexo seguro (*Ang*); **to have** —— tener relaciones (*sexuales*)

sex-linked *adj* ligado al sexo

sexual *adj* sexual

sexuality *n* sexualidad *f*

shake *vi* (*pret* **shook**; *pp* **shaken**) (*to tremble*) temblar; (*to shiver*) estremecerse, tiritar; **Shake well before using**..Agítese bien antes de usarse.

shame *n* vergüenza

shampoo *n* (*pl* **-poos**) champú *m*; *vt* (*pret & pp* **-pooed**) lavarse el pelo *or* la cabeza

shape *n* forma, condición *f*; **in** —— en forma

shark *n* tiburón *m*

sharp *adj* (*pain*) agudo; (*instrument*) afilado, filoso

shave *vt, vi* afeitar(se), rasurar(se)

shaver *n* rasuradora eléctrica, máquina de afeitar

shed *vt* (*pret & pp* **shed**; *ger* **shedding**) (*viruses, parasites, etc.*) eliminar, liberar, botar, tirar (*esp Mex*), echar

sheepskin *n* piel *f* de oveja

sheet *n* (*for a bed*) sábana

shellfish *n* (*pl* **-fish** *o* **-fishes**) marisco(s)

shell shock *n* neurosis *f* de guerra

shelter *n* refugio; **women's** ——, **homeless** ——, **etc.** refugio para mujeres, refugio para personas sin hogar, etc.

Shigella Shigella

shigellosis *n* shigelosis *f*

shin *n* espinilla, canilla; —— **guard** espinillera, canillera; —— **splints** dolor *m* de espinilla debido a ejercicio excesivo

shinbone *n* (*anat*) tibia (*form*), espinilla, canilla

shingles *n* herpes *m* zoster, zona

shirt *n* camisa

shiver *n* escalofrío; *vi* tiritar, estremecerse

shock *n* choque *m*, shock *m* (*Ang*); **ana-phylactic** —— choque anafiláctico; **cardiogenic** —— choque cardiogénico *or* cardiógeno; **electric** —— choque eléctrico, descarga eléctrica; **hypovolemic** —— choque hipovolémico; **neurogenic** —— choque neurogénico *or* neurógeno; **septic** —— choque séptico

shoe *n* zapato

shook *pret de* **shake**

shooter *n* (*vulg*) persona que se inyecta drogas

shooting *adj* (*pain*) punzante

short *adj* (*stature*) bajo, chaparro; (*dimension*) corto; (*time*) breve; —— **of breath** V. **breath**.

short-acting *adj* de acción corta

shorten *vt* acortar, hacer más corto

shortening *n* manteca (*para mezclar con la masa*)

short-term *adj* a corto plazo

shot (*fam*) *n* inyección *f*

shoulder *n* hombro; —— **blade** omóplato, paleta

shower *n* ducha, baño de regadera (*Mex*); **to take a** —— tomar una ducha, ducharse, bañarse (*en la ducha*)

shrimp *n* camarón *m*

shrink *n* (*vulg*) psiquiatra *mf*; *vt, vi* (*pret* **shrank**; *pp* **shrunk**) (*tumor, etc.*) reducir(se)

shunt *n* (*physio*) cortocircuito; (*surg*) derivación *f*; **portacaval** —— derivación portocava; **ventriculoperitoneal** —— derivación ventriculoperitoneal

shy *adj* (*comp* **shyer** *o* **shier**; *super* **shyest** *o* **shiest**) tímido

shyness *n* timidez *f*

Siamese twins *npl* hermanos -nas siameses

sibling *n* hermano -na *mf*; —— **rivalry** rivalidad *f* entre hermanos; *npl* hermanos

sick *adj* enfermo, malo; **to get** —— enfermarse, ponerse enfermo

sickly *adj* (*comp* **-lier**; *super* **-liest**) enfermizo

sickness *n* enfermedad *f*, mal *m*; **decom-pression** —— enfermedad por descompresión; **morning** —— náuseas *or* vómitos del embarazo; **motion** —— mareo (*producido por el movimiento*); **mountain** —— mal de montaña, soroche *m* (*SA*);

serum —— enfermedad del suero;
sleeping —— enfermedad del sueño
side *n* lado, (*anat*) costado; **on your father's
side.**.por el lado de su padre
sideache *n* dolor *m* de costado (*esp al hacer
ejercicio después de comer*)
side rail (*of a bed*) barandal *m*, baranda
SIDS *abbr* **sudden infant death syndrome.**
V. **syndrome.**
sieve *n* colador *m*
sigh *n* suspiro; *vi* suspirar
sight *n* vista, visión *f*
sighted *adj* que puede ver
sigmoid *adj* sigmoideo; —— **colon** colon *m*
sigmoide
sigmoidoscope *n* sigmoidoscopio
sigmoidoscopy *n* (*pl* **-pies**) sigmoidoscopia
or (*esp spoken*) sigmoidoscopía; **flexible**
—— sigmoidoscopia flexible
sign *n* (*of an illness*) signo; **vital signs**
signos vitales; **warning** —— signo de
advertencia, señal *f* de alarma; *vt, vi*
(*one's name*) firmar; (*deaf language*)
hablar por señas
signature *n* firma
silica *n* sílice *f*
silicone *n* silicona
silicosis *n* silicosis *f*
silk *n* seda
silver *n* plata; —— **nitrate** nitrato de plata
simethicone *n* simeticona
simvastatin *n* simvastatina
single *adj* (*unmarried*) soltero
sinoatrial (S-A) *adj* sinoauricular *or* sinoatrial (SA)
sinus *n* seno; —— **tract** fístula
sinusitis *n* sinusitis *f*
sip *n* sorbo; *vt* (*pret & pp* **sipped**; *ger*
sipping) sorber
sister-in-law *n* (*pl* **sisters-in-law**) cuñada
sister *n* hermana
sit *vi* (*pret & pp* **sat**; *ger* **sitting**) sentarse; **to**
—— **down** sentarse; **to** —— **up** (*from a
supine position*) sentarse
sit-up *n* abdominal *m*
size *n* tamaño, talla, medida, dimensiones *fpl*
skeleton *n* esqueleto
skill *n* destreza, habilidad *f*

skin *n* piel *f*; (*of the face*) cutis *m*;
(*complexion*) tez *f*; (*of banana, orange*)
cáscara; —— **tag** acrocordón *m* (*form*),
fibroma *m* pendular (*form*), verruga (*fam*);
vt raspar; **Did you skin your knee?**..¿Se
raspó la rodilla?
skinny *adj* (*fam*) flaco (*fam*), delgado
skirt *n* falda
skull *n* cráneo
skullcap *n* (*bot*) escutelaria
skunk *n* zorrillo
sleep *n* sueño; (*eye secretions*) legaña (*form*),
lagaña; —— **apnea** apnea del sueño; **to
go to** —— dormirse; **Do you have trouble going to sleep?**..¿Tiene problemas
para dormirse?**...Does your arm go to
sleep?**..¿Se le duerme el brazo? **to go
without** —— desvelarse; **to put to** ——
dormir, anestesiar; **We will put you to
sleep for the operation.**.Vamos a dormir-
lo para la operación; *vi* (*pret & pp* **slept**)
dormir
sleeper *V.* **sleeping pill.**
sleeping pill *n* somnífero (*form*), pastilla
para dormir
sleeping sickness *n* enfermedad *f* del sueño
sleepless *adj* desvelado
sleepwalk *vi* caminar dormido
sleepwalking *n* sonambulismo (*form*), (el)
caminar dormido
sleepy *adj* (*comp* **-ier**; *super* **-iest**) **to be**
—— tener sueño; **to make** —— dar sue-
ño; **This medicine makes her sleepy.**.
Esta medicina le da sueño.
slept *pret & pp de* **sleep**
sliding scale *n* escala flexible *or* móvil
slight *adj* leve, ligero
sling *n* cabestrillo
slip *n* resbalón *m*; *vi* (*pret & pp* **slipped**; *ger*
slipping) resbalar(se)
slitlamp *n* lámpara de hendidura
sliver *n* astilla
slouch *vi* sentarse o pararse con mala
postura, encorvarse
slough *vi* (*también* **to** —— **off**) desprenderse, caerse
slur *vi* (*pret & pp* **slurred**; *ger* **slurring**)
hablar con la lengua pesada, arrastrar la

voz, balbucear

small *adj* pequeño, chico; **to get smaller** ponerse más pequeño, reducir(se), disminuir(se); *n* —— **of the back** parte baja de la espalda

smallpox *n* viruela

smart *vi* doler de una manera aguda e intensiva

smear *n* (*micro*) frotis *m*; **Papanicolaou** —— frotis de Papanicolaou

smell *n* olor *m*; *vt, vi* oler; **to** —— **bad** oler mal; **to** —— **like** oler a

smile *n* sonrisa; *vi* sonreír(se); **Smile..Sonría.**

smog *n* aire contaminado, esmog *m* (*Ang*)

smoke *n* humo; *vt, vi* fumar

smoke detector *n* detector *m* de humo

smoker *n* fumador -ra *mf*

smoking *n* (el) fumar (*tabaco*); **No smoking..No fumar**

smooth *adj* liso, suave

smother *vt, vi* ahogar(se), sofocar(se)

snack *n* bocadillo, refrigerio, botana (*Mex*); *vi* comer entre comidas

snail *n* caracol *m*

snake *n* serpiente *f*, culebra

sneeze *n* estornudo; *vi* estornudar

Snellen chart *n* carta de Snellen, (*pocket size*) tarjeta de Snellen

sniff *vt* (*cocaine, glue, etc.*) inhalar, oler (*cocaína, cemento, etc.*); *vi* aspirar por la nariz

sniffle *n* **to have the sniffles** tener secreciones por la nariz, fluirle la naríz, tener mocosidad, tener moquera (*fam*); *vi* aspirar moco líquido por la nariz

snore *vi* roncar

snort *vt* (*vulg, cocaine*) inhalar, oler (*cocaína*)

snot *n* (*vulg*) moquera, moco

snow *n* nieve *f*

snuff *n* (*tobacco*) rapé *m*

soak *vt* (*dressing, etc.*) remojar; (*body part*) meter al agua (*por un tiempo*)

soap *n* jabón *m*

sober *adj* sobrio, no intoxicado; *vi* **to** —— **up** desemborracharse, desembriagarse

soccer *n* fútbol *m*

social service *n* servicio social

social worker *n* trabajador -ra *mf* social

sock *n* calcetín *m*

socket *n* (*of a tooth*) alveolo *or* alvéolo; (*of an eye*) cuenca

soda *n* soda

sodium *n* sodio; —— **bicarbonate** bicarbonato de sodio; —— **chloride** cloruro de sodio; —— **hydroxide** hidróxido de sodio

soft *adj* blando, suave

soft drink *n* refresco

soften *vt* (*skin*) suavizar

softening *adj* (*lotion, etc.*) suavizador, suavizante

soil *vt* ensuciar; **to** —— **oneself** ensuciarse

solar *adj* solar; —— **plexus** plexo solar

soldier *n* soldado

sole *n* (*of the foot*) planta; (*of a shoe*) suela

soleus *n* sóleo

solid *adj & n* sólido

soluble *adj* soluble

solution *n* solución *f*; **normal saline** —— solución salina isotónica

solvent *n* solvente *m*

somatic *adj* somático

somatostatin *n* somatostatina

son *n* hijo

son-in-law *n* (*pl* **sons-in-law**) yerno

sonogram *n* sonograma *m*

soothe *vt* aliviar, calmar

sorbitol *n* sorbitol *m*

sore *adj* adolorido *or* dolorido; —— **throat** dolor *m* de garganta; *n* úlcera, llaga; **pressure** —— escara de presión, úlcera por presión, llaga (*debida a permanecer mucho tiempo sin cambiar de posición*)

sorry *adj* **to be** —— sentir; **I'm sorry you had to wait so long..Siento que haya tenido que esperar tanto tiempo...I'm sorry..Lo siento.**

sound *n* sonido

soup *n* sopa, caldo

sour *adj* agrio

source *n* origen *m*, fuente *f*

South American *adj & n* sudamericano -na *mf*

soybean *n* soya *or* soja

space *n* espacio

spaced out *adj* distraído, bajo el efecto de

drogas

Spaniard *n* español -la *mf*

spasm *n* espasmo

spasmodic *adj* espasmódico

spastic *adj* espástico

spasticity *n* espasticidad *f*

spat *pret & pp de* **spit**

speak *vt, vi* (*pret* **spoke**; *pp* **spoken**) hablar

spearmint *n* (*bot*) menta verde

specialist *n* especialista *mf*

specialty *n* (*pl* -**ties**) especialidad *f*

species *n* (*pl* -**cies**) especie *f*

specific *adj* específico

specimen *n* espécimen *m*, muestra

spectacles *npl* anteojos, gafas

spectinomycin *n* espectinomicina

spectrum *n* (*pl* -**tra** *o* -**trums**) espectro

speculum *n* (*pl* -**la** *o* -**lums**) espéculo

speech *n* habla; —— **development** desarrollo del habla

speed *n* (*vulg*) anfetamina

spell *n* acceso, periodo *or* período (*de mareo, tos, etc.*)

sperm *n* (*with semen*) esperma; (*individual spermatozoon*) espermatozoide *m*

spermatocele *n* espermatocele *m*

spermatozoon *n* espermatozoide *m*

spermicidal, spermatocidal *adj* espermaticida, espermicida

spermicide, spermatocide *n* espermaticida *m*, espermicida *m*

SPF *abbr* **solar protection factor**. *V.* **factor**.

sphincter *n* esfínter *m*

spice *n* especia, condimento

spicy *adj* (*comp* -**ier**; *super* -**iest**) picante

spider *n* araña

spider angioma *n* telangiectasia aracniforme (*form*), araña vascular, nevo en araña

spina bifida *n* espina bífida

spinach *n* espinacas

spinal *adj* espinal, raquídeo; —— **column** columna vertebral, espina dorsal; —— **cord** médula espinal

spine *n* espina dorsal, columna vertebral, columna (*fam*); (*thorn*) espina; **cervical** —— columna cervical; **lumbar** —— columna lumbar; **sacral** —— columna sacra; **thoracic** —— columna torácica *or*

dorsal

spirochete *n* espiroqueta

spirometer *n* espirómetro

spirometry *n* espirometría; **incentive** —— ejercicio respiratorio postquirúrgico

spironolactone *n* espironolactona

spit *n* saliva; *vt, vi* (*pret & pp* **spat** *o* **spit**; *ger* **spitting**) escupir; **to** —— **up** (*fam, esp ped*) vomitar, arrojar, devolver

spleen *n* bazo

splenectomy *n* (*pl* -**mies**) esplenectomía

splenic *adj* esplénico

splint *n* férula (*form*), tablilla; *vt* colocar una férula, entablillar

splinter *n* astilla

split *adj* partido, quebrado; *n* quebradura, fisura; *vt, vi* (*pret & pp* **split**; *ger* **splitting**) partir(se), quebrar(se)

spoil (*pret & pp* **spoiled** *o* **spoilt**) *vt* (*a child*) consentir, mimar; *vi* (*food, etc.*) echarse a perder

spoke *pret de* **speak**

spoken *pp de* **speak**

spondylitis *n* espondilitis *f*; **ankylosing** —— espondilitis anquilosante

spondylosis *n* espondilosis *f*

sponge *n* esponja

spontaneous *adj* espontáneo

spoonful *n* cucharada

sporadic *adj* esporádico

spore *n* espora

sporotrichosis *n* esporotricosis *f*

spot *n* mancha

spotting *n* sangrado vaginal ligero (*que deja manchas en la ropa interior*)

spouse *n* esposo -sa *mf*, cónyuge *mf*

sprain *n* torcedura; *vt* torcer(se); **I sprained my wrist**..Me torcí la muñeca..Se me torció la muñeca.

spray *n* aerosol *m*, espray *m* (*Ang*); **nasal** —— aerosol nasal

spread *n* diseminación *f* (*form*), propagación *f*; *vt, vi* (*pret & pp* **spread**) diseminar(se) (*form*), propagar(se), pasar(se) (*fam*)

spring, springtime *n* primavera

sprue *n* esprue *m&f*; **celiac** *o* **nontropical** —— esprue celiaco *or* no tropical; **tropical** —— esprue tropical

spur *n* (*ortho*) espolón *m*
sputum *n* esputo (*form*), flema
squamous *adj* escamoso
square *adj* cuadrado; —— **meter** metro
cuadrado
squared *adj* cuadrado; **meter** —— metro
cuadrado
squat *vi* ponerse en cuclillas
squeal *vi* chillar
squeeze *vt* apretar; **Squeeze my hand**..
Apriete mi mano.
squint *vt, vi* entrecerrar (*los ojos*), fruncir
(*los ojos, la vista*)
squirrel *n* ardilla
stabbing *adj* (*pain*) punzante
stability *n* estabilidad *f*
stabilization *n* estabilización *f*
stabilize *vt, vi* estabilizar(se)
stabilizer *n* estabilizador *m*
stable *adj* estable
stage *n* (*disease, cancer*) estadío *or* (*esp spoken*) estadio, etapa; (*sleep*) etapa
stagger *vi* tambalear(se)
stain *n* mancha; (*micro*) coloración *f*;
Gram's —— coloración de Gram; **port-wine** —— mancha de vino oporto
stainless steel *n* acero inoxidable
stamina *n* vigor *m*, resistencia
stammer *vi* tartamudear
stance *n* postura
stanch *vt* restañar
stand *vt* (*pret & pp* **stood**) (*to endure*) soportar, aguantar, tolerar; *vi* pararse; **to** —— **up** levantarse, pararse; **Stand here, please**..Párese aquí, por favor...**Stand up**..
Levántese.
standard *adj* estándar; *n* norma, estándar *m*
standing *adj* de pie, parado
staphylococcus *n* estafilococo
Staphylococcus Staphylococcus
staple *n* (*surg*) grapa
starch *n* almidón *m*
stare *vi* fijar la vista; **Stare at that point on the wall**..Fije la vista en ese punto en la pared.
starvation *n* inanición *f*
starve *vi* morir de hambre
stasis *n* estasis *f*; **venous** —— estasis venosa

state *n* estado, condición *f*
station *n* estación *f*; **nursing** —— estación de enfermeras
statistic *n* estadística
status *n* status *m*, estado; —— **asthmaticus** status asthmaticus; —— **epilepticus** status epilepticus
staunch *See* **stanch**.
stay *vi* **to** —— **in bed** guardar cama
STD *abbr* **sexually transmitted disease**. *V.* **disease**.
steadiness *n* firmeza
steady *adj* (*comp* **-ier**; *super* **-iest**) (*pain*) constante; (*hands, gait*) firme; (*gaze*) fijo
steak *n* bistec *m*
steam *n* vapor *m*; *vt* (*cook*) cocer al vapor
steamed *adj* cocido al vapor
steel *n* acero; **stainless** —— acero inoxidable
stenosis *n* (*pl* **-ses**) estenosis *f*
stenotic *adj* estenótico
stent *n* férula (*para mantener permeable un conducto*)
step *n* paso; *vi* (*pret & pp* **stepped**; *ger* **stepping**) (*también* **to take a** ——) dar un paso
stepbrother *n* hermanastro
stepchild *n* (*pl* **-children**) hijastro -tra *mf*
stepdaughter *n* hijastra
stepfather *n* padrastro
stepmother *n* madrastra
stepsister *n* hermanastra
stepson *n* hijastro
sterile *adj* estéril
sterility *n* esterilidad *f*
sterilization *n* esterilización *f*
sterilize *vt* esterilizar
sternum *n* (*pl* **-na**) esternón *m*
steroid *adj & n* esteroide *m*
stethoscope *n* estetoscopio
stick *n* (*of a needle, cactus spine, etc.*) pinchazo, piquete *m* (*esp Mex*), picadura; **You are going to feel a stick**..Va a sentir un pinchazo..Va a sentir un piquete; *vt* (*pret & pp* **stuck**) pinchar(se), picar(se) (*esp Mex*); **How did you stick yourself?**.. ¿Cómo se pinchó? **to** —— **out one's tongue** sacar la lengua; **Stick out your**

tongue..Saque la lengua.

sticker *n* (*bot*) espina, cadillo

sticky *adj* (*comp* **-ier**; *super* **-iest**) pegajoso

sties *pl de* **sty**

stiff *adj* rígido, tieso; **Do your hands feel stiff in the morning?**..¿Siente sus manos rígidas en la mañana?

stiffness *n* rigidez *f*

stillbirth *n* nacimiento de un niño muerto

stillborn *adj* nacido muerto

stimulant *n* estimulante *m*

stimulate *vt* estimular

stimulating *adj* estimulante

stimulation *n* estimulación *f*

stimulus *n* (*pl* **-li**) estímulo

sting *n* piquete *m*, picadura; **Did you feel a sting?**..¿Sintió un piquete? **bee ——** picadura de abeja; *vt* (*pret & pp* **stung**) picar; *vi* arder; **The numbing medication will sting a little bit**..El anestésico le va a arder un poco.

stingray *n* raya

stink *vi* (*pret* **stank** *o* **stunk**; *pp* **stunk**) apestar

stirrup *n* estribo

stitch *n* punto (*de sutura*); (*pain in side*) dolor *m* de costado, punzada; *vt* (*también* **to —— up**) suturar (*form*), coser, poner puntos

stocking *n* media

stoic, stoical *adj* estoico

stoma *n* abertura artificial entre un órgano y el exterior del cuerpo, estoma *m* (*Ang*)

stomach *n* estómago; (*fam*) abdomen *m*; **pit of the ——** boca del estómago; **to be sick to one's ——** (*fam*) tener náusea(s)

stomachache *n* dolor *m* de estómago

stomatitis *n* estomatitis *f*

stone *n* cálculo (*form*), piedra; **kidney ——** cálculo renal (*form*), piedra del riñón

stood *pret & pp de* **stand**

stool *n* excremento, popó *or* pupú *m* (*fam*), caca (*esp Carib, fam*)

stoop *vi* doblarse (*hacia adelante*), agacharse

stooped *adj* encorvado

stop *vi* (*a habit, etc.*) dejar de; **You should stop smoking**..Debería dejar de fumar; **to —— up** obstruir, tapar; **My nose is**

stopped up..Tengo la nariz tapada.

stopper *n* tapón *m*

store *n* reserva, depósito; *vt* almacenar

strabismus *n* estrabismo

straight *adj* derecho, recto

straighten *vt* (*teeth, etc.*) enderezar; (*one's leg, arm*) estirar, extender, poner derecho; **Straighten your leg**..Estire la pierna; *vi* enderezarse

strain *n* tensión *f*; (*of bacteria, etc.*) cepa; (*muscle, ligament, etc.*) dolor debido a uso excesivo o incorrecto; *vt* (*a muscle or ligament*) lastimar(se) por uso excesivo o incorrecto; (*one's eyes, one's voice*) forzar (*la vista, la voz*); (*urine for stones*) filtrar, colar (*la orina para buscar piedras*); *vi* (*at stool*) pujar

strainer *n* colador *m*

straitjacket *n* camisa de fuerza

strangle *vt, vi* estrangular(se)

strangulate *vt* estrangular

strangulation *n* estrangulación *f*

strap *n* correa, tira

strawberry *n* fresa

streak *n* raya, línea

stream *n* (*of urine*) chorro

strength *n* fuerza, potencia; **double ——** fuerza doble; **extra ——** fuerza extra

strengthen *vt* fortalecer, reforzar

strenuous *adj* fuerte, vigoroso; **You should avoid strenuous activity for one week**.. Debe evitar actividades fuertes por una semana.

streptococcus *n* estreptococo

Streptococcus Streptococcus

streptokinase *n* estreptoquinasa

streptomycin *n* estreptomicina

stress *n* tensión *f*, estrés *m*; **under ——** bajo tensión, presionado

stressed *adj* bajo tensión, presionado

stretch *vt, vi* estirar(se)

stretcher *n* camilla

stretch mark *n* estría

strict *adj* estricto

stricture *n* estenosis *f* (*form*), estrechez *f*

strike *vt* golpear, pegar; **The board struck me here**..La tabla me golpeó aquí.

strip *V.* **test strip.**

stroke n (*blow*) golpe m; (*cerebrovascular event*) derrame m cerebral, embolia
strong adj fuerte, potente
Strongyloides Strongyloides
strongyloidiasis n estrongiloidiasis f
strychnine n estricnina
stub vt (*pret & pp* **stubbed;** *ger* **stubbing**) **to ——— one's foot against** tropezar con
stuck *pret & pp de* **stick**
student n estudiante mf
study n (*pl* **-dies**) estudio; **double-blind ———** estudio doble ciego
stuffy, stuffed up adj tapado; **I have a stuffy nose**..Tengo la nariz tapada.
stumble vi tropezar, dar un traspié
stump n (*anat*) muñón m
stun vt (*pret & pp* **stunned;** *ger* **stunning**) atarantar, aturdir; **to become stunned** atarantarse, aturdirse
stung *pret & pp de* **sting**
stupor n estupor m
stutter vi tartamudear
sty, stye n (*pl* **sties, styes**) orzuelo, perrilla (*Mex, fam*)
subacute adj subagudo
subarachnoid adj subaracnoideo
subclavian adj subclavio
subclinical adj subclínico
subconscious adj subconsciente; n subconsciencia
subconsciousness n subconsciencia
subcutaneous adj subcutáneo
subdural adj subdural
sublimation n (*psych*) sublimación f
sublingual adj sublingual
subluxation n subluxación f
subspecialty n subespecialidad f
substance n substancia
substitute n substituto; vt substituir; **You can substitute tortillas for bread**..Puede substituir el pan por las tortillas (*Note that the two objects* tortillas *and* bread *are inverted when translating to Spanish. Observe que los dos objetos* pan y tortillas *se invierten al traducir al inglés.*)
subtract vt, vi (*arith*) restar, quitar; **Subtract seven from one hundred**..Réstele siete a cien.

suck vt chupar, (*at mother's breast*) mamar; **to ——— one's thumb** chuparse el dedo
suckle vt amamantar; vi mamar
sucralfate n sucralfato
suction n succión f
sudden adj repentino, súbito
suddenly adv de repente
sue vt, vi demandar
suffer vt, vi sufrir, padecer; **to ——— from** padecer de
suffering n sufrimiento
sufficient adj suficiente
suffocate vt, vi sofocar(se), asfixiar(se), ahogar(se)
suffocation n sofocación f, asfixia
sugar n azúcar m&f
sugar-coated adj con capa de azucar
sugarless adj sin azúcar
suicidal adj (*act, idea, etc.*) suicida, (*person*) con tendencias suicidas
suicide n suicidio; **——— attempt** intento de suicidio; **——— gesture** intento de suicidio sin mucha posibilidad de lograrlo; **to commit ———** suicidarse
suit n demanda (*legal*)
sulfacetamide n sulfacetamida
sulfadiazine n sulfadiacina
sulfa drug n medicamento a base de sulfas
sulfamethoxazole n sulfametoxazol m
sulfasalazine n salazosulfapiridina
sulfate n sulfato
sulfisoxazole n sulfisoxazol m
sulfite n sulfito
sulfonamide n sulfonamida
sulfur n azufre m; **——— dioxide** bióxido *or* dióxido de azufre
sulindac n sulindaco
sumatriptan n sumatriptan m
summer n verano
sun n sol m; **to get ——— asolearse,** tomar el sol; **the sun's rays** los rayos del sol, los rayos solares
sunburn n quemadura de sol; vi (*también* **to get sunburned** *o* **sunburnt**) quemarse por el sol; **Do you sunburn easily?**..¿Se quema fácilmente por el sol?
sunglasses npl lentes mpl para el sol, lentes *or* anteojos oscuros, gafas de sol

sunlamp *n* lámpara solar *or* bronceadora
sunlight *n* luz *f* del sol
sunscreen *n* filtro *or* protector *m* solar
sunstroke *n* insolación *f*
suntan *n* bronceado; **to get a** —— broncearse
superego *n* (*pl* **-gos**) (*psych*) superego
superficial *adj* superficial
superior *adj* (*anat*) superior
supine *adj* supino, acostado boca arriba
supper *n* cena
supple *adj* flexible
supplement *n* suplemento
supplementary, supplemental *adj* suplementario
supply *n* surtido, suministro; *vt* (*pret & pp* **-plied**) suministrar, proporcionar
support *n* apoyo; (*physical*) soporte *m*; —— **group** grupo de apoyo, amigos y familiares que apoyan a uno; **arch** —— soporte para el arco del pie; *vt* apoyar
suppository *n* (*pl* **-ries**) supositorio
suppress *vt* suprimir
suppressant *n* supresor *m*; **appetite** —— supresor del apetito
suppression *n* supresión *f*
sure *adj* seguro, cierto; **We have to make sure you don't have tuberculosis**..Tenemos que estar seguros que no tiene tuberculosis.
surface *n* superficie *f*
surfactant *n* surfactante *m*
surgeon *n* cirujano -na *mf*
surgery *n* (*pl* **-ries**) cirugía; **cosmetic** —— cirugía cosmética *or* estética; **elective** —— cirugía electiva; **general** —— cirugía general; **major** —— cirugía mayor; **minor** —— cirugía menor; **open heart** —— cirugía de corazón abierto; **oral** —— cirugía oral; **orthopedic** —— cirugía ortopédica; **plastic** —— cirugía plástica; **radical** —— cirugía radical; **reconstructive** —— cirugía reconstructiva
surgical *adj* quirúrgico
surrogate mother *n* madre subrogada
survival *n* supervivencia
survive *vt, vi* sobrevivir
survivor *n* sobreviviente *mf*, superviviente *mf*
susceptibility *n* susceptibilidad *f*
susceptible *adj* susceptible, sensible
suspend *vt* suspender
suspenders *npl* tirantes *mpl*
suspension *n* suspensión *f*
sustained-release *adj* (*pharm*) de liberación sostenida
suture *n* sutura; *vt* suturar, coser (*fam*)
swab *n* hisopo, aplicador *m*
swaddle *vt* envolver con ropa apretadita
swallow *vt* tragar, pasar (*esp Mex*); *vi* tragar, tragar saliva, pasar saliva; **Swallow, please**..Trague, por favor..Trague saliva, por favor..Pase saliva, por favor.
swam *pret de* **swim**
swathe *vt* (*to swaddle*) envolver con ropa apretadita; (*to bandage*) vendar
sweat *n* sudor *m*; *vi* (*pret & pp* **sweat** *o* **sweated**) sudar
sweater *n* suéter *m*
sweaty *adj* sudoroso
sweet *adj* dulce; *n* **sweets** dulces *mpl*
sweetener *n* dulcificante *m*
swell *vi* (*pret* **swelled**; *pp* **swelled** *o* **swollen**) hincharse; **Do your feet swell?**..¿Se le hinchan los pies?
swelling *n* hinchazón *f*
swim *vi* (*pret* **swam**; *pp* **swum**; *ger* **swimming**) nadar
swimmer's itch *n* dermatitis *f* de los bañistas, anquilostomiasis *f* (*form*)
swimming *n* natación *f*
swollen (*pp de* **swell**) *adj* hinchado
swum *pp de* **swim**
symmetrical, symmetric *adj* simétrico
symmetry *n* simetría
sympathectomy *n* simpatectomía
sympathetic *adj* compasivo, comprensivo; (*neuro*) simpático; —— **nervous system** sistema nervioso simpático
sympathy *n* compasión *f*
symphysis *n* (*pl* **-ses**) sínfisis *f*
symptom *n* síntoma *m*
synapse *n* sinapsis *f*
synchronize *vt* sincronizar
syncope *n* síncope *m*
syndrome *n* síndrome *m*; **acquired immune**

deficiency —— (AIDS) síndrome de inmunodeficiencia adquirida (SIDA); **adult respiratory distress** —— (ARDS) síndrome de insuficiencia respiratoria del adulto; **Asherman's** —— síndrome de Asherman; **attention deficit** —— síndrome del niño hiperactivo; **battered child** —— síndrome del niño maltratado; **carcinoid** —— síndrome carcinoide; **carpal tunnel** —— síndrome del túnel carpiano; **Cushing's** —— síndrome de Cushing; **DiGeorge** —— síndrome de DiGeorge; **Down's** —— síndrome de Down; **Ehlers-Danlos** —— síndrome de Ehlers-Danlos; **Felty's** —— síndrome de Felty; **fetal alcohol** —— síndrome alcohólico fetal; **Gilbert's** —— enfermedad *f* de Gilbert; **Gilles de la Tourette** —— síndrome de Gilles de la Tourette; **Guillain-Barré** —— síndrome de Guillain-Barré; **hemolytic-uremic** —— síndrome hemolítico-urémico; **hepatorenal** —— síndrome hepatorrenal; **irritable bowel** —— síndrome del intestino irritable; **Kawasaki's** —— síndrome de Kawasaki; **Klinefelter's** —— síndrome de Klinefelter; **Korsakoff's** —— síndrome de Korsakoff; **malabsorption** —— síndrome de malabsorción; **Mallory-Weiss** —— síndrome de Mallory-Weiss; **Marfan's** —— síndrome de Marfan; **Ménière's** —— síndrome de Ménière; **nephrotic** —— síndrome nefrótico; **organic brain** —— síndrome cerebral orgánico; **Osler-Rendu-Weber** —— síndrome de Osler-Rendu-Weber; **Peutz-Jeghers** —— síndrome de Peutz-Jeghers; **Pickwickian** —— síndrome de Pickwick; **postconcussional** —— síndrome de cefalea postraumática; **premenstrual** —— síndrome premenstrual; **Reiter's** —— síndrome de Reiter; **restless legs** —— síndrome de piernas inquietas; **Reye's** —— síndrome de Reye; **Sheehan's** —— síndrome de Sheehan; **sick sinus** —— síndrome del seno enfermo; **Sjögren's** —— síndrome de Sjögren; **staphylococcal scalded skin** —— síndrome estafilocócico de piel escaldada; **Stevens-Johnson** —— síndrome de Stevens-Johnson; **sudden infant death** —— (SIDS) síndrome de muerte súbita infantil; **toxic shock** —— síndrome del choque tóxico; **Turner's** —— síndrome de Turner; **von Willebrand's** —— enfermedad *f* de von Willebrand

synergy *n* sinergia
synovial *adj* sinovial
synovitis *n* sinovitis *f*
synthesize *vt* sintetizar
synthetic *adj* sintético
syphilis *n* sífilis *f*
syphilitic *adj* sifilítico
syringe *n* jeringa, jeringuilla (*esp Carib*); **bulb** —— perilla, pera
syringomyelia *n* siringomielia
syrup *n* jarabe *m*; **cough** —— jarabe para la tos
system *n* sistema *m*; **autonomic nervous** —— sistema nervioso autónomo; **cardiovascular** —— sistema cardiovascular; **central nervous** —— (CNS) sistema nervioso central (SNC); **digestive** —— sistema digestivo; **endocrine** —— sistema endocrino; **immune** —— sistema inmunitario; **musculoskeletal** —— sistema musculoesquelético; **parasympathetic nervous** —— sistema nervioso parasimpático; **peripheral nervous** —— sistema nervioso periférico; **reproductive** —— sistema reproductor; **respiratory** —— sistema respiratorio; **skeletal** —— sistema esquelético; **sympathetic nervous** —— sistema nervioso simpático
systemic *adj* sistémico
systolic *adj* sistólico

tab   85   tem

T

table *n* mesa; **examining** —— mesa de exploración (*form*), mesa de exámenes; **operating** —— mesa de operaciones, mesa de cirugía

tablespoonful *n* cucharada, cucharada grande

tablet *n* tableta

taboo *n* (*pl* **taboos**) tabú *m*

tachycardia *n* taquicardia

taenia, tenia *n* tenia

tailbone *n* (*fam*) cóccix *m* (*form*), colita

take *vt* (*pret* **took**; *pp* **taken**) tomar; **to** —— **off** (*clothing, etc.*) quitarse; **Take off your shirt**..Quítese la camisa; **to** —— **out** extraer (*form*), sacar; **We have to take out your appendix**..Tenemos que sacarle el apéndice.

talc *n* talco

talcum powder *n* talco, polvos de talco

tall *adj* alto; **How tall are you?**..¿Qué altura tiene?

tamoxifen *n* tamoxifén *m*

tampon *n* tampón *m*

tamponade *n* taponamiento; **cardiac** —— taponamiento cardiaco

tan *adj & n* bronceado; *vi* (*pret & pp* **tanned**; *ger* **tanning**) (*también* **to get a** ——) broncearse

tannin *n* tanino

tantrum *n* berrinche *m*

tap *n* (*procedure to extract fluid*) punción *f*; **spinal** —— punción lumbar; *vt* (*pret & pp* **tapped**; *ger* **tapping**) puncionar (*form*), hacer una punción

tape *n* (*for dressings*) tela, cinta; —— **measure** *o* **measuring** —— cinta métrica

tapeworm *n* tenia, solitaria

tar *n* alquitrán *m*

tarantula *n* tarántula

tardive dyskinesia *n* discinesia tardía

tarsal *adj* tarsal

tartar *n* tártaro (*form*), sarro (*dental*)

tartaric acid *n* ácido tartárico

taste *n* sabor *m*, gusto; —— **bud** papila gustativa; *vt* (*to try*) probar; **Taste it**..Pruébelo...**Can you taste all right?**..¿Distingue bien los sabores? *vi* saber; **This medicine doesn't taste bad**..Esta medicina no sabe mal; **to** —— **like** saber a

tattoo *n* (*pl* **-toos**) tatuaje *m*

taught *pret & pp de* **teach**

tea *n* té *m*

teach *vt* (*pret & pp* **taught**) enseñar

teacher *n* maestro -tra *mf*

team *n* (*of health workers, etc.*) equipo

tear *n* (*muscle, ligament, etc.*) desgarro, desgarre *m*, desgarramiento; *vt, vi* (*pret* **tore**; *pp* **torn**) desgarrar(se)

tear *n* (*from crying*) lágrima

teaspoonful *n* (*pl* **-fuls**) cucharadita, cucharada chica

technician *n* técnico -ca *mf*

technique *n* técnica, método

technology *n* tecnología

teenager *n* joven *mf* de 13 a 19 años

teeth *pl de* **tooth**

teethe *vi* salirle los dientes; **Is he teething yet?**..¿Le están saliendo los dientes ya?

teething *n* dentición *f* (*form*), salida de los dientes

telangiectasia *n* telangiectasia

telemetry *n* telemetría

telephone *n* teléfono; **to call by** —— llamar por teléfono, telefonear

temperament *n* temperamento

temperature *n* temperatura; (*fam*) fiebre;

Did you take your temperature at home?..¿Se tomó la temperatura en la casa? **room** —— temperatura ambiente

temple n (*anat*) sien f

temporal *adj* temporal

temporary *adj* temporal, transitorio; **This bandage is only temporary**..Este vendaje es solo temporal.

temporomandibular *adj* temporomandibular

tendency n (*pl* -**cies**) tendencia

tender *adj* (*sore, painful*) adolorido *or* dolorido, doloroso

tenderness n dolor m (*al tocar*)

tendinitis n tendonitis f

tendon n tendón m; **Achilles** —— tendón de Aquiles

tendonitis *See* **tendinitis**.

tennis n tenis m

tennis elbow n codo de tenista

tenosynovitis n tenosinovitis f

tense *adj* tenso; *vt* (*one's muscles*) poner tenso (*los músculos*); *vi* **to** —— **up** ponerse tenso; **Try not to tense up**..Trate de no ponerse tenso.

tension n tensión f; **nervous** —— tensión nerviosa

tent n tienda; **oxygen** —— tienda de oxígeno

tepid *adj* tibio

teratoma n teratoma m

terazosin n terazosina

terbutaline n terbutalina

terfenadine n terfenadina

term n término; **at** —— a término

terminal *adj* terminal

tertiary *adj* del tercer nivel

test n prueba, examen m; **blood** —— prueba de sangre; **exercise stress** —— prueba de esfuerzo; **eye** —— examen de la vista; **glucose tolerance** —— prueba de tolerancia a la glucosa; **hearing** —— prueba de la audición; **patch** —— prueba del parche; **pregnancy** —— prueba de embarazo; **pulmonary function** —— prueba de función pulmonar; **skin** —— prueba cutánea; **TB** —— prueba de la tuberculosis; **urine** —— prueba de la orina; *vt* examinar, probar

testicle n testículo, huevo (*vulg, usually pl*), bola (*vulg, usually pl*); **undescended** —— testículo no descendido

testosterone n testosterona

test strip n tira reactiva

test tube n tubo de ensayo

tetanus n tétanos m

tetracycline n tetraciclina

tetrahydrocannabinol (THC) n tetrahidrocanabinol m

tetralogy of Fallot n tetralogía de Fallot

texture n textura

thalamus n tálamo

thalassemia n talasemia, talasanemia

thallium n talio

THC *V*. **tetrahydrocannabinol**.

theophylline n teofilina

theory n (*pl* -**ries**) teoría

therapeutic *adj* terapéutico

therapist n terapista mf, terapeuta mf (*form*); (*fam*) psicoterapista mf

therapy n (*pl* -**pies**) terapia, terapéutica (*form*); **electroconvulsive** —— **(ECT)** terapia electrochoque *or* electroconvulsiva (TEC); **group** —— terapia de grupo; **occupational** —— terapia ocupacional; **physical** —— terapia física; **radiation** —— radioterapia; **respiratory** —— terapia respiratoria; **speech** —— terapia del habla

thermal *adj* termal

thermometer n termómetro; **oral** —— termómetro bucal *or* oral; **rectal** —— termómetro rectal

thiabendazole n tiabendazol m

thiamine n tiamina

thick *adj* (*dimension*) grueso; (*consistency*) espeso

thickness n (*dimension*) espesor m, grosor m; (*consistency*) espesura, espesor m, viscosidad f

thigh n muslo

thin *adj* (*comp* **thinner**; *super* **thinnest**) delgado, flaco; (*hair*) ralo, escaso; **to become** —— enflaquecerse

think *vt*, *vi* (*pret* & *pp* **thought**) pensar

thinner n tíner m; **blood** —— (*fam*) anticoagulante m

thioridazine *n* tioridacina
thirst *n* sed *f*
thirsty *adj* **to be** —— tener sed
thistle *n* cardo
thoracic *adj* torácico
thoracotomy *n* (*pl* **-mies**) toracotomía
thorax *n* tórax *m*
thorn *n* espina
thought (*pret & pp de* **think**) *n* pensamiento
three-day measles *n* sarampión *m* alemán, rubeola *or* rubéola (*form*)
threonine *n* treonina
threshold *n* umbral *m*
threw *pret de* **throw**
throat *n* garganta; **sore** —— dolor *m* de garganta
throb *vi* (*pret & pp* **throbbed**; *ger* **throbbing**) latir, pulsar; **Is your head throbbing?**..¿Le late la cabeza?..¿Le pulsa la cabeza?
throbbing (*ger de* **throb**) *adj* pulsante, pulsátil, que late
thrombectomy *n* (*pl* **-mies**) trombectomía
thrombocytopenia *n* trombocitopenia
thrombocytosis *n* trombocitosis *f*
thromboembolism *n* (*pl* **-li**) tromboembolia
thrombolytic *adj & n* trombolítico
thrombophlebitis *n* tromboflebitis *f*
thrombosis *n* (*pl* **-ses**) trombosis *f*
thrombus *n* (*pl* **-bi**) trombo
throw *vt, vi* (*pret* **threw**; *pp* **thrown**) **to** —— **up** arrojar, devolver, deponer (*Mex*), tener basca, vomitar
thrush *n* algodoncillo, sapo (*PR, SD*), infección en la boca producida por hongos
thumb *n* pulgar *m*, dedo gordo
thumbnail *n* uña del pulgar
thump *n* **precordial** —— golpe precordial *or* torácico
thymectomy *n* (*pl* **-mies**) timectomía
thymoma *n* timoma *m*
thymus *n* (*pl* **-muses** *o* **-mi**) timo
thyroglobulin *n* tiroglobulina
thyroid *adj* tiroideo; —— **storm** crisis tiroidea; *n* (*gland*) tiroides *m&f*
thyroidectomy *n* (*pl* **-mies**) tiroidectomía
thyroiditis *n* tiroiditis *f*; **Hashimoto's** —— tiroiditis de Hashimoto; **subacute** ——

tiroiditis subaguda
thyrotoxic *adj* tirotóxico
thyrotoxicosis *n* tirotoxicosis *f*
thyrotropin (TSH) *n* tirotropina
thyroxine *n* tiroxina
tibia *n* tibia
tic *n* tic *m*; —— **douloureux** tic doloroso
tick *n* garrapata
tickle *n* cosquilleo; *vt* causar cosquillas, dar *or* hacer cosquillas; **Am I tickling you?**.. ¿Le causo cosquillas?
tickling *n* cosquillas, cosquilleo
ticklish *adj* cosquilloso
tight *adj* apretado
time *n* tiempo, vez *f*; (*by the clock*) hora; **all the time** todo el tiempo; **a long** —— mucho tiempo; **a short** —— un rato, poco tiempo; **at times** a veces; **each** —— *o* **every** —— cada vez; **four times a day** cuatro veces al día; **from** —— **to** —— de vez en cuando; **in** —— (*eventually*) con el tiempo; **one** —— una vez; **next** —— la próxima vez; **partial thromboplastin** —— **(PTT)** tiempo parcial de tromboplastina; **prothrombin** —— **(PT)** tiempo de protrombina; **the first** —— la primera vez; **the last** —— la última vez
timed release *n* (*pharm*) difusión regulada
timid *adj* tímido
timolol *n* timolol *m*
tincture *n* tintura
tinea *n* tiña *or* tinea; —— **capitis** tiña de la cabeza; —— **corporis** tiña del cuerpo; —— **cruris** tiña inguinal; —— **pedis** tiña del pie; —— **versicolor** tiña versicolor
tingle *vi* hormiguear
tingling *n* hormigueo
tip *n* (*tongue, finger, etc.*) punta
tiptoe *n* **to walk on tiptoes** caminar de puntillas
tire *vt, vi* (*también* **to** —— **out**) cansar(se); **Just walking to the bathroom tires him out**..Con solo caminar al baño se cansa.
tired *adj* (*también* —— **out**) cansado; **to get** —— cansarse
tiredness *n* cansancio, fatiga
tireless *adj* incansable, infatigable
tiring *adj* fatigoso

tirosine *n* tirosina

tissue *n* tejido; (*for blowing one's nose*) pañuelo de papel; **connective** —— tejido conectivo *or* conjuntivo; **granulation** —— tejido de granulación; **soft** —— tejido blando

tissue plasminogen activator (tPA) *n* activador *m* del plasminógeno tisular

titer *n* título

toast *n* pan tostado

tobacco *n* (*pl* **-cos** *o* **-coes**) tabaco; —— **use** tabaquismo

tocopherol *n* tocoferol *m*

today *adv* hoy

toe *n* dedo (*del pie*); **big** —— dedo gordo (del pie); **little** —— dedo chico (del pie)

toenail *n* uña (*de un dedo del pie*)

toilet *n* inodoro, excusado; —— **bowl** taza del inodoro *or* excusado; —— **paper** papel sanitario *or* higiénico; —— **training** (*ped*) (el) enseñar a usar el baño

tolbutamide *n* tolbutamida

tolerance *n* tolerancia

tolerant *adj* tolerante

tolerate *vt* tolerar, aguantar

toluene *n* tolueno

tomato *n* (*pl* **-toes**) tomate *m*

tomogram *n* tomograma *m*, tomografía

tomography *n* tomografía; **computed** —— **(CT)** tomografía computada (TC); **computerized axial** —— **(CAT)** tomografía axial computarizada (TAC); **positron emission** —— **(PET)** tomografía por emisión de positrones (TEP)

tomorrow *adv* mañana

tone *n* tono; **muscle** —— tono muscular; *vt* tonificar

tongue *n* lengua; —— **depressor** *o* **blade** bajalenguas *m*, depresor *m*, abatelenguas *m* (*Mex*), paleta (*fam*)

tonic *adj* & *n* tónico

toning *adj* tonificador

tonsil *n* amígdala

tonsillectomy *n* (*pl* **-mies**) amigdalectomía

tonsillitis *n* amigdalitis *f*

took *pret de* **take**

tooth *n* (*pl* **teeth**) diente *m*, muela; **baby** —— diente de leche; **back** —— muela;

canine —— diente canino, colmillo (*fam*); **false teeth** dientes postizos, dentaduras postizas; **front** —— diente, diente incisivo (*form*); **set of teeth** dentadura; **wisdom** —— muela del juicio

toothache *n* dolor *m* de muelas, (*front tooth*) dolor de dientes

toothbrush *n* cepillo de dientes

toothpaste *n* pasta dental

tophus *n* (*pl* **-phi**) tofo

topical *adj* tópico

tore *pret de* **tear**

torn *pp de* **tear**

torsion *n* torsión *f*; **ovarian** —— torsión ovárica; **testicular** —— torsión testicular

torso *n* torso

torticollis *n* tortícolis *or* torticolis *f*

torture *n* tortura; *vt* torturar

torus *n* torus *m*; —— **palatinus** torus palatino

total *adj* & *n* total *m*

touch *n* (*sense*) tacto; (*fam, light case*) caso leve; **a touch of flu**..un caso leve de gripe; *vt* tocar

tough *adj* duro, correoso

tourniquet *n* torniquete *m*

towel *n* toalla

toxemia *n* toxemia

toxemic *adj* toxémico

toxic *adj* tóxico; —— **epidermal necrolysis** necrólisis tóxica epidérmica

toxicity *n* toxicidad *f*

toxicologist *n* toxicólogo -ga *mf*

toxicology *n* toxicología

toxin *n* toxina

toxocariasis *n* toxocariasis *f*

toxoid *n* toxoide *m*; **diphtheria** —— toxoide diftérico; **tetanus** —— toxoide tetánico

toxoplasmosis *n* toxoplasmosis *f*

tPA *V.* **tissue plasminogen activator**.

TPN *abbr* **total parenteral nutrition**. *V.* **nutrition**.

trace *n* trazas; **There is a trace of protein in your urine**..Hay trazas de proteína en su orina.

trachea *n* (*pl* **-cheae**) tráquea

tracheitis *n* traqueítis *f*

tracheobronchitis *n* traqueobronquitis *f*

tracheostomy *n* (*pl* -**mies**) traqueostomía
tracheotomy *n* (*pl* -**mies**) traqueotomía
trachoma *n* tracoma *m*
tracing *n* (*EKG, etc.*) trazo, registro
tracks *npl* (*from drug addiction*) marcas
tract *n* tracto, vía, fascículo, haz *m*; **biliary**
—— vías biliares; **corticospinal** —— vía
corticospinal; **gastrointestinal** —— tubo
digestivo; **pyramidal** —— vía piramidal;
respiratory —— tracto respiratorio;
spinothalamic —— vía espinotalámica;
urinary —— tracto urinario
traction *n* tracción *f*
train *vt, vi* entrenar(se)
training *n* entrenamiento
trait *n* característica
trance *n* trance *m*
tranquilize *vt* tranquilizar
tranquilizer *n* tranquilizante *m*
transcutaneous *adj* transcutáneo
transfer *vt* (*a patient*) trasladar
transference *n* (*psych*) transferencia
transferrin *n* transferrina
transfuse *vt* transfundir (*form*), hacer una
transfusión, poner sangre (*fam*)
transfusion *n* transfusión *f*; **to give a** ——
hacer una transfusión, poner sangre (*fam*);
I need to give you a transfusion..Tengo
que hacerle una transfusión..Tengo que
ponerle sangre...**Have you ever had a**
transfusion before?..¿Le han hecho una
transfusión alguna vez antes?..¿Le han
puesto sangre alguna vez antes?
transient *adj* transitorio, pasajero
transition *n* transición *f*
transitional *adj* transicional
translate *vt* traducir
translocation *n* translocación *f*
transmission *n* transmisión *f*
transmit *vt* (*pret & pp* -**mitted**; *ger*
-**mitting**) transmitir
transparent *adj* transparente
transplant *n* trasplante *m*; *vt* trasplantar
transport *n* transporte *m*; *vt* transportar
transsexual *adj & n* transexual *mf*
transurethral *adj* transuretral; —— **resec-**
tion of the prostate (TURP) resección *f*
transuretral de la próstata

transvestite *n* transvestista *mf*
trapezius *n* trapecio
trauma *n* traumatismo, trauma *m*; (*psych*)
trauma
traumatic *adj* traumático
traumatize *vt* traumatizar
tray *n* bandeja, charola (*Mex*)
trazodone *n* trazodona
treat *vt* (*illness, patient*) tratar
treatment *n* tratamiento
tremble *vi* temblar
tremor *n* temblor *m*; **familial** —— temblor
familiar
tremulous *adj* tembloroso
trench mouth *n* angina *or* enfermedad *f* de
Vincent
trend *n* tendencia
treponeme *n* treponema
tretinoin *n* tretinoína
triage *n* evaluación *f* inicial de pacientes de
emergencia para establecer prioridades
trial *n* ensayo, prueba
triamcinolone *n* triamcinolona
triamterene *n* triamtereno
triazolam *n* triazolam *m*
triceps *n* tríceps *m*
trichinosis *n* triquinosis *f*
Trichomonas Trichomonas
trichomoniasis *n* tricomoniasis *f*
tricuspid *adj* tricúspide
tried *pret de* **try**
tries *pl de* **try**
trifluoperazine *n* trifluoperacina
trigeminal *adj* trigémino; —— **neuralgia**
neuralgia del trigémino
trigger *vt* provocar
trigger finger *n* dedo de gatillo
trigger point *n* punto doloroso
triglyceride *n* triglicérido
trimester *n* trimestre *m*
trimethoprim *n* trimetoprim *m*
trip *vi* tropezar, dar un traspié
triplet *n* trillizo -za *mf*
trismus *n* trismo
trisomy *n* trisomía; —— **21** trisomía 21
trivalent *adj* trivalente
trochanter *n* trocánter *m*
troche *n* trocisco, pastilla para chupar

tropical *adj* tropical

trouble *n* molestia; **Do you have trouble with your back?**..¿Tiene molestias con su espalda?

trousers *npl* pantalón *m* (*frec pl*)

trunk *n* (*anat*) tronco

truss *n* faja abdominal

trust *n* confianza; *vt* tener confianza en, confiar en

trypanosomiasis *n* tripanosomiasis *f*

trypsin *n* tripsina

tryptophan *n* triptófano

TSH *abbr* **thyroid-stimulating hormone.** *V.* **hormone.**

TTP *abbr* **thrombotic thrombocytopenic purpura.** *V.* **purpura.**

tube *n* tubo, sonda, manguera, trompa, conducto; **auditory** —— conducto auditivo; **drainage** —— tubo de drenaje; **endotracheal** —— tubo endotraqueal; **Eustachian** —— trompa de Eustaquio; **fallopian** —— trompa de Falopio; **feeding** —— sonda para alimentación; **nasogastric** —— sonda nasogástrica; **ventilating** —— tubo de ventilación

tuberculosis *n* tuberculosis *f*

tuberous sclerosis *n* esclerosis tuberosa

tubing *n* tubería

tubular *adj* tubular

tubule *n* túbulo

tularemia *n* tularemia

tummy *n* (*ped*) estomaguito, barriguita

tumor *n* tumor *m*; **benign** —— tumor benigno; **Ewing's** —— tumor de Ewing; **malignant** —— tumor maligno; **Wilms'** —— tumor de Wilms

tuna *n* atún *m*

tuning fork *n* diapasón *m*

tunnel *n* túnel *m*

turbid *adj* turbio

turkey *n* pavo

turn *n* vuelta; *vi* darse vuelta; **to** —— **around** darse media vuelta; **to** —— **blue, stiff, numb, etc.** ponerse azul, tieso, dormido, etc.; **Did he turn blue?**..¿Se puso azul? **to** —— **out** resultar, salir; **The tests turned out negative**..Las pruebas resultaron negativas; **to** —— **over** voltearse, darse vuelta; **Turn over faceup**.. Voltéese boca arriba.

TURP *abbr* **transurethral resection of the prostate.** *V.* **transurethral.**

turpentine *n* trementina

tweezers *npl* pinzas

twin *adj* & *n* gemelo -la *mf*, mellizo -za *mf*; **conjoined twins** gemelos siameses; **fraternal twins** gemelos fraternos, gemelos que no se parecen; **identical twins** gemelos idénticos; **Siamese twins** (*ant*) gemelos siameses

twinge *n* punzada, dolor agudo y repentino

twist *vt*, *vi* (*one's ankle, etc.*) torcer(se); **Did you twist your neck?**..¿Se le torció el cuello?

twitch *n* contracción espasmódica, sacudida repentina; *vi* contraer espasmódicamente

tympanectomy *n* (*pl* **-mies**) timpanectomía

tympanic *adj* timpánico; —— **membrane** membrana timpánica

tympanoplasty *n* (*pl* **-ties**) timpanoplastia

type *n* tipo; **blood** —— grupo sanguíneo (*form*), tipo de sangre

typhus *n* tifus *m*, tifo

typical *adj* típico

tyramine *n* tiramina

tyrosine *n* tirosina

U

ugly *adj* feo

ulcer *n* úlcera, llaga; **decubitus** —— úlcera de decúbito; **duodenal** —— úlcera duodenal; **gastric** —— úlcera gástrica; **stress** —— úlcera de estrés

ulcerated *adj* ulcerado

ulceration *n* ulceración *f*

ulna *n* cúbito

ulnar *adj* cubital

ultrasonography *n* ultrasonografía

ultrasound *n* ultrasonido

ultraviolet *adj* ultravioleta

umbilical cord *n* cordón *m* umbilical

umbilicus *n* (*pl* **-ci**) ombligo

unable *adj* incapaz

unavoidable *adj* inevitable

unbearable *adj* insoportable, intolerable

unbreakable *adj* irrompible

unbuckle *vt* desabrochar(se), desabotonar(se)

unbutton *vt* desabrochar(se), desabotonar(se); **Unbutton your shirt**..Desabróchese la camisa.

uncle *n* tío

uncomfortable *adj* incómodo

uncommon *adj* poco común

unconscious *adj* inconsciente

underachiever *n* persona que no logra su potencial

undercooked *adj* insuficientemente cocinado

underdeveloped *adj* insuficientemente desarrollado

undernourished *adj* desnutrido, mal alimentado

undernourishment *n* desnutrición *f*, subalimentación *f*

underpants *npl* (*men's*) calzoncillos; (*women's*) calzón *m* (*frec pl*), pantaletas (*Mex*), bloomer *m* (*esp CA*), panties *mpl* (*esp Carib*)

undershirt *n* camiseta

underwear *n* ropa interior

undesirable *adj* indeseable

undifferentiated *adj* indiferenciado

uneasy *adj* (*comp* **-ier**; *super* **-iest**) inquieto

unexpected *adj* inesperado

unfriendly *adj* poco amistoso, hostil

unhappy *adj* infeliz

uniform *adj* uniforme; *n* uniforme *m*

union *n* unión *f*

unit *n* unidad *f*; **coronary care** —— unidad de cuidado coronario; **intensive care** —— **(ICU)** unidad de cuidados intensivos (UCI), unidad de terapia intensiva; **international** —— unidad internacional

unite *vt, vi* unir(se)

unmarried *adj* soltero

Unna's paste boot *n* bota de pasta de Unna

unpleasant *adj* desagradable

unresponsive *adj* que no responde

unsaturated *adj* no saturado, insaturado

unstable *adj* inestable

untiring *adj* incansable, infatigable

unusual *adj* raro, extraño

upper *adj* (*anat*) superior, de arriba

upset *adj* alterado, trastornado, agitado; (*stomach*) revuelto; **I have an upset stomach**..Tengo revuelto el estómago; **to become** —— alterarse, trastornarse, agitarse; *vt* (*pret & pp* **upset**; *ger* **upsetting**) alterar, trastornar, agitar

uptake *n* captación *f*

upward *adv* hacia arriba

urban *adj* urbano

urea *n* urea

uremia *n* uremia

uremic *adj* urémico

ureter *n* uréter *m*

ureteral *adj* ureteral, uretérico

urethra *n* uretra
urethral *adj* uretral
urethritis *n* uretritis *f*; **non-gonococcal** —— uretritis no gonocócica
urgent *adj* urgente
uric acid *n* ácido úrico
urinal *n* (*hand-held*) orinal *m*, pato
urinalysis *n* (*pl* **-ses**) examen *m* general de orina, prueba de la orina
urinary *adj* urinario
urinate *vi* orinar, (*ped*) hacer pipí
urine *n* orina
urodynamics *n* urodinámica
urogenital *adj* urogenital
urogram *n* urograma *m*, urografía
urography *n* urografía; **excretory** —— urografía excretoria; **retrograde** —— urografía retrógrada
urokinase *n* urokinasa
urologist *n* urólogo -ga *mf*

urology *n* urología
urosepsis *n* urosepsis *f*
urticaria *n* urticaria
Uruguayan *adj* & *n* uruguayo -ya *mf*
use *n* uso; *vt* usar; **to** —— **up** usar todo, agotar
useless *adj* inútil
user *n* usuario -ria *mf*
usual *adj* usual; **as** —— como de costumbre, como siempre; **Are you taking your insulin as usual?**..¿Está tomando su insulina como de costumbre? **than** —— que de costumbre; **Are you drinking more liquids than usual?**..¿Está tomando más líquidos que de costumbre?
uterus *n* (*pl* **-ri**) útero, matriz *f*
utilize *vt* utilizar
uvea *n* úvea
uveitis *n* uveítis *f*
uvula *n* (*pl* **-las** *o* **-lae**) úvula, campanilla

V

vaccinate *vt* vacunar; **Have you been vaccinated against tetanus?**..¿Se ha vacunado contra el tétano?
vaccination *n* vacunación *f*
vaccine *n* vacuna; **BCG** ——, **DPT** ——, **Salk** ——, **etc.** vacuna BCG, vacuna DPT, vacuna Salk, etc.; **mumps** ——, **rabies** ——, **etc.** vacuna contra las paperas, vacuna contra la rabia, etc.
vacuum *n* vacío
vagal *adj* vagal
vagina *n* vagina
vaginal *adj* vaginal
vaginitis *n* vaginitis *f*
vagotomy *n* (*pl* **-mies**) vagotomía; **selective** —— vagotomía selectiva
vagus *n* (*pl* **vagi**) vago
valerian *n* (*bot*) valeriana
valgus *adj* valgus, valgo

valine *n* valina
valproic acid *n* ácido valproico
value *n* valor *m*
valve *n* válvula; **aortic** —— válvula aórtica; **mitral** —— válvula mitral; **pulmonic** —— válvula pulmonar; **pyloric** —— válvula pilórica; **tricuspid** —— válvula tricúspide
valvuloplasty *n* (*pl* **-ties**) valvuloplastia *or* (*esp spoken*) valvuloplastía
vancomycin *n* vancomicina
vapor *n* vapor *m*
vaporizer *n* vaporizador *m*
variable *adj* & *n* variable *f*
variant *adj* & *n* variante *f*
variation *n* variación *f*
varicella *n* varicela
varices *pl de* **varix**
varicocele *n* varicocele *m*

varicose *adj* varicoso; —— **vein** vena varicosa
varix *n* (*pl* -**ices**) várice *f* (*en inglés se emplea casi siempre la forma plural:* **varices**)
varus *adj* varus, varo
vary *vi* variar
vascular *adj* vascular
vasculitis *n* vasculitis *f*; **hypersensitivity** —— vasculitis por hipersensibilidad; **necrotizing** —— vasculitis necrosante
vas deferens *n* conducto deferente
vasectomy *n* (*pl* -**mies**) vasectomía
vasoconstriction *n* vasoconstricción *f*
vasoconstrictor *n* vasoconstrictor *m*
vasodilation *n* vasodilatación *f*
vasodilator *n* vasodilatador *m*
vasopressin *n* vasopresina
vasospasm *n* vasospasmo *or* vasoespasmo
vasovagal *adj* vasovagal
VD *abbr* **venereal disease.** *V.* **disease.**
VDRL *n* VDRL *m*
vector *n* vector *m*
vegetable *n* vegetal *m*, verdura; —— **oil** aceite *m* de vegetal
vegetarian *adj* & *n* vegetariano -na *mf*
vegetarianism *n* vegetarianismo
vegetation *n* vegetación *f*
vegetative *adj* vegetativo
vehicle *n* vehículo
vein *n* vena; **antecubital** —— vena antecubital; **external jugular** —— vena yugular externa; **femoral** —— vena femoral; **internal jugular** —— vena yugular interna; **portal** —— vena porta; **saphenous** —— vena safena; **subclavian** —— vena subclavia; **varicose** —— vena varicosa
vein stripping *n* extracción *f* de várices *or* venas varicosas
vena cava *n* vena cava; **inferior** —— —— vena cava inferior; **superior** —— —— vena cava superior
venereal *adj* (*ant*) venéreo
Venezuelan *adj* & *n* venezolano -na *mf*
venogram *n* flebografía, flebograma *m*, venograma *m*
venography *n* flebografía
venom *n* veneno
venous *adj* venoso

ventilate *vt* ventilar
ventilation *n* ventilación *f*
ventilator *n* ventilador *m*
ventral *adj* ventral
ventricle *n* ventrículo
ventricular *adj* ventricular
venule *n* vénula
verapamil *n* verapamil *m*
vermicide *n* vermicida *m*
vermifuge *n* vermífugo
vernix caseosa *n* vérnix caseosa
vertebra *n* (*pl* -**brae** *o* -**bras**) vértebra
vertebral column *n* columna vertebral, columna (*fam*)
vertigo *n* vértigo
vesicle *n* vesícula
vessel *n* vaso; **blood** —— vaso sanguíneo
veteran *n* veterano -na *mf*
veterinarian *n* veterinario -ria *mf*
veterinary *adj* veterinario
viable *adj* viable
vibration *n* vibración *f*
vice *n* vicio
victim *n* víctima, (*of an accident*) accidentado -da *mf*
vigorous *adj* vigoroso
vinblastine *n* vinblastina
vincristine *n* vincristina
vinegar *n* vinagre *m*
violence *n* violencia
violent *adj* violento
violet *adj* violeta
viper *n* víbora
viral *adj* viral, vírico
virgin *adj* & *n* virgen *mf*
virginity *n* virginidad *f*
virile *adj* viril
virility *n* virilidad *f*
virilization *n* virilización *f*
virology *n* virología
virulence *n* virulencia
virulent *adj* virulento
virus *n* (*pl* **viruses**) virus *m*; **Epstein-Barr** —— **(EBV)** virus de Epstein-Barr; **human immunodeficiency** —— **(HIV)** virus de inmunodeficiencia humana (VIH)
visceral *adj* visceral
viscosity *n* viscosidad *f*
viscous *adj* viscoso
visible *adj* visible

vision *n* vista, visión *f*; **blurred** —— vista empañada, visión borrosa; **double** —— visión *or* vista doble; **nocturnal** *o* **night** —— vista *or* visión nocturna; **peripheral** —— visión periférica; **tunnel** —— visión en túnel

visit *n* visita; *vt, vi* visitar

visiting hours *npl* horas de visita

visitor *n* visita, visitante *mf*

visual *adj* visual

visualization *n* formación de una imagen mental

visualize *vt* formar una imagen mental

vital *adj* vital

vitality *n* vitalidad *f*

vitalize *vt* vitalizar

vitamin *adj* vitamínico; *n* vitamina; —— A, B₁₂, etc. vitamina A, B₁₂, etc.; **fat-soluble** —— vitamina liposoluble; **water-soluble** —— vitamina hidrosoluble

vitiligo *n* vitíligo

vitreous *adj* vítreo

vocal *adj* vocal; —— **cord** cuerda vocal

voice *n* voz *f*

void *vi* vaciar la vejiga, orinar

volt *n* voltio

volume *n* volumen *m*

voluntary *adj* voluntario

volunteer *n* voluntario -ria *mf*

volvulus *n* vólvulo

vomit *n* vómito; *vt, vi* vomitar, arrojar (*fam*), devolver (*fam*), deponer (*Mex, fam*), tener basca (*fam*); **Did you vomit blood?**.. ¿Vomitó sangre?

vomiting *m* vómito (*frec pl*); **Have you had vomiting?**..¿Ha tenido vómito(s)?

voodoo *n* vudú *m*

voyeurism *n* voyeurismo

VSD *abbr* **ventricular septal defect.** *V. defect.*

vulnerable *adj* vulnerable

vulva *n* (*pl* **-vae**) vulva

W

waist *n* cintura; **from the** —— **up** de la cintura para arriba

wait *vi* esperar; **to** —— **for** esperar

waiting list *n* lista de espera

waiting room *n* sala de espera

wake *vt, vi* (*pret* **waked** *o* **woke**; *pp* **waked**) (*también* **to** —— **up**) despertar(se)

walk *n* paseo, caminata; **to take a** —— *o* **to go for a** —— dar un paseo; *vi* caminar, andar; **to** —— **in one's sleep** caminar dormido

walker *n* andadera

wall *n* (*anat*) pared *f*

war *n* guerra; **nuclear** —— guerra nuclear

ward *n* (*of a hospital*) sala; —— **clerk** secretaria de sala

warfarin *n* warfarina

warm *adj* caliente; **to be** *o* **feel** —— tener *or* sentir calor; *vt, vi* (*también* **to** —— **up**) calentar(se); **to** —— **up** (*sports*) hacer ejercicios de calentamiento

warmth *n* calor *m*

warmup *n* (ejercicios de) calentamiento

wart *n* verruga; **genital** —— verruga genital; **plantar** —— verruga plantar

wash *vt* lavar; (*to bathe*) bañar; **to** —— **one's hair, face, hands, etc.** lavarse la cabeza *or* el pelo, la cara, las manos, etc.; *vi* bañarse

washable *adj* lavable

wasp *n* avispa

wastes *npl* desechos, desperdicios; **hazardous** —— desechos peligrosos; **metabolic** —— desechos metabólicos

water *n* agua; —— **on the lung, knee, etc.** agua en el pulmón, la rodilla, etc.; **boiling**

—— agua hirviendo; **distilled** —— agua destilada; **drinking** —— agua potable; **fresh** —— agua dulce; **hard** —— agua dura (*con alto contenido de minerales*); **mineral** —— agua mineral; **purified** —— agua purificada; **running** —— agua corriente; **salt** —— agua salada; **soft** —— agua con escaso contenido de minerales; **tap** —— agua de la llave *or* del grifo

water-borne *adj* transmitido por el agua

wave *n* onda; **brain** —— onda cerebral

wavelength *n* longitud *f* de onda

wax *n* cera

weak *adj* débil

weaken *vt, vi* debilitar(se)

weakening *n* debilitación *f*, decaimiento

weakness *n* debilidad *f*

wean *vt* destetar

weaning *n* destete *m*

weapon *n* arma; **sharp** —— arma blanca

wear *vt* (*pret* **wore**; *pp* **worn**) llevar; *vi* —— **off** pasar; **The numbness will wear off in a couple hours.**.Lo dormido se le va a pasar en un par de horas.

weather *n* tiempo, clima *m*

web *n* membrana; **esophageal** —— membrana esofágica

wedge *n* cuña

week *n* semana

weekend *n* fin *m* de semana

weep *vi* (*pret & pp* **wept**) llorar; (*lesion*) secretar líquido claro

weigh *vt, vi* pesar; **How much did you weigh six months ago?**..¿Cuánto pesaba hace seis meses?...¿**Did the nurse weigh you?**..¿Lo pesó la enfermera?

weight *n* peso; **excess** —— sobrepeso

welfare *n* bienestar *m*, bien *m*; asistencia social, asistencia pública

well *adj & adv* (*comp* **better**; *super* **best**) bien; **to get** —— aliviarse, curarse

well-being *n* bienestar *m*

wen *n* quiste sebáceo

wet *adj* (*comp* **wetter**; *super* **wettest**) mojado; **to get** —— mojarse; *vt* (*pret & pp* **wet** *o* **wetted**; *ger* **wetting**) mojar; **to** —— **the bed** orinarse en la cama

wet dream *n* sueño húmedo *or* mojado

wet nurse *n* nodriza

wheal *n* roncha

wheat *n* trigo

wheelchair *n* silla de ruedas

wheeze *n* sibilancia (*form*), chillido, silbido; *vi* chillarle *or* silbarle el pecho, tener chillidos *or* silbidos; **Are you wheezing?**.. ¿Le chilla el pecho?..¿Tiene silbidos?

whiplash *n* lesión *f* por latigazo

whipworm *n* tricocéfalo

whiskers *npl* pelitos de la cara del hombre que no se ha afeitado

white *adj* blanco; *n* (*of an egg*) clara (*del huevo*)

whitlow *n* panadizo

whole *adj* entero; —— **wheat** trigo integral *or* entero

whooping cough *n* tos ferina, coqueluche *m&f*

wick *n* mecha

wide *adj* ancho

widen *vt* ensanchar, hacer más ancho

widow *n* viuda

widowed *adj* viudo

widower *n* viudo

wife *n* (*pl* **wives**) esposa

wig *n* peluca

wiggle *vt, vi* mover(se); **Wiggle your toes.**. Mueva sus dedos del pie.

will *n* voluntad *f*; —— **power** fuerza de voluntad; **against one's** —— contra la voluntad de uno; **of one's own free** —— por voluntad propia

wind *n* viento

windburn *n* resequedad de la piel debida al viento

windpipe *n* gaznate *m*, tráquea

wine *n* vino; **red** —— vino tinto; **white** —— vino blanco

winter *n* invierno

wipe *vt* enjugar; **to** —— (**oneself**) (*after moving bowels*) limpiarse, asearse

wire *n* alambre *m*

wired *adj* (*vulg*) acelerado

witchcraft *n* brujería

witch hazel *n* agua de hamamelis

withdrawal *n* síndrome *m* de abstinencia (*form*), síntomas sufridos por el adicto al suspender drogas o alcohol

wives *pl de* **wife**

woman *n* (*pl* **women**) mujer *f*

womb *n* matriz *f*, útero

women *pl de* **woman**
women's room *n* baño para mujeres
wood alcohol *n* alcohol *m* de madera
wool *n* lana
wore *pret de* **wear**
work *n* trabajo; *vi* trabajar; (*to function*) funcionar, trabajar; **Your kidneys have stopped working**..Sus riñones han dejado de funcionar; **to —— out** hacer ejercicio, levantar pesas
worker *n* obrero -ra *mf*, trabajador -ra *mf*
workout *n* sesión *f* de ejercicio
worm *n* gusano; (*intestinal*) lombriz *f*
worn *pp de* **wear**
worry *vi* (*pret & pp* **worried**) preocuparse; **Don't worry**..No se preocupe.
worse *adj & adv* (*comp de* **bad** *y* **poorly**) peor; **to get —— empeorar(se), agravarse, ponerse peor; **to make —— agravar, empeorar; **Is there anything that makes the pain worse?**..¿Hay algo que le agrave el dolor?
worsening *n* empeoramiento
wound *n* herida; **gunshot —— balazo, herida de bala; **knife —— cuchillada; **puncture —— herida punzante; **stab —— puñalada; *vt* herir
wounded *adj & n* herido
wrap *vt* (*pret & pp* **wrapped**; *ger* **wrapping**) envolver
wrinkle *n* arruga; *vt, vi* arrugar(se)
wrist *n* muñeca; **—— drop** mano péndula
writer's cramp *n* calambre *m* del escritor
writhe *vi* retorcerse

X

xanthoma *n* xantoma *m*
xiphoid process *n* apófisis *f* xifoides
X-linked *adj* ligado al cromosoma X, ligado al X

x-ray *n* (*single ray*) rayo X; (*film*) radiografía, rayos X (*fam*); **the —— department** el departamento de rayos X; *vt* tomar una radiografía (de)

Y

yarrow *n* (*bot*) milenrama
yawn *n* bostezo; *vi* bostezar
yaws *n* pián *m*, frambesia
year *n* año
yeast *n* clase *f* de hongo, hongos (*fam*)
yellow *adj* amarillo
yellowish *adj* amarillento
yellow jacket *n* especie *f* de avispa

yesterday *adv* ayer
yoga *n* yoga
yogurt *n* yogur *m*
yohimbine *n* yohimbina
yolk *n* yema; **egg —— yema del huevo
young *adj* joven
youth *n* juventud *f*
yucca *n* (*bot*) yuca

Z

zalcitabine *n* zalcitabina
zidovudine *n* zidovudina
zinc *n* cinc *or* zinc *m*; —— **oxide** óxido de cinc

zip code *n* código postal
zipper *n* cierre *m*
zone *n* zona

ESPAÑOL-INGLÉS

SPANISH-ENGLISH

A

abajo *adv* de —— lower

abandonar *vt* (*un tratamiento, etc.*) to give up on

abanico *m* fan

abatelenguas *m* (*Mex*) tongue depressor *o* blade

abatido -da *adj* depressed

abdomen *m* abdomen, belly, stomach (*fam*)

abdominal *adj* abdominal; *m* sit-up

abeja *f* bee; —— **africanizada** *or* **asesina** Africanized *o* killer bee

abertura *f* opening

abierto -ta (*pp of* **abrir**) *adj* open

abortar *vt* to abort; *vi* (*con intención*) to have an abortion; (*sin intención*) to miscarry, to have a miscarriage

aborto *m* (*inducido*) abortion; (*espontáneo*) miscarriage; —— **accidental** accidental abortion; —— **espontáneo** spontaneous abortion; —— **habitual** *or* **de repetición** habitual abortion; —— **incompleto** incomplete abortion; —— **terapéutico** therapeutic abortion; **amenaza de** —— threatened abortion

abotagado -da *adj* bloated

abotonar *vt, vr* to button (up)

abrasión *f* abrasion

abrasivo -va *adj & m* abrasive

abrazar *vt* to embrace, hug

abrazo *m* embrace, hug

abrigo *m* coat, overcoat

abrir *vt, vr* (*pp* **abierto**) to open

abrochar *vt, vr* to button (up), buckle

absceso *m* abscess

absorbente *adj* absorbent

absorber *vt* to absorb

absorbible *adj* absorbable; **no** —— nonabsorbable

absorción *f* absorption

abstenerse *vr* to abstain; —— **de la cerveza** to abstain from beer

abstinencia *f* abstinence

abuelo -la *m* grandfather, grandparent; *f* grandmother

abultamiento *m* swelling

aburrirse *vr* to become bored

abusador -ra *mf* abuser

abusar *vt* to abuse; **Abusó de ella..**He abused her...**Ella abusa de las drogas..** She abuses drugs.

abuso *m* abuse; —— **de drogas** drug abuse; —— **de substancias intoxicantes** substance abuse; —— **infantil** child abuse

acabarse *vr* to run out; **Se me acabaron las pastillas..**My pills ran out.

acalasia *f* achalasia

acalenturado -da *adj* feverish

acarbosa *f* acarbose

acariciar *vt* to caress, to fondle

ácaro *m* mite

acaso, por si just in case

acatarrado -da *adj* (*fam*) having a cold; **Estoy acatarrado..**I have a cold.

acatarrarse *vr* to catch a cold

acceso *m* attack, fit, spell; access; —— **para sillas de rueda** wheelchair access

accidentado -da *adj* injured (*in an accident*); *mf* accident victim

accidentarse *vr* to have an accident

accidente *m* accident

acción *f* action; **de** —— **corta** short-acting; **de** —— **prolongada** long-acting; **de** —— **rápida** fast-acting, (*insulina*) regular

acedía *f* heartburn

aceite *m* oil; —— **de cacahuate** peanut oil; —— **de cártamo** safflower oil; —— **de coco** coconut oil; —— **de hígado de bacalao** cod-liver oil; —— **de maíz** corn oil; —— **de oliva** olive oil; —— **de palma** palm oil; —— **de ricino** castor oil;

—— **mineral** mineral oil; —— **vegetal** vegetable oil

acelerado -da *adj* nervously energetic

acero *m* steel; —— **inoxidable** stainless steel

acetaminofén *m* acetaminophen

acetazolamida *f* acetazolamide

acético -ca *adj* acetic

acetilcefuroxima *f* cefuroxime axetil

acetona *f* acetone

achacoso -sa *adj* sickly, having many ailments

achaque *m* mild illness, ailment, affliction

aciclovir *m* acyclovir

acidez *f* acidity; (*estomacal*) heartburn

ácido -da *adj & m* acid; —— **acético** acetic acid; —— **ascórbico** ascorbic acid; —— **bórico** boric acid; —— **clorhídrico** hydrochloric acid; —— **desoxirribonucleico (ADN** *or* **DNA)** deoxyribonucleic acid (DNA); —— **fólico** folic acid; —— **gástrico** gastric acid; —— **glutámico** glutamic acid; —— **graso** fatty acid; —— **láctico** lactic acid; —— **linoleico** linoleic acid; —— **nalidíxico** nalidixic acid; —— **nicotínico** nicotinic acid; —— **pantoténico** pantothenic acid; —— **ribonucleico** ribonucleic acid; —— **salicílico** salicylic acid; —— **tartárico** tartaric acid; —— **úrico** uric acid; —— **valproico** valproic acid

acné *f* acne

acojinamiento *m* cushioning

acojinar *vt* to pad, cushion

acolchar *vt* to pad, cushion

acomodar *vt* (*los huesos*) to set (*a bone*), to reduce (*a fracture or dislocation*), to adjust, perform an adjustment

acondicionador *m* conditioner

acondroplasia *f* achondroplasia

acordarse *vr* (*also* —— **de**) to remember

acortar *vt* to shorten

acostarse *vr* to lie down; to go to bed

acrílico -ca *adj* acrylic

acrocordón *m* (*form*) skin tag

acrofobia *f* acrophobia

acromegalia *f* acromegaly

acta de nacimiento *f* birth certificate

actinomicosis *f* actinomycosis

actitud *f* attitude

activador *m* activator; —— **del plasminógeno tisular** tissue plasminogen activator (tPA)

activar *vt* to activate

actividad *f* activity; —— **fuerte** strenuous activity, exertion

activo -va *adj* active

acto *m* act; —— **sexual** sexual intercourse, intercourse; **durante el acto sexual**..during sexual intercourse

acumulación *f* buildup

acumular *vt, vr* to accumulate, build up

acumulativo -va *adj* cumulative

acuoso -sa *adj* aqueous

acupresión *f* acupressure

acupuntura *f* acupuncture

acústico -ca *adj* acoustic

adaptación *f* adaptation

adaptar *vt, vr* to adapt

adecuado -da *adj* adequate; appropriate

adelante *adv* hacia —— forward

adenitis *f* adenitis

adenocarcinoma *m* adenocarcinoma

adenoidectomía *f* adenoidectomy

adenoiditis *f* adenoiditis

adenoma *m* adenoma; —— **velloso** villous adenoma

adentro *adv* inside

adherencia *f* adhesion

adhesivo -va *adj* adhesive; **cinta** *or* **tela adhesiva** adhesive tape

adicción *f* addiction

adictivo -va *adj* addictive

adicto -ta *mf* addict

aditivo -va *adj & m* additive

administración *f* administration

admisión *f* (*al hospital*) admission

Admisión *f* Admissions

admitir *vt* (*al hospital*) to admit

ADN *abbr* **ácido desoxirribonucleico.** *See* **ácido.**

adolescencia *f* adolescence

adolescente *adj & mf* adolescent

adolorido -da *adj* sore, painful, tender

adopción *f* adoption

adoptar *vt* to adopt

adoptivo -va *adj* adoptive
adormecedor -ra *adj* numbing
adormecer *vt* to numb (up); *vr* to become numb, to go to sleep (*fam*)
adormecido -da *adj* numb, asleep (*fam*)
adormecimiento *m* numbness
adormilado -da *adj* drowsy
adquirido -da *adj* acquired
adquirir *vt* to acquire
adrenal *adj* adrenal; *f* adrenal gland
adrenalina *f* adrenaline
adsorbente *adj* adsorbent
adulto -ta *adj* & *mf* adult
adyuvante *adj* (*quimioterapia*) adjuvant
aeróbico -ca *adj* aerobic; *mpl* aerobics
aerosol *m* aerosol; (*nasal*) nasal inhaler, nasal spray; —— **dosificador** metered dose inhaler; **en** —— aerosolized
afasia *f* aphasia
afección *f* affection
afectar *vt* to affect
afecto *m* affection; (*psych*) affect
afectuoso -sa *adj* affectionate
afeitar *vt*, *vr* to shave
afeminado -da *adj* effeminate
afilado -da *adj* sharp
afinidad *f* affinity
aflicción *f* grief, distress
afligirse *vr* to grieve
aflojar *vt* to loosen; (*fam*) to relax; **Afloje la pierna**..Relax your leg; *vr* to relax
afrecho *m* bran
afta *f* canker sore; thrush
agachar *vt* (*la cabeza*) to bend down (*one's head*); **Agache la cabeza**..Bend your head down; *vr* to bend over, bend down, stoop; to squat
agammaglobulinemia, agamaglobulinemia *f* agammaglobulinemia
agarrar *vt* to grasp, grip; (*una enfermedad*) to catch; —— **aire** to catch one's breath
agarrotarse *See* **engarrotarse**.
agencia *f* agency
agente *m* (*pharm*) agent
ágil *adj* agile
agitado -da *adj* agitated, upset
agitar *vt* to agitate; **Agítese bien antes de usarse**..Shake well before using; *vr* to

become agitated, upset
agorafobia *f* agoraphobia
agotado -da *adj* exhausted, run-down; depleted, used up
agotador -ra *adj* fatiguing
agotamiento *m* extreme fatigue, exhaustion; depletion
agotar *vt* to deplete, use up; *vr* to become fatigued; to become depleted
agrandar *vt* to enlarge
agravar *vt* to aggravate, make worse; *vr* to get worse; **Se agravó**..He got worse.
agregar *vt* to add; **No agregue sal**..Don't add salt.
agresión *f* aggression
agresivo -va *adj* aggressive
agrietado -da *adj* cracked
agrietarse *vr* to crack, to chap, get chapped
agrio -ria *adj* sour
agruras *fpl* heartburn
agua *f* water; —— **con alto contenido de minerales** *or* —— **dura** hard water; —— **con escaso contenido de minerales** soft water; —— **corriente** running water; —— **de hamamelis** witch hazel; —— **de la llave** *or* **del grifo** tap water; —— **destilada** distilled water; —— **dulce** fresh water; —— **en el pulmón, la rodilla, etc.** water on the lung, the knee, etc.; —— **mineral** mineral water; —— **oxigenada** hydrogen peroxide; —— **purificada** purified water; —— **salada** salt water
aguacate *m* avocado
aguado -da *adj* flabby, flaccid, weak; runny
aguamala *f* jellyfish
aguantar *vt* to tolerate, endure, stand, bear; —— **la respiración** *or* **el resuello** to hold one's breath; **Aguante la respiración**.. Hold your breath.
aguas negras *fpl* sewage, sewer water
aguas termales *fpl* hot springs
agudeza *f* acuity; —— **visual** visual acuity
agudo -da *adj* (*enfermedad*) acute; (*dolor*) sharp; (*tono*) high-pitched
agüita *f* (*esp Mex, CA*) serum, body fluid
aguja *f* needle; —— **hipodérmica** hypodermic needle
agujero *m* hole

ahogar *vt, vr* to suffocate, smother; to drown; **¿Siente que se ahoga?**..Do you feel as though you are suffocating?..Do you feel short of breath?

ahogo *m* choking sensation, shortness of breath

ahorcar *vt* to hang (*by the neck*); *vr* to hang oneself

ai *interj* Ouch!

aire *m* air; —— **acondicionado** air conditioning; —— **contaminado** air pollution, smog; **al —— libre** outdoors; **tener ——** (*en el pecho, abdomen, etc.*) to have air (*in one's chest, abdomen, etc.*) (*refers to a popular belief that pain in the chest or abdomen may be due to trapped air*)

aislado -da *adj* isolated; (*emocionalmente*) alienated

aislamiento *m* isolation

aislar *vt* to isolate

ajo *m* garlic

ajustable *adj* adjustable

ajustador *m* (*Carib*) brassiere

ajustar *vt* to adjust, correct, to fit

ajuste *m* adjustment, correction, fitting

alacrán *m* scorpion

alambre *m* wire; —— **de púas** barbed wire

alanina *f* alanine

albendazol *m* albendazole

albinismo *m* albinism

albino -na *adj & mf* albino

albúmina *f* albumin

albuterol *m* albuterol

álcali *m* alkali

alcalino -na *adj* alkaline

alcalosis *f* alkalosis

alcance *m* reach; **fuera del —— de los niños** out of reach of children

alcanfor *m* camphor

alcanzar *vt, vi* to reach

alcaptonuria *f* alkaptonuria

alcohol *m* alcohol, liquor; —— **de madera** wood alcohol; —— **desnaturalizado** denatured alcohol; —— **etílico** ethyl alcohol; —— **metílico** methyl alcohol; —— **para fricciones** rubbing alcohol

alcohólico -ca *adj & mf* alcoholic

Alcohólicos Anónimos *m* Alcoholics Anonymous (AA)

alcoholismo *m* alcoholism

aldosterona *f* aldosterone

aldosteronismo *m* aldosteronism

alegre *adj* cheerful

alergeno *m* allergen

alergia *f* allergy

alérgico -ca *adj* allergic; **¿Es Ud. alérgico a la penicilina?**..Are you allergic to penicillin?

alergista *mf* (*Ang*) allergist

alergólogo -ga *mf* allergist

alerta *adj* alert

aleteo *m* flutter; —— **auricular** atrial flutter

alfa *f* alpha; —— **feto proteína** alpha fetoprotein; —— **metildopa** alpha methyldopa

alfalfa *f* (*bot*) alfalfa

alfiler *m* pin, safety pin; —— **de seguridad** safety pin

algas *fpl* algae

algodón *m* cotton

algodoncillo *m* thrush

alguate *m* (*Mex*) fine cactus spine

aliento *m* breath; **mal ——** bad breath

alimentación *f* feeding, nourishment

alimentar *vt* to feed

alimentario -ria *adj* alimentary

alimenticio -cia *adj* nutritional

alimento *m* (*frec pl*) food; **alimentos enlatados** canned food; **alimentos procesados** processed food

alineamiento *m* alignment

alinear *vt, vr* to align, line up

aliviar *vt* to alleviate, soothe, relieve; *vr* to recover, get well; (*Mex, fam*) to give birth, deliver

alivio *m* relief

almacén *m* store

almacenar *vt* to store

almidón *m* starch; —— **de maíz** cornstarch

almohada *f* pillow, cushion

almohadilla *f* small pillow, small cushion, pad

almorrana *f* hemorrhoid

almorzar *vi* to have lunch

almuerzo *m* lunch

áloe *m* aloe

alojarse *vr* to lodge

alopático -ca *adj* allopathic
alopurinol *m* allopurinol
alprazolam *m* alprazolam
alquitrán *m* tar; —— **de hulla** coal tar
alteración *f* disturbance
alterado -da *adj* upset
alterar *vt* to upset; *vr* to become upset
alternar *vt, vi* to alternate
alterno -na *adj* alternate; **días alternos** alternate days
altitud *f* altitude
alto -ta *adj* high, tall; **Su glucosa está muy alta..**Your glucose is very high...**¿Es muy alto su papá?..**Is your father very tall?
altura *f* height; altitude, elevation; **¿Qué altura tiene Ud.?..**How tall are you?
alucinación *f* hallucination
alumbramiento *m* childbirth; (*form*) delivery of the placenta
alumbrar *vi* to give birth
aluminio *m* aluminum
alveolo, alvéolo *m* alveolus; (*dent*) socket
amable *adj* friendly, kind
ama de casa *f* housewife, homemaker
amalgama *f* (*dent*) amalgam
amamantar *vt* (*form*) to breast-feed, to nurse
Amanita Amanita
amantadina *f* amantadine
amar *vt, vi* to love
amargo -ga *adj* bitter
amargón *m* (*bot*) dandelion
amarillento -ta *adj* yellowish
amarillo -lla *adj* yellow
ambidextro -tra *adj* ambidextrous
ambiental *adj* environmental
ambiente *m* surroundings, environment
ambrosia *f* (*bot*) ragweed
ambulancia *f* ambulance
ambulatorio -ria *adj* ambulatory
ameba *f* ameba
amebiano -na *adj* amebic
amebiasis *f* amebiasis
amenorrea *f* amenorrhea
americano -na *adj* & *mf* American
amiba *f* ameba
amibiano -na *adj* amebic
amibiasis *f* amebiasis
amígdala *f* tonsil

amigdalectomía *f* tonsillectomy
amigdalitis *f* tonsillitis
amigo -ga *mf* friend
amikacina *f* amikacin
amilasa *f* amylase
amiloidosis *f* amyloidosis
amilorida *f* amiloride
aminoácido *m* amino acid
aminofilina *f* aminophylline
aminoglucósido *m* aminoglycoside
aminorar *vt, vr* to diminish, reduce
amistad *f* friendship
amistoso -sa *adj* friendly
amitriptilina *f* amitriptyline
amlodipina *f* amlodipine
amnesia *f* amnesia
amniocentesis *f* (*pl* -**sis**) amniocentesis
amnionitis *f* amnionitis
amodorrado -da *adj* drowsy
amoniaco, amoníaco *m* ammonia
amontonamiento *m* buildup
amor *m* love; —— **propio** self-esteem
amoratado -da *adj* bruised, black-and-blue; cyanotic
amortiguado -da *adj* buffered
amortiguador *m* buffer; **solución amortiguadora** buffer solution
amortiguamiento *m* cushioning
amortiguar *vt* to cushion
amoxacilina *f* amoxacillin
ampicilina *f* ampicillin
ampolla *f* blister
ampolleta *f* ampule
ámpula *f* ampule
amputación *f* amputation
amputar *vt* to amputate
anabólico -ca *adj* anabolic
anaerobio -bia *adj* anaerobic
anafiláctico -ca *adj* anaphylactic
anafilaxis *f* anaphylaxis
anal *adj* anal
analfabetismo *m* illiteracy
analfabeto -ta *adj* illiterate
analgesia *f* analgesia
analgésico -ca *adj* & *m* analgesic
análisis *m* (*pl* -**sis**) analysis, test
analizar *vt* to analyze
anatomía *f* anatomy

anatómico -ca *adj* anatomical, anatomic
ancho -cha *adj* wide
anciano -na *adj* old, elderly; *m* old man, old person; *f* old woman
andadera *f* walker
andar *vi* to walk
andrógeno *m* androgen
anemia *f* anemia; —— **aplásica** aplastic anemia; —— **de células falciformes** *or* —— **drepanocítica** sickle cell anemia; —— **ferropriva, ferropénica,** *or* **por deficiencia de hierro** iron deficiency anemia; —— **hemolítica** hemolytic anemia; —— **perniciosa** pernicious anemia; —— **sideroblástica** sideroblastic anemia
anémico -ca *adj* anemic
anencefalia *f* anencephaly
anergia *f* anergy
anestesia *f* anesthesia; —— **general** general anesthesia; —— **local** local anesthesia; —— **regional** regional anesthesia
anestesiar *vt* to anesthetize, numb up, put to sleep (*fam*)
anestésico -ca *adj & m* anesthetic
anestesiología *f* anesthesiology
anestesiólogo -ga *mf* anesthesiologist
anestesista *mf* anesthetist
aneurisma *m* aneurysm; —— **disecante** dissecting aneurysm; —— **micótico** mycotic aneurysm
anfetamina *f* amphetamine
anfotericina B *f* amphotericin B
angélica *f* (*bot*) angelica
angiitis *f* angiitis
angina *f* (*de pecho*) angina; **anginas** (*esp Mex, fam*) tonsils; —— **de Prinzmetal** Prinzmetal's angina; —— **de Vincent** Vincent's angina, trench mouth; —— **inestable** unstable angina; **tener anginas** (*Mex, fam*) to have tonsillitis
angiodisplasia *f* angiodysplasia
angioedema *m* angioedema
angiografía *f* angiography; angiogram
angiograma *m* angiogram
angioma *m* angioma
angioplastia *f* angioplasty; —— **translumi-nal percutánea coronaria** percutaneous transluminal coronary angioplasty
angiosarcoma *m* angiosarcoma
ángulo *m* angle, bend; —— **del ojo** angle *o* corner of the eye
angustia *f* anxiety
anilina *f* aniline
anillo *m* ring
animal *m* animal; —— **doméstico** pet
animalito (*fam*) *m* bug, insect; parasite
ano *m* anus
anoche *adv* last night
anomalía *f* anomaly
anorexia *f* anorexia; —— **nerviosa** anorexia nervosa
anormal *adj* abnormal
anormalidad *f* abnormality
anovulación *f* anovulation
anovulatorio -ria *adj* anovulatory
anquilosis *f* ankylosis
anquilostomiasis *f* ancylostomiasis
ansia *f* (*frec pl*) anxiety; (*fam*) asthma, shortness of breath
ansiedad *f* anxiety
ansioso -sa *adj* anxious
anteanoche *adv* night before last
anteayer *adv* the day before yesterday
antebrazo *m* forearm
anteojos *mpl* glasses, eyeglasses; —— **oscuros** sunglasses
antepasado *m* ancestor
anterior *adj* anterior; previous
antiácido -da *adj & m* antacid
antiarrítmico -ca *adj & m* antiarrhythmic
antibacteriano -na *adj* antibacterial
antibiótico -ca *adj & m* antibiotic; —— **de amplio espectro** broad spectrum antibiotic
anticoagulante *adj & m* anticoagulant, blood thinner (*fam*)
anticoagular *vt* to anticoagulate
anticolinérgico -ca *adj* anticholinergic
anticoncepción *f* contraception
anticonceptivo -va *adj & m* contraceptive
anticongelante *m* antifreeze
anticonvulsivo -va *adj & m* anticonvulsant
anticuerpo *m* antibody
antidepresivo -va *adj & m* antidepressant; —— **tricíclico** tricyclic antidepressant
antidiarreico -ca *adj* antidiarrheal

antídoto *m* antidote
antiemético -ca *adj & m* antiemetic
antier *See* **anteayer**.
antiespasmódico -ca *adj & m* antispasmodic
antiespástico -ca *adj & m* antispasmodic
antígeno *m* antigen; —— **carcinoembrió-nico** carcinoembryonic antigen
antihelmíntico -ca *adj & m* anthelminthic
antihipertensivo -va *adj* antihypertensive
antihistamínico *m* antihistamine
antiinflamatorio -ria *adj* antiinflammatory; *m* antiinflammatory agent; —— **no este-roide** nonsteroidal antiinflammatory drug (NSAID)
antimicrobiano -na *adj & m* antimicrobial
antipático -ca *adj* unfriendly
antiperspirante *adj & m* antiperspirant
antipirético -ca *adj & m* antipyretic
antipsicótico -ca *adj & m* antipsychotic
antiséptico -ca *adj & m* antiseptic
antisocial *adj* antisocial
antisuero *m* antiserum
antitoxina *f* antitoxin
antitranspirante *m* antiperspirant
antojo *m* (*obst*) craving
ántrax *m* anthrax
anual *adj* annual
anular *adj* annular
anzuelo *m* fishhook
año *m* year; **¿Cuántos años tiene Ud.?**.. How old are you?
aorta *f* aorta
aórtico -ca *adj* aortic
apachurrar *vt* to mash, press down
aparato *m* apparatus, device; (*cardiovascular, etc.*) system; (*fam, obst*) intrauterine device (IUD); —— **ortopédico** brace
apariencia *f* appearance
apatía *f* apathy
apático -ca *adj* apathetic
apellido *m* last name
apenarse *vr* to grieve
apéndice *m* appendix
apendicectomía *f* appendectomy
apendicitis *f* appendicitis
apestar *vi* to stink, smell bad
apetito *m* appetite
apio *m* celery

aplastante *adj* (*sensación, dolor*) crushing
aplastar *vt* to crush
aplazar *vt* to postpone
aplicación *f* application
aplicador *m* applicator, swab
aplicar *vt* to apply; *vr* to apply to oneself
apnea *f* apnea; —— **del sueño** sleep apnea
apófisis *f* (*pl* -sis) (*anat*) process; —— **mastoides** mastoid process; —— **xifoides** xiphoid process
apoplejía *f* (*form*) stroke
apósito *m* large gauze dressing, dressing
apoyar *vt* to support
apoyo *m* support; **grupo de** —— support group
apraxia *f* apraxia
aprendizaje *m* learning; **dificultad** *f* *or* **problema** *m* **del** —— learning disability
apretado -da *adj* tight; (*el pecho*) tight (*as with asthma*)
apretar *vt* to press; to squeeze; to constrict; (*ropa, calzado*) to pinch, to be too tight for; —— **la mano** to make a fist; —— **los dientes** to bite down; *vi* (*ropa, calzado*) to bind, to be too tight
apropiado -da *adj* appropriate
aproximadamente *adv* approximately
aptitud *f* aptitude
aquejar *vt* to bother; **Me aqueja un dolor de rodilla**..A pain in my knee is bothering me.
araña *f* spider; —— **vascular** spider angioma
arañar *vt* to scratch (*esp with claws*)
arañazo *m* scratch (*esp by claws*)
arco *m* arch; —— **de Hawley** (*orthodontia*) retainer; —— **del pie** arch of the foot
arder *vi* to burn; **Esto le va a arder un poco**..This will burn a little bit.
ardiente *adj* burning
ardilla *f* squirrel
ardor *m* (*sensación*) burning, burning sensation; **Siento ardor en el pecho**..I feel burning in my chest.
área *f* area
arete *m* earring
argentino -na *adj & mf* Argentine *o* Argentinean

arginina *f* arginine

arma *f* weapon; —— **blanca** sharp weapon; —— **de fuego** firearm

armazón *m* (*para lentes*) frames

árnica *f* (*bot*) arnica

aros *mpl* (*fam*) frames (*for eyeglasses*)

arrastrar *vt* —— **la voz** *or* **la lengua** to slur

arrebatado -da *adj* (*vulg*) high (*on drugs*)

arreglar *vt* to repair, fix

arriba *adv* **de** —— upper; **hacia** —— upward

arriesgar *vt* to risk; *vr* to take a risk

arritmia *f* arrhythmia

arrojar *vt* to throw up, to vomit; (*esp Mex, fam*) to cough up; (*Mex*) to pass, to shed; —— **gases** *or* **vientos** to pass gas; —— **una piedra** (*Mex*) to pass a stone; *vi* to throw up, to vomit

arrollar *vt* (*con un vehículo*) to run over

arroz *m* rice

arruga *f* wrinkle

arrugar *vt, vr* to wrinkle

arrullar *vi, vr* to coo

arsénico *m* arsenic

arteria *f* artery; —— **braquial** brachial artery; —— **carótida** carotid artery; —— **coronaria** coronary artery; —— **femoral** femoral artery; —— **iliaca** iliac artery; —— **radial** radial artery; —— **subclavia** subclavian artery

arterial *adj* arterial

arteriosclerosis *f* arteriosclerosis

arteriovenoso -sa *adj* arteriovenous

arteritis *f* arteritis; —— **temporal** temporal arteritis

articulación *f* joint; —— **de la cadera** hip-joint

artificial *adj* artificial

artrítico -ca *adj* arthritic

artritis *f* arthritis; —— **juvenil** juvenile arthritis; —— **reumatoide** rheumatoid arthritis

artrografía *f* arthrography; arthrogram

artrograma *m* arthrogram

artroscopia, artroscopía *f* arthroscopy

asado -da *adj* roasted, grilled; —— **a la parilla** grilled, broiled

asaltar *vt* to assault

asalto *m* assault

asar *vt* to roast, to grill; —— **a la parrilla** to grill, broil

asbesto *m* asbestos

ascariasis, ascaridiasis *f* ascariasis

ascáride *m* roundworm

Ascaris Ascaris

ascendente *adj* ascending

ascitis *f* ascites

asco *m* (*Mex, CA*) nausea; **dar** —— to make nauseated; **tener** —— to be nauseated

ascórbico -ca *adj* ascorbic

asearse *vr* (*después de defecar*) to wipe (*oneself*)

aseo *m* hygiene; —— **oral** *or* **bucal** oral hygiene

aséptico -ca *adj* aseptic

asfixia *f* asphyxia

asfixiar *vt, vr* to asphyxiate, suffocate

asientos *mpl* **tener** —— (*CA, fam*) to have diarrhea

asilo *m* asylum, nursing home; —— **de ancianos** nursing home

asistencia *f* assistance; —— **social** *or* **pública** welfare

asistente *mf* assistant, aide; —— **de enfermera** nursing assistant, nurse's aide

asistir *vt* to assist, aid; (*una clínica, clase, etc.*) to attend

asma *f* asthma

asmático -ca *adj & mf* asthmatic

asociación *f* association

asolearse *vr* to get sun

asparagina *f* asparagine

aspecto *m* appearance

aspereza *f* roughness

aspergilosis *f* aspergillosis

áspero -ra *adj* rough, harsh

aspiración *f* aspiration; —— **articular** joint aspiration; —— **con aguja** needle aspiration

aspirar *vt* to aspirate, to inhale

aspirina *f* aspirin

asqueroso -sa *adj* nauseating

astemizol *m* astemizole

astigmatismo *m* astigmatism

astilla *f* sliver, splinter, chip, fragment

astillar *vt, vr* to chip
astringente *adj & m* astringent
atacar *vt* to attack
ataque *m* attack, bout, fit, convulsion, seizure; —— **cardiaco** *or* **al corazón** heart attack; —— **de nervios** (*fam*) anxiety attack, panic attack; —— **de pánico** panic attack; **darle** *or* **pegarle un** —— to have an attack, to have a seizure
atarantado -da *adj* dazed, in a daze, stunned
atarantar *vt* to daze, stun; *vr* to become dazed, to become stunned
ataxia *f* ataxia
atáxico -ca *adj* ataxic
atención *f* attention; —— **del tercer nivel** tertiary care; —— **médica** healthcare; —— **prenatal** prenatal care; —— **primaria** *or* **del primer nivel** primary care
atender *vt* (*un paciente*) to take care of, to treat; (*un parto*) to deliver; **La Dra. Ng atendió seis partos anoche**..Dr. Ng delivered six babies last night...**Atendió a la señora Reid**..She delivered Mrs. Reid... **Atendió a los gemelos**..She delivered the twins.
atenolol *m* atenolol
atenuado -da *adj* attenuated
aterosclerosis *f* atherosclerosis
atípico -ca *adj* atypical
atleta *mf* athlete; **pie** *m* **de** —— athlete's foot
atlético -ca *adj* athletic
atmósfera *f* atmosphere
atolondrado -da *adj* confused
atópico -ca *adj* atopic
atorar *vr* to stick, get stuck; **¿Siente que se le atora la comida?**..Does it feel as though food sticks in your throat?
atragantarse *vr* —— **con** to choke on
atrás *adv* back, ago; **hacia** —— backward; **la parte de** —— the back part; **tres días atrás** three days ago, three days earlier
atravesar *vt* to pierce
atrioventricular (AV) *adj* atrioventricular (A-V)
atrofia *f* atrophy

atrofiarse *vr* to atrophy
atropellar *vt* to run over
atropina *f* atropine
atún *m* tuna
aturdido -da *adj* dazed, in a daze, stunned
aturdimiento *m* daze, dizziness
aturdir *vt* to stun, daze, make dizzy; *vr* to become stunned, dazed, dizzy
audición *f* hearing, sense of hearing
audífono *m* hearing aid; *mpl* headset, headphones
audiograma *m* audiogram
audiología *f* audiology
audiólogo -ga *mf* audiologist
audiometría *f* audiometry
audiómetro *m* audiometer
auditivo -va *adj* auditory
aumentar *vt, vi* to increase, enlarge, (*de peso*) to gain (*weight*); —— **las defensas** to build up (*one's*) resistance
aumento *m* increase, gain, rise
aura *f* aura
aurícula *f* (*del corazón*) atrium
auricular *adj* atrial
auriculoventricular (AV) *adj* atrioventricular (A-V)
ausencia *f* absence
ausente *adj* absent
autismo *m* autism
autista *mf* autist (*form*), autistic person
autístico -ca *adj* autistic
autoayuda *f* self-help
autoclave *m* autoclave
autodestructivo -va *adj* self-destructive
autodisciplina *f* self-discipline
autoestima *f* self-esteem
autoevaluación *f* self-examination
autoexamen *m* self-examination
autoinmune *adj* autoimmune
autoinmunidad *f* autoimmunity
autolimitado -da *adj* self-limited
autólogo -ga *adj* autologous
automóvil *m* automobile, car
autoprescribirse *vr* (*pp* **-scrito**) to self-prescribe
autopsia *f* autopsy
autorrecetarse *vr* to self-prescribe
autorrespeto *m* self-respect

autosómico -ca *adj* autosomal
autotratamiento *m* self-treatment
auxiliar *mf* assistant, aide
auxilio *interj* Help! *m* help, aid; **primeros auxilios** first aid
AV *See* **auriculoventricular.**
avance *m* advance, progress
avena *f* oats, oatmeal; **hojuelas de —** oatmeal
aversión *f* aversion
aves de corral *fpl* poultry
avispa *f* wasp, yellow jacket
avispón *m* hornet
axila *f* axilla, armpit (*fam*)
axilar *adj* axillary
ay *interj* Ouch!
ayer *adv* yesterday

ayuda *f* help, aid, assistance
ayudante *mf* assistant, aide
ayudar *vt, vi* to help, aid, assist
ayunar *vi* to fast
ayunas, en fasting; **glucosa en ayunas** fasting glucose
ayuno *m* fast, fasting; **glucosa en —** fasting glucose
azarcón *m* lead oxide, toxic Mexican folk remedy
azatioprina *f* azathioprine
azitromicina *f* azithromycin
azúcar *m&f* sugar; **sin —** sugarless
azufre *m* sulfur
azul *adj* blue
azulado -da *adj* bluish

B

baba *f* drool
babear *vi* to drool
babero *m* bib
bacilo *m* bacillus, rod; **— de Calmette-Guérin (BCG)** Calmette-Guérin bacillus (BCG)
bacín *m* basin
bacinica *f* bedpan
bacinilla *f* bedpan
bacitracina *f* bacitracin
bacteria *f* bacterium (*en inglés se emplea casi siempre la forma plural:* bacteria)
bacteriano -na *adj* bacterial
bactericida *adj* bactericidal
Bacteroides Bacteroides
baja *f* fall, drop
bajalenguas *m* tongue depressor *o* blade
bajar *vt* to lower; *vi* to go down, fall, drop; **Le bajó el potasio.**.Your potassium went down; **— de peso** to lose weight; **bajarle la regla** (*fam*) to have one's period

bajo -ja *adj* low; (*anat*) lower; (*de estatura*) short; **Su potasio está bajo.**.Your potassium is low...**una dieta baja en fibra**..a low-fiber diet...**la parte baja**..the lower part
bala *f* bullet
balanceado -da *adj* balanced
balanitis *f* balanitis
balanza *f* balance scale, scale
balazo *m* gunshot wound
balbucear *vi* to slur; (*ped*) to babble
balbuceo *m* slurring; (*ped*) babble
balón *m* (*de una sonda Foley, etc.*) balloon
baloncesto *m* basketball
bálsamo *m* balm
banco de sangre *m* blood bank
banda *f* band
bandeja *f* tray
banquito *m* footstool
bañadera *f* (*Cub*) bathtub
bañar *vt* to wash, bathe; *vr* wash oneself, bathe, take a bath; to go swimming

bañera _f_ bathtub
baño _m_ bath; bathroom, rest room; —— **de asiento** sitz bath; —— **de esponja** sponge bath; —— **de regadera** (_Mex_) shower; —— **de vapor** steam bath; —— **para hombres** men's room; —— **para mujeres** women's room; **hacer del** —— (_Mex, fam_) to have a bowel movement; **ir al** —— to go to the bathroom
baranda _f_ bedrail, side rail
barandal _m_ bedrail, side rail
barba _f_ beard, whiskers; chin
barbero _m_ barber
barbilla _f_ chin
barbitúrico _m_ barbiturate
bardana _f_ (_bot_) burdock
bario _m_ barium
barrera _f_ barrier
barriga _f_ belly, stomach (_fam_)
barrigón -na _adj_ potbellied
barriguita _f_ (_ped_) tummy
barril _m_ (_de una jeringa_) barrel
barrio _m_ neighborhood
barro _m_ pimple (_due to acne_)
basal _adj_ baseline
basca _f_ (_frec pl_) nausea, vomiting; vomit; **dar** —— to make sick _o_ nauseated; **tener** —— to be nauseated, to vomit
báscula _f_ scale (_for weighing_)
base _f_ (_chem, pharm_) base; —— **libre de cocaína** freebase; **a** —— **de aceite** oil-based; **a** —— **de agua** water-based
básico -ca _adj_ basic
basketball _m_ (_Ang_) basketball
basquear _vi_ (_esp Mex_) to vomit
bastón _m_ cane; (_del ojo_) rod
bata _f_ gown
batata _f_ (_PR, SD; fam_) calf
baumanómetro _m_ blood pressure cuff
bazo _m_ spleen
BCG _abbr_ **bacilo de Calmette-Guérin**. See **bacilo**.
bebé _m_ (_pl_ **bebés**) baby
bebedero _m_ drinking fountain
bebedor -ra _mf_ drinker
beber _vt, vi_ to drink
bebida _f_ drink
beclometasona _f_ beclomethasone

béisbol _m_ baseball
belcho _m_ (_bot_) ephedra
belladona _f_ belladonna
benazepril _m_ benazepril
bencedrina _f_ benzedrine
benceno _m_ benzene
beneficio _m_ benefit; **por su** —— for your benefit
benéfico -ca _adj_ beneficial
benigno -na _adj_ benign
benjuí _m_ benzoin
benzodiacepina _f_ benzodiazepine
benzoína _f_ benzoin
berenjena _f_ eggplant
beriberi _m_ beriberi
berrinche _m_ tantrum
besar _vt_ to kiss
beso _m_ kiss
beta _f_ beta; —— **bloqueador** _m_ beta blocker
betahemolítico -ca _adj_ beta hemolytic
biberón _m_ nursing bottle, baby's bottle
bicarbonato _m_ bicarbonate; —— **de sodio** sodium bicarbonate
bíceps _m_ (_pl_ **bíceps**) biceps
bicho _m_ bug, tiny animal
bicicleta _f_ bicycle; —— **fija** stationary bicycle; **ir** _or_ **montar en** —— to ride a bicycle
bicúspide _adj & m_ bicuspid
bien _adj & adv_ well; **Estoy bien**..I'm well...**Estoy comiendo bien**..I'm eating well; —— **parecido** good-looking; _m_ good, welfare, benefit; **por su** —— for your benefit; **por su propio** —— for your own good
bienestar _m_ well-being, welfare
bifocal _adj_ bifocal; **lentes** _mpl_ **bifocales** bifocal eyeglasses; **bifocales** _mpl_ (_fam_) bifocals (_fam_)
bigote _m_ moustache
biliar _adj_ biliary
bilingüe _adj_ bilingual
bilirrubina _f_ bilirubin
bilis _f_ bile
biodegradable _adj_ biodegradable
bioestadística _f_ biostatistics
biología _f_ biology
biológico -ca _adj_ biological, biologic

biometría hemática *f* blood count
biopsia *f* biopsy; —— **abierta** open biopsy; —— **con aguja** needle biopsy
bioquímico -ca *adj* biochemical; *f* biochemistry
biorretroalimentación *f* biofeedback
bióxido *m* dioxide; —— **de azufre** sulfur dioxide; —— **de carbono** carbon dioxide
bíper *m* (*Ang*) beeper, pager
bipolar *adj* bipolar
bisabuelo -la *m* great-grandfather, great-grandparent; *f* great-grandmother
bisexual *adj* bisexual
bismuto *m* bismuth
bisnieto -ta, biznieto -ta *m* great-grandson, great-grandchild; *f* great-granddaughter
bistec *m* steak, beefsteak
bisturí *m* (*pl* **-ríes**) scalpel
bizco -ca *adj* cross-eyed; *mf* cross-eyed person
blanco -ca *adj* white, (*tez*) fair
blando -da *adj* soft
blanqueador *m* bleach
blanquillo *m* (*Mex, fam*) egg
blastomicosis *f* blastomycosis
blefaritis *f* blepharitis
bleomicina *f* bleomycin
bloomer *m* (*esp CA*) panties, (*women's*) underpants
bloqueador *m* blocker; —— **de los canales de calcio** calcium channel blocker; —— **de los receptores H₂** H₂-blocker; **beta** —— beta blocker
bloquear *vt* (*pharm, physio*) to block
bloqueo *m* block; obstruction, blockage; —— **cardiaco** heart block; —— **de rama** bundle branch block; —— **nervioso** nerve block
blusa *f* blouse
bobito *m* gnat
bobo *m* (*PR*) pacifier
boca *f* mouth; —— **abajo** facedown; —— **arriba** faceup; —— **del estómago** pit of the stomach; **por la** —— by mouth
bocadillo *m* snack
bocado *m* mouthful
bochorno *m* flush, hot flash
bocio *m* goiter

bola *f* lump, bump
bolita *f* small lump *o* bump
boliviano -na *adj & mf* Bolivian
bolsa *f* pouch; bursa; bag; **bolsas bajo los ojos** bags under one's eyes; —— **de agua caliente** hot-water bottle *o* bag; —— **de hielo** ice pack; —— **de las aguas** bag of waters
bomba *f* pump; bomb; (*esp CA, fam*) blister; —— **atómica** atomic bomb
bombear *vt* to pump
bombero *m* fireman
boquera *f* dryness and fissures at the corners of the mouth; cold sore, fever blister
boquilla *f* mouthpiece
borde *m* border, edge, margin
bordón *m* cane
bórico -ca *adj* boric
borrachera *f* binge
borracho -cha *adj & mf* drunk
borrarse *vr* (*la vista*) to blur; **Se me borra la vista**..My vision blurs.
borroso -sa *adj* blurred; **visión borrosa** blurred vision
bostezar *vi* to yawn
bostezo *m* yawn
bota *f* boot; —— **de pasta de Unna** Unna's paste boot
botana *f* (*Mex*) snack
botanear *vi* (*Mex*) to snack
botanica, botánica *f* herb shop
botar *vt* to eliminate, expel, pass, shed; —— **aire** to breathe out; —— **una piedra** (*al orinar*) to pass a stone
bote *m* can
botella *f* bottle
botica *f* pharmacy, drugstore
boticario -ria *mf* pharmacist, druggist
botiquín *m* medicine chest *o* cabinet; —— **de primeros auxilios** first-aid kit
botulismo *m* botulism
bovino -va *adj* bovine
bradicardia *f* bradycardia
braguero *m* truss
bragueta *f* fly (*of trousers*)
Braille *m* Braille
brasileño -ña *adj & mf* Brazilian
brassiere *m* brassiere

brazalete de identificación *m* identification bracelet

brazo *m* arm

breve *adj* brief, short

brincar *vi* to hop

brinco *m* hop

bromocriptina *f* bromocriptine

bromuro de ipratropio *m* ipratropium bromide

bronceado -da *adj* tan; *m* suntan, tan

broncearse *vr* to tan, to get a suntan

broncodilatador *m* bronchodilator

broncogénico -ca, broncógeno -na *adj* bronchogenic

bronconeumonía *f* bronchopneumonia

broncoscopia, broncoscopía *f* bronchoscopy

broncoscopio *m* bronchoscope

broncospasmo, broncoespasmo *m* bronchospasm

bronquial *adj* bronchial

bronquiectasia *f* bronchiectasis

bronquio *m* bronchus

bronquiolitis *f* bronchiolitis

bronquiolo *m* bronchiole

bronquitis *f* bronchitis

brotar *vi* **brotarle los dientes** (*esp Mex*) to teethe; **brotarle granos** (*esp Mex*) to break out (*one's skin*); **Le brotaron granos.**.His skin broke out.

brote *m* outbreak

brucelosis *f* brucellosis

brujería *f* witchcraft

bruxismo *m* bruxism

bubón *m* bubo

bubónico -ca *adj* bubonic

bucal *adj* oral; **por vía ——** by mouth

buen *See* **bueno.**

bueno -na *adj* (**buen** *before masculine singular nouns*) good; **un buen médico**..a good doctor

buffer *m* buffer

bulbo *m* bulb; **—— raquídeo** medulla

bulimia *f* bulimia

bulímico -ca *adj* bulimic

bulto *m* large lump *o* bump, swelling

bumetanida *f* bumetanide

burbuja *f* bubble

bursitis *f* bursitis

buspirona *f* buspirone

busto *m* bust, female breast

busulfán *m* busulfan

bypass *m* (*Ang*) bypass

C

cabecera *f* head (*of a bed*)

cabello *m* hair (*head only*)

cabestrillo *m* sling

cabeza *f* head; **—— or cabecita de vena** (*fam*) venous star, telangiectasia

cabra *f* goat

caca *f* (*esp Carib, fam*) stool, (*ped*) poopoo

cacahuate, cacahuete *m* peanut

cacao *m* cocoa

cacarizo -za *adj* having pockmarks

cacto, cactus *m* cactus

cadáver *m* cadaver

cadera *f* hip

cadillo *m* (*bot*) burr, sticker

cadmio *m* cadmium

caducado -da *adj* outdated, out of date

caerse *vr* to fall, fall down, collapse; (*los párpados, etc.*) to droop, sag; (*una costra, tejido necrótico, etc.*) to slough

café *adj* brown; *m* (*pl* **cafés**) coffee

cafeína *f* caffeine

caída *f* fall; **—— del pelo** hair loss; **—— de mollera** (*Mex, CA*) sunken fontanel; pediatric folk illness manifest by a sunken fontanel and other signs and symptoms of dehydration, believed to be caused by improper handling of the infant and said to be cured by massage of the upper palate

caja *f* —— **de dientes** (*esp Carib*) denture; —— **torácica** *or* **de las costillas** rib cage

calambre *m* cramp; —— **del escritor** writer's cramp

calamina *f* calamine

calcetín *m* sock

calcificar *vt, vr* to calcify

calcio *m* calcium

calcitonina *f* calcitonin

cálculo *m* stone; —— **biliar** gallstone; —— **renal** *or* **del riñón** kidney stone

caldo *m* broth, soup

calefacción *f* heating

calentador *m* heater

calentamiento *m* warmup; **hacer ejercicios de** —— to warm up (*before exercise*)

calentar *vt, vr* to warm (up), to heat (up)

calentura *f* fever

calibrar *vt* to calibrate

calidad *f* quality; —— **de vida** quality of life

caliente *adj* warm, hot; (*vulg, sexual*) horny (*vulg*), sexually aroused

calistenia *f* calisthenics

callejero -ra *adj* pertaining to the street, street; **droga callejera** street drug

callo *m* callus

callosidad *f* callus, hardened skin

calma *f* calm

calmante *adj & m* sedative

calmar *vt* to calm, soothe; *vr* to calm down, quiet down

calomel *m* calomel

calor *m* heat, warmth; hot flash; —— **corporal** body heat; **tener** *or* **sentir** —— to be *o* feel hot; **Tengo mucho calor**..I'm really hot.

caloría *f* calorie

calostro *m* colostrum

calvicie *f* baldness

calvo -va *adj* bald

calzado *m* footwear; —— **ortopédico** orthopedic shoes

calzón *m* (*frec pl*) panties, (*women's*) underpants

calzoncillos *mpl* underpants

cama *f* bed

cámara *f* chamber; —— **hiperbárica** hyperbaric chamber

camarón *m* shrimp

cambiar *vt, vi* to change

cambio *m* change; —— **de vida** change of life

camilla *f* stretcher, litter

caminar *vi* to walk; —— **dormido** to sleepwalk, walk in one's sleep

caminata *f* long walk, hike

camisa *f* shirt; —— **de fuerza** straitjacket

camiseta *f* undershirt

camisón *m* gown

campanilla *f* uvula

campaña *f* campaign

campo *m* field; rural area, country; —— **visual** visual field

Campylobacter Campylobacter

cana *f* gray hair

canadillo *m* (*bot*) ephedra

canal *m* canal; —— **auditivo** auditory tube *o* canal; —— **del parto** birth canal

cancelar *vt* to cancel

cáncer *m* cancer; —— **de la mama, del seno** *or* **del pecho** breast cancer; —— **del pulmón, de la próstata, etc.** lung cancer, prostate cancer, etc.

cancerología *f* oncology, study of cancer

cancerólogo -ga *mf* oncologist, cancer specialist

canceroso -sa *adj* cancerous

Candida Candida

candidiasis *f* candidiasis

canilla *f* shin, leg, thin leg, calf

canillera *f* shin guard

canino *m* (*diente*) cuspid, canine tooth

cansado -da *adj* tired

cansancio *m* tiredness, fatigue; —— **visual** eyestrain

cansar *vt* to tire (out), make tired; *vr* to tire (out), get tired

canto negro *m* (*PR, fam*) bruise

canturrear *vt, vi* to hum (*a note*)

cánula *f* cannula; —— **nasal** nasal cannula

caño *m* (*fam*) prick (*fam*), penis

capa *f* coating, layer, film

capacidad *f* ability, capacity
capar *vt* (*fam*) to castrate
capaz *adj* (*pl* capaces) capable
capilar *m* capillary
cápsula *f* capsule
captación *f* uptake
captopril *m* captopril
capuchón cervical *m* cervical cap
cara *f* face
caracol *m* snail
característico -ca *adj* characteristic; *f* characteristic, trait
carbamazepina, carbamacepina *f* carbamazepine
carbidopa *f* carbidopa
carbohidrato *m* carbohydrate
carbón *m* coal, charcoal; —— activado activated charcoal
carbonatado -da *adj* carbonated
carbonato *m* carbonate; —— de calcio calcium carbonate
carbono *m* carbon (*element*)
carbunco *m* carbuncle
cárcel *f* jail; prison
carcinoide *adj* & *m* carcinoid
carcinoma *m* carcinoma; —— basocelular basal cell carcinoma; —— de células en avena oat cell carcinoma; —— de células pequeñas small cell carcinoma; —— espinocelular *or* de células escamosas squamous cell carcinoma
cardenal *m* bruise
cardiaco -ca, cardíaco -ca *adj* cardiac
cardiogénico -ca, cardiógeno -na *adj* cardiogenic
cardiología *f* cardiology
cardiólogo -ga *mf* cardiologist
cardiomiopatía *f* cardiomyopathy; —— dilatada dilated cardiomyopathy; —— hipertrófica hypertrophic cardiomyopathy; —— restrictiva restrictive cardiomyopathy
cardiopatía *f* cardiopathy; —— reumática rheumatic heart disease
cardiopulmonar *adj* cardiopulmonary
cardiovascular *adj* cardiovascular
cardioversión *f* cardioversion
carditis *f* carditis

cardo *m* thistle
carecer *vt* —— de to lack
carencia *f* lack, deficiency
careta *f* face mask, shield
caridad *f* charity
caries *f* caries, tooth decay
cariño *m* affection, love
cariñoso -sa *adj* affectionate, loving
carne *f* flesh; meat; —— de cerdo pork; —— de cordero lamb; —— de puerco pork; —— de res beef; —— viva raw flesh
carnicero -ra *mf* butcher
carnosidad *f* pterygium (*form*), benign growth on the eye
carnoso -sa *adj* fleshy
carótido -da *adj* carotid
carpiano -na *adj* carpal
carpintero -ra *mf* carpenter
carraspear *vi* to clear one's throat
carraspera *f* irritation of the throat
carrillo *m* inside wall of mouth, cheek
carro *m* car, automobile
carta *f* chart; —— del examen visual eye chart; —— de Snellen Snellen chart
cartílago *m* cartilage
casa *f* home; —— de cuna orphanage; en —— at home
cáscara sagrada *f* (*bot*) cascara sagrada
casco *m* helmet
casero -ra *adj* homemade, home; remedio —— home remedy
caso *m* case; en nueve de diez casos..in nine out of ten cases
caspa *f* dandruff
castañetear *vi* (*los dientes*) to chatter
castración *f* castration
castrar *vt* to castrate
cataplasma *f* plaster (*medicinal*)
catarata *f* cataract
catarro *m* cold; runny nose
catatonía *f* catatonia
catatónico -ca *adj* catatonic
catéter *m* catheter; —— central central line; —— Foley Foley catheter; —— Hickman Hickman catheter; —— Tenckhoff Tenckhoff catheter
cateterismo *m* catheterization; ——

cardiaco cardiac catheterization
catgut *m* catgut
causa *f* cause
causalgia *f* causalgia
causar *vt* to cause
cáustico -ca *adj* caustic
cauterización *f* cauterization
cauterizar *vt* to cauterize
cavidad *f* cavity
cc. *abbr* **centímetro cúbico.** *See* **centímetro.**
cebolla *f* onion
cecear *vi* to lisp
ceceo *m* lisp
cefaclor *m* cefaclor
cefadroxil *m* cefadroxil
cefalea *f* (*form*) headache; —— **en grupos** cluster headache; —— **por tensión** *or* **tensional** tension headache; —— **postraumática** postconcussional syndrome; —— **vascular** vascular headache
cefalexina *f* cephalexin
cefálico -ca *adj* cephalic
cefalosporina *f* cephalosporin
cefalotina *f* cephalothin
cefixima *f* cefixime
cefotaxima *f* cefotaxime
cefprozil *m* cefprozil
ceftriaxona *f* ceftriaxone
ceguera *f* blindness; —— **nocturna** night blindness
ceja *f* eyebrow
celíaco -ca, celíaco -ca *adj* celiac
célula *f* cell; —— **B** B cell; —— **plasmática** plasma cell; —— **T** T cell
celulitis *f* cellulitis; (*depósitos de grasa debajo de la piel*) cellulite
cena *f* dinner, supper
centígrado -da *adj* centigrade
centímetro (cm.) *m* centimeter (cm.); —— **cúbico (cc.)** centimeter cubed *o* cubic centimeter (cc.)
central *adj* central
centro *m* center; —— **de salud** healthcare center
cepa *f* strain (*of bacteria, etc.*)
cepillado *m* brushing
cepillar *vt* to brush; *vr* **cepillarse el pelo** to brush one's hair; **cepillarse los dientes** to brush one's teeth
cepillo *m* brush; —— **de dientes** toothbrush
cera *f* wax
cerclaje *m* cerclage
cerda *f* bristle; **cepillo de cerdas duras** brush with stiff bristles
cerdo *m* pork
cereal *m* cereal, grain
cerebelo *m* cerebellum
cerebral *adj* cerebral
cerebro *m* cerebrum (*form*), brain; (*fam*) back of head or neck; —— **medio** midbrain
cerebrovascular *adj* cerebrovascular
cerilla *f* earwax
cerrar *vt* to close; —— **la mano** to make a fist; *vi, vr* to close
certificado *m* certificate; —— **de defunción** death certificate; —— **de nacimiento** birth certificate; —— **para no trabajar** work excuse
cerveza *f* beer
cervical *adj* cervical
cervicitis *f* cervicitis
cérvix *f* (*pl* **-vix**) cervix
cetoacidosis *f* ketoacidosis
cetona *f* ketone
cetónico -ca *adj* ketotic; **no** —— nonketotic
chalazión *m* chalazion
chamaco -ca *m* boy, child; *f* girl
chamarra *f* (*Mex*) jacket
chamorro *m* (*Mex, fam*) calf (*of leg*)
champú *m* (*pl* **-púes**) shampoo
chancro *m* chancre; —— **blando** soft chancre
chancroide *f* chancroid
chaparro -ra *adj* short (*stature*)
chaqueta *f* jacket; (*dent*) cap
charlatán -na *mf* charlatan, quack
charola *f* (*Mex*) tray
chasquido *m* (*card*) click
chata *f* bedpan
chato *m* (*Mex, fam*) crab louse, crab (*fam*)
chequear *vt* (*Ang*) to check
chequeo *m* checkup
chichi, chiche, chicha *f* (*vulg*) breast
chichón *m* lump, bump (*due to trauma, esp about the head*)

chicle *m* chewing gum

chico -ca *adj* small, little; *m* boy, child; *f* girl

chiflar *vi* **chiflarle el pecho** to wheeze

chiflido *m* wheeze

chile *m* chili

chileno -na *adj & mf* Chilean

chillar *vi* to squeal; (*el pecho*) to wheeze; **Me chilla el pecho cuando hace frío..**I wheeze when the weather is cold.

chillido *m* wheeze; **Tengo chillidos..**I have wheezing.

chimpinilla *f* (*CA, fam*) shin

china *f* (*PR, fam*) orange

chinche *f* bedbug; (*vector de la enfermedad de Chagas*) kissing bug

chipote *m* (*Mex, CA; fam*) lump, bump (*due to trauma*)

chiva *f* (*Mex, vulg*) heroin; (*PR, fam*) jaw

chivola *f* (*ES*) bump, lump

Chlamydia Chlamydia

chocho -cha *adj* senile

chocolate *m* chocolate

choque *m* shock; automobile accident; —— **anafiláctico** anaphylactic shock; —— **cardiogénico** *or* **cardiógeno** cardiogenic shock; —— **eléctrico** electric shock; —— **hipovolémico** hypovolemic shock; —— **nervioso** nervous breakdown; —— **neurogénico** *or* **neurógeno** neurogenic shock; —— **séptico** septic shock

choquezuela *f* kneecap

chorizo *m* sausage

chorrear *vi* to flow, run

chorro *m* (*de la orina*) stream; (*Mex, CA; fam*) diarrhea

choyarse *vr* (*Nic*) to graze (*oneself*)

choyón *m* (*Nic*) graze

chucho *m* (*SA*) malaria

chueco -ca *adj* (*SA*) bowlegged; (*Mex*) crooked

chupar *vt* to suck; **chuparse el dedo** to suck one's thumb

chupete *m* pacifier; hickey

chupón *m* pacifier; hickey

CIA *abbr* **comunicación interauricular**. *See* **comunicación**.

cianosis *f* cyanosis

cianótico -ca *adj* cyanotic

cianuro *m* cyanide

ciático -ca *adj* sciatic; *f* sciatica

cicatriz *f* (*pl* **-trices**) scar; **dejar** —— to leave a scar

cicatrizar *vt, vr* to heal (*a wound*)

ciclamato *m* cyclamate

cíclico -ca *adj* cyclic

ciclismo *m* cycling

ciclo *m* cycle; —— **anovulatorio** anovulatory cycle; —— **menstrual** menstrual cycle; —— **ovulatorio** ovulatory cycle; —— **reproductor** reproductive cycle

ciclofosfamida *f* cyclophosphamide

ciclosporina *f* cyclosporin

cicuta *f* (*bot*) hemlock

ciego -ga *adj* blind; *mf* blind person; *m* cecum

ciempiés *m* (*pl* **-piés**) centipede

científico -ca *adj* scientific; *mf* scientist

cierre *m* zipper

cierto -ta *adj* sure

cifoscoliosis *f* kyphoscoliosis

cifosis *f* kyphosis

cigarrillo *m* cigarette

cigarro *m* cigarette, cigar

cilindro urinario *m* urinary cast

cimetidina *f* cimetidine

cinc *m* zinc; **óxido de** —— zinc oxide

cincho *m* belt

cinta *f* tape, band; —— **adhesiva** adhesive tape; —— **de mariposa** butterfly bandage; —— **métrica** measuring tape; —— **reactiva** test strip, dipstick

cinto *m* belt

cintura *f* waist; **de la** —— **para arriba** from the waist up

cinturón *m* belt, wide belt, (*para prevenir hernias*) abdominal supporter, kidney belt; —— **de seguridad** seat belt

ciprofloxacina *f* ciprofloxacin

circadiano -na *adj* circadian

circulación *f* circulation; —— **colateral** collateral circulation; —— **fetal** fetal circulation; —— **pulmonar** pulmonary circulation; —— **sistémica** *or* **mayor** systemic circulation

circular *vi* to circulate

circulatorio -ria *adj* circulatory

círculo *m* circle
circuncidar *vt* (*pp* **-ciso**) to circumcise
circuncisión *f* circumcision
circunciso -sa (*pp of* **circuncidar**) *adj* circumcised
cirrosis *f* cirrhosis
cirrótico -ca *adj & mf* cirrhotic
ciruela *f* plum; —— **pasa** prune
cirugía *f* surgery; —— **cosmética** *or* **estética** cosmetic surgery; —— **de corazón abierto** open heart surgery; —— **electiva** elective surgery; —— **general** general surgery; —— **mayor** major surgery; —— **menor** minor surgery; —— **oral** oral surgery; —— **ortopédica** orthopedic surgery; —— **plástica** plastic surgery; —— **radical** radical surgery; —— **reconstructiva** reconstructive surgery
cirujano -na *mf* surgeon
cisaprida *f* cisapride
cisplatin *m* cisplatin
cistectomía *f* cystectomy
cisteína *f* cysteine
cisticercosis *f* cysticercosis
cístico -ca *adj* cystic (*duct, artery*)
cistinuria *f* cystinuria
cistitis *f* cystitis
cistocele *m* cystocele
cistoscopia, cistoscopía *f* cystoscopy
cistoscopio *m* cystoscope
cita *f* appointment
citología *f* (*exfoliativa*) Papanicolaou smear
citomegalovirus *m* cytomegalovirus
citotóxico -ca *adj* cytotoxic
citrato *m* citrate
cítrico -ca *adj* citric; *mpl* citrus fruits
CIV *abbr* **comunicación interventricular.** *See* **comunicación.**
claritromicina *f* clarithromycin
claro -ra *adj* clear; *f* (*de huevo*) white (*of an egg*)
clase *f* class
clásico -ca *adj* classic
claudicación *f* claudication; —— **intermitente** intermittent claudication
claustrofobia *f* claustrophobia
clavícula *f* clavicle

clavo *m* nail; (*ortho*) pin
clima *m* climate, weather
clímax *m* (*pl* **-max**) (*sexual*) climax, orgasm
clindamicina *f* clindamycin
clínico -ca *adj* clinical; *m* clinician; *f* clinic; **clínica de urgencias** urgent care clinic
clítoris *m* clitoris
clofazimina *f* clofazimine
clofibrato *m* clofibrate
clomifén *m* clomiphene
clona *f* clone
clonacepam *m* clonazepam
clónico -ca *adj* clonic
clonidina *f* clonidine
clonus, clono *m* clonus
cloración *f* chlorination
clorado -da *adj* chlorinated
clorambucilo *m* chlorambucil
cloranfenicol, cloramfenicol *m* chloramphenicol
clordano *m* chlordane
clorfeniramina *f* chlorpheniramine
clorhexidina *f* chlorhexidine
clorhídrico -ca *adj* hydrochloric
cloro *m* chlorine
cloroformo *m* chloroform
cloropromacina *f* chlorpromazine
cloroquina *f* chloroquine
clorpropamida *f* chlorpropamide
cloruro *m* chloride; —— **de sodio** sodium chloride
Clostridium Clostridium
clotrimazol *m* clotrimazole
cm. *See* **centímetro.**
coagulación *f* coagulation; —— **intravascular diseminada** disseminated intravascular coagulation (DIC)
coagular *vt, vr* to clot, coagulate
coágulo *m* clot
coagulopatía *f* coagulopathy
coartación *f* coarctation
cobalto *m* cobalt
cobayo *m* guinea pig
cobertor *m* bedspread; —— **eléctrico** electric blanket
cobertura *f* (*seguros*) coverage
cobija *f* (*esp Mex*) blanket; —— **eléctrica** electric blanket

cobre *m* copper
cobro *m* bill, charge
coca *f* (*bot*) coca; (*fam*) cocaine, coke (*fam*); —— **en pasta** freebase (*cocaine*)
cocaína *f* cocaine
cocainómano -na *mf* cocaine addict
coccidioidomicosis *f* coccidioidomycosis
cóccix *m* coccyx
cocer *vt, vi* to cook; (*carne*) to boil; —— **al horno** to bake; —— **al vapor** to steam
coche *m* automobile, car
cocido -da *adj* cooked, boiled; —— **al horno** baked; —— **al vapor** steamed
cociente de inteligencia (CI) *m* intelligence quotient (IQ)
cocinar *vt, vi* to cook
cocinero -ra *mf* cook
cóclea *f* cochlea
coco *m* (*micro*) coccus; (*bot*) coconut
codeína *f* codeine
código postal *m* zip code
codo *m* elbow; —— **de tenista** tennis elbow
coger *vt* to grasp, grip; (*una enfermedad*) to catch
cohibición *f* inhibition
cohibido -da *adj* inhibited
coito *m* coitus; —— **bucal** *or* **oral** fellatio; —— **interrumpido** coitus interruptus
cojear *vi* to limp
cojín *m* cushion, pad; —— **eléctrico** heating pad
cojincillo *m* small cushion, pad
cojo -ja *adj* lame, crippled; *mf* lame person, crippled person
cojón *m* (*vulg, frec pl*) ball (*vulg, frec pl*), testicle
cola de caballo *f* (*bot*) horsetail
colador *m* sieve, strainer
colágeno, colágena *m* collagen
colangiocarcinoma *m* cholangiocarcinoma
colangiografía *f* cholangiography; cholangiogram; —— **transhepática percutánea** percutaneous transhepatic cholangiography (PTC)
colangiograma *m* cholangiogram
colangiopancreatografía retrógrada endoscópica *f* endoscopic retrograde cholangiopancreatography (ERCP)

colangitis *f* cholangitis
colapso *m* collapse, breakdown; —— **nervioso** nervous breakdown; **sufrir un** —— to collapse
colar *vt* to strain; **Tiene que colar su orina para buscar piedras.** You have to strain your urine for stones.
colateral *adj* collateral
colcha *f* blanket
colchicina *f* colchicine
colchón *m* mattress
colecistectomía *f* cholecystectomy
colecistitis *f* cholecystitis
colectomía *f* colectomy
colega *mf* colleague
colelitiasis *f* cholelithiasis
cólera *m* cholera; *f* anger, rage
colesteatoma *f* cholesteatoma
colesterol *m* cholesterol
colestiramina *f* cholestyramine
colgajo *m* (*surg*) flap
colgar *vt* to hang, to dangle
cólico -ca *adj* pertaining to the colon, (*anat*) colic; *m* colic; —— **menstrual** menstrual cramp(s)
coliflor *f* cauliflower
colirio *m* eyewash
colitis *f* colitis; —— **seudomembranosa** pseudomembranous colitis; —— **ulcerosa** ulcerative colitis
collar cervical *m* (*rígido, blando*) cervical collar (*hard, soft*)
collarín *m* (*rígido, blando*) cervical collar (*hard, soft*)
colmillo *m* cuspid, canine tooth, fang
coloidal *adj* colloidal
coloide *m* colloid
colombiano -na *adj & mf* Colombian
colon *m* colon; —— **ascendente** ascending colon; —— **descendente** descending colon; —— **sigmoide** sigmoid colon; —— **transverso** transverse colon
colónico -ca *adj* colonic, pertaining to the colon
colonización *f* colonization
colonoscopia, colonoscopía *f* colonoscopy
colonoscopio *m* colonoscope
color *m* color

coloración f (*micro*) stain; —— **de Gram** Gram's stain

colorado -da *adj* red

colorante m dye

colostomía f colostomy; **bolsa para** —— colostomy bag

colposcopia, colposcopía f colposcopy

colquicina f colchicine

columna f backbone, spine; —— **cervical** cervical spine; —— **lumbar** lumbar spine; —— **sacra** sacral spine; —— **torácica** or **dorsal** thoracic spine; —— **vertebral** spinal column

coma m coma; **en** —— in a coma

comadrona f midwife (*esp without training*)

comatoso -sa *adj* comatose

combinación f combination

combustible m fuel

comer vt, vi to eat; (*Mex*) to have lunch; **dar de** —— to feed; vr **comerse las uñas** to bite o chew one's nails

comestible m food

comezón f itching, itch; **tener** —— to itch

comida f food, meal; (*Mex*) lunch; —— **balanceada** balanced meal; —— **para niños** baby food

comienzo m onset, beginning

comodidad f comfort

cómodo -da *adj* comfortable; m (*Mex*) bedpan

compañero -ra mf companion

compasión f compassion, sympathy

compasivo -va *adj* sympathetic

compatible *adj* compatible

compensar vt, vi to compensate

complejo m complex; —— **de Edipo** Oedipal complex; —— **relacionado con el SIDA** AIDS-related complex (ARC)

complemento m complement

completo -ta *adj* complete

complexión f build, physique

complicación f complication

componer vt (pp -**puesto**) to fix; vr (*fam*) to get well

comportamiento m behavior

comportarse vr to behave

comprensivo -va *adj* understanding, sympathetic

compresa f compress, pack; —— **de hielo** ice pack

compresión f compression, (*de un nervio*) entrapment; **compresiones torácicas** chest compressions

comprimido m tablet

comprimir vt to compress

comprometer vt to compromise

compuesto m compound

compuesto pp of **componer**

compulsión f compulsion

compulsivo -va *adj* compulsive

computadora f computer

común *adj* common; **poco** —— uncommon

comunicación f communication; —— **interauricular (CIA)** atrial septal defect (ASD); —— **interventricular (CIV)** ventricular septal defect (VSD)

comunidad f community

comunitario -ria *adj* community

cóncavo -va *adj* concave

concebir vi to conceive

concentración f concentration

concentrado -da *adj* concentrated; m (*pharm*) concentrate

concentrar vt, vr to concentrate

concepción f conception

conciencia f consciousness; conscience; —— **culpable** guilty conscience; **perder la** —— to lose consciousness

concusión f concussion

condado m county (*US*)

condición f condition

condicionado -da *adj* conditioned

condimento m spice

condón m condom, rubber (*fam*)

condrosarcoma m chondrosarcoma

conducir vt (*un vehículo*) to drive

conducta f behavior; **modificación** f **de la** —— behavior modification

conducto m duct; canal; —— **arterioso persistente** patent ductus arteriosus (PDA); —— **de Eustaquio** Eustachian tube; —— **deferente** or —— **excretorio del testículo** vas deferens; —— **semicircular** semicircular canal

conectar vt to connect

conejillo de Indias m guinea pig (*esp fig*)

conexión *f* connection

confabulación *f* confabulation

confiable *adj* reliable

confianza *f* confidence, trust; —— **en sí mismo** self-confidence; **tener** —— **(en)** to trust

confiar *vi* to trust; **Confío en Ud...**I trust you.

confidencial *adj* confidential, private

conflicto *m* conflict

confort *m* comfort

confortar *vt* to comfort

confrontar *vt* to confront

confundido -da *adj* confused

confundir *vt* to confuse; *vr* to become confused

confusión *f* confusion

congelación *f* freezing; (*path*) frostbite

congelar *vt, vr* to freeze

congénito -ta *adj* congenital

congestión *f* congestion

congestionado -da *adj* congested

congestivo -va *adj* congestive

conjugado -da *adj* conjugated

conjuntiva *f* conjunctiva

conjuntivitis *f* conjunctivitis, pinkeye (*fam*)

conminuto -ta *adj* comminuted

conmoción *f* concussion

cono *m* cone

conocimiento *m* consciousness; **perder el** —— to lose consciousness

consciencia *See* **conciencia**.

consciente *adj* conscious; —— **de sí mismo** self-conscious

consecuencia *f* consequence

consecutivo -va *adj* consecutive

consejero -ra *mf* counselor

consejo *m* advice, recommendation

consentimiento *m* consent

consentir *vt* to pamper, spoil; *vi* to consent; —— **en** to consent to

conservador -ra *adj* (*medidas, etc.*) conservative

consistencia *f* consistency

consolador *m* (*fam*) dildo

consolar *vt* to console, to comfort

consomé *m* consommé, broth

constante *adj* constant, (*dolor*) steady

constipación *f* (*del intestino*) constipation; (*esp Mex, CA; de la nariz*) congestion, nasal congestion

constipado -da *adj* (*del intestino*) constipated; (*esp Mex, CA; de la nariz*) congested, having nasal congestion

constipar *vt* to constipate; *vr* to become constipated; (*esp Mex, CA; de la nariz*) to become congested

constitución *f* constitution

constricción *f* constriction

consuelda *f* (*bot*) comfrey

consulta *f* consultation; **horas de** —— office hours; **pasar (la)** —— to visit (*a doctor*)

consultar *vt* to consult

consultorio *m* office (*of a doctor*)

consumo *m* consumption

contacto *m* contact

contador *m* meter, measuring device

contagiar *vt* (*una enfermedad*) to give, to spread; **Me contagió la gripe..**He gave me the flu; *vr* to catch, to become infected; **Me contagié con la gripe..**I caught the flu...**Podría contagiarse..**You could become infected.

contagioso -sa *adj* contagious, catching (*fam*)

contaminación *f* contamination, pollution; —— **atmosférica** *or* **del aire** air pollution, smog

contaminar *vt* to contaminate; *vr* to become contaminated

contar *vt, vi* to count

contenido *m* content(s)

contento -ta *adj* happy

continuo -nua *adj* continual

contorno *m* contour

contracción *f* contraction; —— **auricular prematura** premature atrial contraction (PAC); —— **ventricular prematura** premature ventricular contraction (PVC)

contracepción *f* contraception

contraceptivo -va *adj & m* contraceptive

contractura *f* contracture

contraer *vt, vr* to contract

contraindicación *f* contraindication

contrarrestar *vt* to counteract

control *m* control; —— **de la natalidad** birth control; **fuera de** —— out of control

controlar *vt* to control

contusión *f* contusion

convalecencia *f* convalescence

convalecerse *vr* to convalesce

convaleciente *adj* convalescent

conversión *f* conversion; **reacción** *f* **de** —— conversion reaction

convexo -xa *adj* convex

convulsión *f* convulsion, seizure

cónyuge *mf* spouse

cooperar *vi* to cooperate

cooperativo -va *adj* cooperative

coordinación *f* coordination

coprocultivo *m* stool culture

coqueluche *m&f* whooping cough

coraje *m* rage

coral *m* coral

corazón *m* heart; core; **ataque** *m* **al** —— heart attack; **enfermedad** *f* **del** —— heart disease

corcova *f* hump

corcovado -da *mf* humpback

cordal *See* **muela cordal**.

cordero *m* lamb

cordón *m* cord; —— **umbilical** umbilical cord

cordura *f* sanity

corea *f* chorea; —— **de Huntington** Huntington's chorea

coriocarcinoma *m* choriocarcinoma

coriorretinitis *f* chorioretinitis

córnea *f* cornea

corona *f* (*anat, dent*) crown

coronario -ria *adj* coronary

corporal *adj* corporal

corpúsculo *m* corpuscle

correa *f* strap

corrección *f* correction, adjustment

correctivo -va *adj* corrective

correcto -ta *adj* correct

corredor *m* hall, hallway

corregir *vt* to correct; *vi* (*Cub*) to have a bowel movement

correlación *f* correlation

correoso -sa *adj* tough, leathery

correr *vi* to run

corrosivo -va *adj* corrosive

corsé *m* (*pl* **-sés**) girdle; truss

cortada *f* cut

cortadura *f* cut

cortar *vt* to cut; *vr* to cut oneself; **Me corté..**I cut myself...**Me corté la mano..**I cut my hand; **cortarse el pelo** to get a haircut; **cortarse las uñas** to cut one's nails

corte *m* cut; —— **de pelo** haircut; —— **por congelación** frozen section

corteza *f* bark; (*anat*) cortex

cortical *adj* cortical

corticosteroide *m* corticosteroid

cortisol *m* cortisol

cortisona *f* cortisone

corto -ta *adj* short; **a** —— **plazo** short-term; **hacer más** —— to shorten

cortocircuito *m* shunt (*physiological*)

corva *f* back of the knee; ham; **tendón** *m* **de la** —— hamstring

coser *vt* (*una herida*) to sew, stitch (up)

cosmético -ca *adj & m* cosmetic

cosquillas *fpl* tickling; **¿Siente cosquillas?..** Do you feel tickling?..Does that tickle?... **¿Le causo cosquillas?..**Am I tickling you?

cosquilleo *m* tickle, tickling

cosquilloso -sa *adj* ticklish

costado *m* (*anat*) side

costarricense *adj & mf* Costa Rican

costilla *f* rib

costo *m* charge, cost

costocondritis *f* costochondritis

costra *f* scab, crust

costumbre *f* habit; **como de** —— as usual; **¿Está comiendo tanto como de costumbre?..**Are you eating as much as usual; **que de** —— than usual; **¿Está orinando más que de costumbre?..**Are you urinating more than usual?

cotidiano -na *adj* daily, everyday; **rutina** —— daily routine

coyuntura *f* joint

crack *m* (*Ang*) crack (*cocaine*)

craneal *adj* cranial

craneano -na *adj* cranial

cráneo *m* cranium (*form*), skull

craneofaringioma *m* craniopharyngioma

craneotomía f craniotomy

creatinina f creatinine

crecer vi to grow, to get bigger; to grow up

crecimiento m growth

creencia f belief

crema f cream; —— **dental** toothpaste; —— **limpiadora** cold cream; —— **para el sol** suntan lotion; —— **para los labios** lip balm

cresa f maggot

cresta f (Mex) genital wart

cretinismo m cretinism

cretino -na mf cretin

criar vt to raise (a child); to nurture

criatura f infant, baby

crioterapia f cryotherapy

criptorquidia f cryptorchidism

crisis f (pl -sis) crisis; (convulsiva) seizure; —— **blástica** blast crisis; —— **de ausencia** absence seizure; —— **de identidad** identity crisis; —— **de la edad madura** midlife crisis; —— **del lóbulo temporal** temporal lobe seizure; —— **focal** focal seizure; —— **generalizada** generalized seizure; —— **gran mal** gran mal seizure; —— **jacksoniana** Jacksonian seizure; —— **nerviosa** nervous breakdown; —— **parcial compleja** complex partial seizure; —— **pequeño mal** petit mal seizure; —— **psicomotora** psychomotor seizure; —— **tiroidea** thyroid storm; —— **tonicoclónica** tonic-clonic seizure

cristal m crystal

cristalino m lens (of the eye)

crítico -ca adj critical

cromo m chromium

cromoglicato de sodio m cromolyn sodium

cromomicosis f chromomycosis

cromosoma m chromosome

crónico -ca adj chronic

crudo -da adj raw; (Mex) hungover; f (Mex) hangover; **tener una cruda** to have a hangover, to be hungover

cruel adj cruel

crueldad f cruelty

crup m croup

Cruz Roja f Red Cross

cruzar vt (la sangre) to crossmatch (blood); —— **los brazos** to fold one's arms

Cryptococcus Cryptococcus

cuadrado -da adj square, squared; **metro** —— meter squared o square meter

cuadrante m quadrant

cuádriceps m (pl -ceps) quadriceps

cuadril m hip bone, hip

cuadrillizo -za mf quadruplet

cuadriplejía f quadriplegia

cuadripléjico -ca adj & mf quadriplegic

cuadrupleto -ta mf quadruplet

cuajarón m (Mex, fam) clot, large clot

cuarentena f quarantine; (Mex, CA) forty days following childbirth; **poner en** —— to quarantine

cuarto m room, bedroom; (de galón) quart; —— **de baño** bathroom

cuasiorcor m kwashiorkor

cuate -ta mf (Mex, fam) twin

cubano -na adj & mf Cuban

cubierto pp of **cubrir**

cubital adj ulnar

cúbito m ulna

cubreboca m (surg, etc.) mask

cubrir vt (pp **cubierto**) to cover; (el estómago, etc.) to coat

cucaracha f cockroach

cucharada f spoonful, tablespoonful

cucharadita f teaspoonful

cuchillada f knife wound, gash

cuchillo m knife

cuclillas, en squatting

cuello m neck; collar; —— **uterino** or **de la matriz** cervix

cuenca f (del ojo) socket

cuenta f bill, charges

cuentagotas m medicine dropper, eyedropper

cuerda f cord; —— **vocal** vocal cord

cuerdo -da adj sane

cuero cabelludo m scalp

cuerpo m body; —— **de bomberos** fire department; —— **extraño** foreign body

cuestionario m questionnaire

cuidado m care; —— **del primer nivel** primary care; —— **del tercer nivel** tertiary care; **cuidados intensivos** intensive care; **tener** —— to be careful; **Tenga**

cuidado con este medicamento..Be careful with this medication.

cuidador -ra *mf* caregiver, caretaker

cuidar *vt* to care for, take care of; **¿Quién cuida a su abuelo en casa?**..Who cares for your grandfather at home? *vr* to take care of oneself; (*fam*) to use birth control; **Tiene que cuidarse si no quiere quedarse embarasada**..You have to use birth control if you don't want to end up pregnant.

culdocentesis *f* (*pl* -sis) culdocentesis

culdoscopia, culdoscopía *f* culdoscopy

culebra *f* snake

culebrilla *f* (*esp Carib*) shingles

culero *m* (*Carib*) diaper

culpa *f* guilt; **sentimientos de —— guilt** feelings

cultivar *vt* (*micro*) to culture

cultivo *m* (*micro*) culture

cultura *f* culture

cumarina *f* coumarin

cumpleaños *m* birthday; **¡Feliz cumpleaños!**..Happy birthday!

cuna *f* cradle, crib

cunilinguo *m* cunnilingus

cuña *f* wedge

cuñada *f* sister-in-law

cuñado *m* brother-in-law

cura *m* priest; *f* cure

curable *adj* curable

curación *f* cure, treatment; **—— de nervio** (*fam, dent*) root canal

curanderismo *m* folk medicine, faith healing

curandero -ra *mf* folk healer, faith healer

curar *vt* to cure, heal, treat; *vr* to be cured, heal, get well

curativo -va *adj* curative

curetaje *m* curettage

Curita *m&f* Band-Aid (*Los dos términos son marcas. Both terms are trademarks.*)

curso *m* course

curva *f* curve, bend; **—— de crecimiento** growth curve

curvatura *f* curvature

cutáneo -a *adj* cutaneous

cutícula *f* cuticle

cutis *m* complexion

D

dacriocistitis *f* dacryocystitis

daltoniano -na *adj* color-blind

daltonismo *m* color blindness

damiana *f* (*bot*) damiana

danazol *m* danazol

dañado -da *adj* damaged, impaired

dañar *vt* to damage, harm

dañino -na *adj* harmful; **no —— harmless**

daño *m* damage, harm; **hacer —— to hurt,** damage, harm; to be bad for (*one*), to make (*one*) sick; **No le hizo ningún daño la caída**..The fall didn't hurt him at all...**¿Le hace daño la medicina?**..Is the medicine making you sick?

dapsona *f* dapsone

dar *vt* **—— a luz** to give birth to, deliver; **La señora Ruiz dio a luz una niña ayer**..Mrs. Ruiz gave birth to a baby girl yesterday; **—— de alta** to discharge (*from the hospital*); **Voy a darle de alta mañana**..I am going to discharge you tomorrow; **—— de comer** to feed; **—— del cuerpo** (*Carib, fam*) to have a bowel movement; **darle** (*a uno*) to have, to get, to catch; **Le dieron vómitos**..He had vomiting...**Me dio un catarro**..I got a cold; **—— pecho, —— seno,** *or* **—— de mamar** to breast-feed, to nurse; **¿Le va a dar pecho?**..Are you going to breast-feed him? *vi* **—— a luz** to give birth, to deliver; *vr* **darse vuelta** to turn around, to turn over, roll over

dátil *m* date

datos *mpl* data *n o npl*

DDT *See* **diclorodifeniltricloroetano**.

debido -da *adj* proper, appropriate; —— **a** due to

débil *adj* weak, (*el pulso*) faint

debilidad *f* weakness

debilitación *f* debilitation, weakening

debilitado -da *adj* debilitated, run-down

debilitante *adj* debilitating

debilitar *vt* to weaken, make weak; *vr* to weaken, become weak

decaer *vi* to weaken, to get worse; to become depressed

decaído -da *adj* weak, run-down, debilitated; depressed

decaimiento *m* weakening, weakness, debilitation; depression

decibel *m* decibel

decidir *vt, vr* to decide

decilitro *m* deciliter

decisión *f* decision

dedo *m* (*de la mano*) finger; (*del pie*) toe; —— **anular** ring finger; —— **chico** (*del pie*) little toe; —— **de gatillo** trigger finger; —— **de hule** finger cot; —— **del corazón** middle finger; —— **gordo** (*de la mano*) thumb, (*del pie*) big toe; **dedos hipocráticos** *or* **en palillo de tambor** clubbing, clubbed fingers; —— **índice** index finger; —— **medio** middle finger; —— **meñique** little finger

defecación *f* bowel movement

defecar *vi* to defecate, to have a bowel movement

defecto *m* defect; —— **del tubo neural** neural tube defect; —— **de nacimiento** birth defect

deficiencia *f* deficiency, lack

deficiente *adj* deficient

déficit *m* (*pl* **déficits**) deficit

definitivo -va *adj* definitive

deforme *adj* deformed

deformidad *f* deformity

degenerar *vi* to degenerate

degenerativo -va *adj* degenerative

deglutir *vi* to swallow

dejar *vi* —— **de** to quit, stop, give up; ¿**Cuándo dejó de comer?**..When did you quit eating?...**Debe dejar de fumar**..You should give up smoking.

delantal *m* apron; —— **de plomo** lead apron

delantero -ra *adj* front; **la parte delantera del pie**..the front part of the foot

deleción *f* deletion

delgado -da *adj* thin

delicado -da *adj* frail, sickly, delicate; ill, seriously ill; (*condición*) serious

delirante *adj* delirious

delirar *vi* to be delirious, to rave; **Está delirando**..He is delirious.

delirio *m* delirium

delirium tremens *m* delirium tremens, the d.t.'s (*fam*)

delta *f* delta

deltoides *m* (*pl* **-des**) deltoid

demacrado -da *adj* emaciated

demandar *vt* to sue

demencia *f* dementia

demente *adj* demented

demostrar *vt* to demonstrate

dengue *m* dengue fever, dengue

denso -sa *adj* dense

dentadura *f* teeth, set of teeth; (*postiza*) denture, false teeth (*fam*); —— **parcial** partial denture

dental *adj* dental

dentario -ria *adj* dental

dentición *f* (*form*) teething

dentina *f* dentin

dentista *mf* dentist

dentro *adv* inside; **dentro de su cuerpo**..inside your body

departamento *m* department; —— **de salud** Health Department

dependencia *f* dependence

dependiente *adj* dependent

depilatorio -ria *adj & m* depilatory

deponer *vt, vi* (*pp* **depuesto**) (*Mex, fam*) to throw up, vomit

deposición *f* (*SA*) bowel movement

depositar *vt, vr* to deposit

depósito *m* deposit, buildup; store; **de** —— (*pharm*) depot

depresión *f* depression

depresivo -va *adj* depressive

depresor -ra *adj* (*pharm, physio*) depressant; *m* depressant; tongue depressor *o* blade

deprimido -da *adj* depressed

deprimirse *vr* to get depressed

depuesto *pp of* **deponer**

depurador *m* purifier

depurar *vt* to purify

derecho -cha *adj* straight; right; right-handed; *m* right (*legal, moral*); *f* right, right-hand side

derivación *f* (*surg*) shunt, bypass; —— **portacava** portacaval shunt; —— **ventriculoperitoneal** ventriculoperitoneal shunt

dermatitis *f* dermatitis; —— **atópica** atopic dermatitis; —— **de los bañistas** swimmer's itch; —— **por contacto** contact dermatitis; —— **por estasis**; —— **por pañal** diaper rash; —— **seborreica** seborrheic dermatitis

dermatología *f* dermatology

dermatólogo -ga *mf* dermatologist

dermatomiositis *f* dermatomyositis

derrame *m* effusion, bleed; —— **cerebral** cerebral hemorrhage, hemorrhagic stroke, (*fam*) stroke (*of any type*); —— **pericárdico** *or* **pericardiaco** pericardial effusion; —— **pleural** pleural effusion

DES *See* **dietilestilbestrol**.

desabotonar *vt, vr* to unbutton

desabrochar *vt, vr* to unbutton, to unbuckle

desagradable *adj* unpleasant

desagüe *m* sewer

desahogo *m* (*psych*) relief, outlet

desalentado -da *adj* discouraged, despondent

desalentar *vt* to discourage; *vr* to become discouraged

desanimado -da *adj* discouraged, despondent

desanimar *vt* to discourage; *vr* to become discouraged

desaparecerse *vr* to disappear

desarrollar *vt, vr* to develop

desarrollo *m* development

desatender *vt* to neglect

desayunarse *vr* to have breakfast

desayuno *m* breakfast

desbaratar *vt* (*una tableta, etc.*) to crush

desbridamiento *m* debridement

descafeinado -da *adj* decaffeinated

descalabrar *vt* to injure the head of (*someone*); **Lo descalabraron**..They injured his head; *vr* to injure (*one's*) head; **Me descalabré**..I injured my head.

descalzo -za *adj* barefoot

descamarse *vr* (*form*) to peel, flake

descansar *vt, vr* to rest

descanso *m* rest

descarga *f* discharge; —— **eléctrica** electric shock; —— **nasal posterior** postnasal drip

descartar *vt* to rule out; **Tenemos que descartar el cáncer**..We need to rule out cancer.

descendente *adj* descending

descendiente *mf* descendant

descongestionante *adj & m* decongestant

descongestivo -va *adj & m* decongestant

descontaminar *vt* to decontaminate

descontinuar *vt* to discontinue

describir *vt* to describe

descuidado -da *adj* careless; neglected

descuidar *vt* to neglect

descuido *m* neglect, carelessness

desde *prep* **¿Desde cuándo tiene diabetes?**.. How long have you had diabetes?

desear *vt* to desire

desecado -da *adj* dried, dessicated

desecante *adj & m* desiccant

desecativo -va *adj & m* desiccant

desechable *adj* disposable

desecho *m* (*frec pl*) waste; (*Mex, fam*) vaginal discharge; **desechos metabólicos** metabolic wastes; **desechos peligrosos** hazardous wastes

desemborracharse *vr* to sober up

desembriagarse *vr* to sober up

desensibilización *f* desensitization

desensibilizar *vt* to desensitize

deseo *m* desire; —— **sexual** sexual desire, libido

desequilibrio *m* imbalance

desesperación *f* desperate feeling, severe anxiety

desesperado -da *adj* hopeless, desperate

desesperarse *vr* to lose hope; to become desperate

desfibrilación *f* defibrillation

desfibrilar *vt* to defibrillate

desgarradura *f* (*de un músculo, ligamento, etc.*) tear

desgarramiento *m* (*de un músculo, ligamento, etc.*) tear

desgarrar *vt, vr* (*un músculo, ligamento, etc.*) to tear; (*flema*) to cough up; **Se me desgarró el músculo**..I tore my muscle... **¿Está desgarrando flema?**..Are you coughing up phlegm?

desgarre *m* (*de un músculo, ligamento, etc.*) tear

desgarro *m* (*de un músculo, ligamento, etc.*) tear

desguanzado -da *adj* (*Mex, fam*) tired, run-down, lightheaded

desguanzarse *vr* (*Mex, fam*) to become tired, to become run-down, to feel faint

deshacerse *vr* —— **de** to get rid of

deshidratación *f* dehydration

deshidratado -da *adj* dehydrated

deshidrogenasa láctica *f* lactic dehydrogenase

deshumanizante *adj* dehumanizing

deshumedecer *vt* to dehumidify

deshumidificador *m* dehumidifier

desinfectante *adj & m* disinfectant

desinfectar *vt* to disinfect

desintoxicación *f* detoxification

desmayarse *vr* to faint, pass out

desmayo *m* faint, blackout

desmielinizante *adj* demyelinating

desmoralizar *vt* to demoralize; *vr* to become demoralized

desnudo -da *adj* naked

desnutrición *f* malnutrition

desnutrido -da *adj* malnourished, undernourished

desodorante *m* deodorant

desorden *m* disorder

desorientado -da *adj* disoriented

despellejarse *vr* (*fam*) to peel

desperdicios *mpl* wastes

despersonalización *f* (*psych*) depersonalization

despertar *vt* (*pp* **-tado** *or* **-pierto**) to wake (up), arouse; *vr* to wake up

despierto -ta (*pp of* **despertar**) *adj* awake

despigmentación *f* depigmentation

desplomarse *vr* to collapse

despostillarse *vr* to chip (*a tooth*)

desprenderse *vr* to slough, slough off

destetar *vt* to wean

destete *m* weaning

destilado -da *adj* distilled

destreza *f* skill

destructivo -va *adj* destructive

destruir *vt* to destroy

desvanecerse *vr* to faint

desvariar *vi* to rave, talk nonsense

desvelado -da *adj* sleepless, lacking sleep

desvelarse *vr* to go without sleep

desvelo *m* period without sleep

desventaja *f* disadvantage

detección *f* screening, detection

detectar *vt* to detect

detector de humo *m* smoke detector

detener *vt* —— **la respiración** *or* **el resuello** to hold one's breath; **Detenga la respiración**..Hold your breath.

detergente *adj & m* detergent

deteriorarse *vr* to deteriorate

deterioro *m* deterioration

devolver *vt, vi* (*pp* **devuelto**) to throw up, vomit

dexametasona *f* dexamethasone

dextrometorfán *m* dextromethorphan

día *m* day; **cada dos días** every other day; **el —— anterior** the day before; **el —— siguiente** the day after, the following day; **todos los días** every day

diabetes *f* diabetes; —— **insípida** diabetes insipidus; —— **mellitus** diabetes mellitus

diabético -ca *adj & mf* diabetic

diablos azules *mpl* (*fam*) the d.t.'s (*fam*), delirium tremens

diacepam *m* diazepam

diafragma *m* (*anat, gyn*) diaphragm

diagnosis *f* (*pl* **-sis**) diagnosis

diagnosticar *vt* to diagnose

diagnóstico -ca *adj* diagnostic; *m* diagnosis

diagrama *m* diagram

diálisis f dialysis; —— **peritoneal** peritoneal dialysis

diámetro m diameter

diapasón m tuning fork

diariamente adv daily

diario -ria adj daily; **a** —— daily, every day

diarrea f diarrhea; —— **del viajero** traveler's diarrhea

diastólico -ca adj diastolic

diclofenaco m diclofenac

diclorodifeniltricloroetano (DDT) m dichlorodiphenyltrichloroethane (DDT)

dicloxacilina f dicloxacillin

dieldrín m dieldrin

diente m tooth, front tooth; —— **canino** canine tooth, cuspid; —— **de leche** baby tooth; —— **incisivo** incisor, front tooth; —— **molar** molar; —— **picado** decayed tooth, tooth with a cavity; **Tiene un diente picado..**You have a cavity; **dientes postizos** false teeth; **dientes salidos** buckteeth

diente de león m (bot) dandelion

dieta f diet; —— **baja en grasas** low-fat diet; —— **alta en fibra** high-fiber diet; **estar a** —— to be on a diet, to diet

dietético -ca adj dietary

dietilamida del ácido lisérgico (LSD) f lysergic acid diethylamide (LSD)

dietilestilbestrol (DES) m diethylstilbestrol (DES)

dietista mf dietician

difenhidramina f diphenhydramine

difteria f diphtheria

difunto -ta adj & mf deceased

difusión f diffusion; **de** —— **regulada** (pharm) timed-release

digerible adj digestible

digerir vt to digest

digestión f digestion

digestivo -va adj digestive

digital adj digital; f (pharm) digitalis

digoxina f digoxin

dilatación f dilation

dilatador m dilator

dilatar vt, vr to dilate

diltiazem m diltiazem

diluido -da adj dilute

diluir vt to dilute

diluvio m flood

dimensión f dimension

dimetilsulfóxido m dimethyl sulfoxide (DMSO)

dimetiltriptamina (DMT) f dimethyltryptamine (DMT)

dinitrato de isosorbide m isosorbide dinitrate

dióxido m dioxide; —— **de azufre** sulfur dioxide; —— **de carbono** carbon dioxide

diplococo m diplococcus

dirección f direction; address

discinesia tardía f tardive dyskinesia

disciplina f discipline

disciplinar vt to discipline

disco m disk; —— **desplazado** slipped disk; —— **herniado** herniated disk

discrasia f dyscrasia; —— **sanguínea** blood dyscrasia

diseminación f spread

diseminado -da adj disseminated

diseminar vt, vr to disseminate, spread

disentería f dysentery

disfasia f dysphasia

disfunción f dysfunction

disgregación f (psych) disintegration

dislexia f dyslexia

dislocación f dislocation

dislocar vt, vr to dislocate, to become dislocated; **¿Se le había dislocado el hombro antes?**..Had you dislocated your shoulder before?

disminución f decrease

disminuir vt to reduce, decrease; vi, vr to decrease, to get smaller

disociación f (psych) dissociation

disolvente m solvent

disolver vt, vr (pp **disuelto**) to dissolve

disopiramida f disopyramide

dispensar vt (pharm) to dispense

displasia f dysplasia

disponible adj available

dispositivo m device; —— **intrauterino (DIU)** intrauterine device (IUD)

distender vt to distend; vi, vr to become distended; **distendérsele el estómago** to get bloated; **Se me distiende el estóma-go.**.My stomach gets bloated.

distensión *f* distention *o* distension

distinguir *vt* to distinguish

distraído -da *adj* absent-minded

distrofia muscular progresiva *f* muscular dystrophe

disuelto *pp of* **disolver**

disulfiramo *m* disulfiram

disvariar *See* **desvariar**.

DIU *abbr* **dispositivo intrauterino.** *See* **dispositivo.**

diuresis *f* diuresis

diurético -ca *adj & m* diuretic

diván *m* (*psych*) couch

diverticulitis *f* diverticulitis

divertículo *m* diverticulum

diverticulosis *f* diverticulosis

divorciar *vt, vr* to divorce

divorcio *m* divorce

DMT *See* **dimetiltriptamina.**

doblar *vt* to bend, flex; to double; **Doble la pierna.**.Bend your leg; *vr* to bend, bend over, bend down; to sprain, twist; **Dóblese.**.Bend over...**Me doblé el tobillo.**. I sprained my ankle.

doble *adj & adv* double

dobutamina *f* dobutamine

doctor -ra *mf* doctor, physician

dolencia *f* ache, pain, ailment

doler *vi* to hurt; **¿Le duele?**..Does it hurt?...**¿Le duele el pie?**..Does your foot hurt?...**¿Dónde le duele?**..Where does it hurt?...**El procedimiento no duele.**.The procedure doesn't hurt.

dolor *m* pain, ache; —— **de barriga** bellyache; —— **de cabeza** headache; —— **de dientes** toothache; —— **de espalda** backache; —— **de estómago** stomachache; —— **de garganta** sore throat; —— **de hambre** hunger pang *o* pain; —— **del parto** labor pain, contraction; —— **de muelas** toothache; —— **de oído** earache; —— **menstrual** menstrual cramp; **sin** —— painless

dolorido -da *adj* sore, tender

doloroso -sa *adj* painful, sore, tender

domicilio *m* home; address

dominante *adj* dominant

dominicano -na *adj & mf* Dominican

dominio de sí mismo *m* self-control

donado -da *adj* donated, donor; **sangre donada** donated blood, donor blood

donador -ra *mf* donor

donante *mf* donor

donar *vt* to donate

dopamina *f* dopamine

Doppler *m* Doppler

dormido -da *adj* asleep; (*adormecido*) numb, asleep; **Tengo dormido el brazo.**. My arm is numb..My arm is asleep.

dormir *vt* to put to sleep; to numb (up); **¿Me van a dormir el pie?**..Are you going to numb up my foot? *vi* to sleep; **¿Duerme bien?**..Do you sleep well? *vr* to go to sleep, to fall asleep; (*adormecerse*) to become numb, to go to sleep, to fall asleep; **Se me duerme el brazo.**.My arm gets numb.

dormitar *vi* doze

dormitorio *m* bedroom

dorsal *adj* dorsal

dorso *m* (*de la mano*) back (*of the hand*)

dosificación *f* dosage

dosis *f* (*pl* **dosis**) dose; —— **excesiva** overdose

doxiciclina *f* doxycycline

dren *m* drain

drenaje *m* drain, drainage; sewer

drenar *vt, vr* to drain

drepanocitemia *f* sickle cell disease

droga *f* drug

drogadicto -ta *mf* drug abuser, drug addict

drogado -da *adj* drugged, high (*fam*)

drogar *vt* to drug; *vr* to take drugs, to become intoxicated

ducha *f* shower; douche; **darse** *or* **tomarse una** —— to take a shower

ducharse *vr* to take a shower; to douche

duela *f* fluke

dulce *adj* sweet; *m* piece of candy; **dulces** candy, sweets

dulcificante *m* sweetener

duodenal *adj* duodenal

duodenitis *f* duodenitis

duodeno *m* duodenum

duración *f* duration
duradero -ra *adj* durable
durar *vi* to last; **Los vómitos me duraron toda la noche.**.The vomiting lasted all night.
duro -ra *adj* hard, tough; stiff; **Se me puso duro el brazo.**.My arm got stiff;—— **de oído** hard of hearing

E

eccema *m&f* eczema
ECG *See* **electrocardiograma**.
echar *vt* to pass, to shed; —— **de menos** to miss; **¿Echa de menos a su hija?**..Do you miss your daughter? *vr* **echarse a perder** to spoil (*food, etc.*); **echarse vientos** *or* **gases** to pass gas
Echinococcus Echinococcus
eclampsia *f* eclampsia
ecocardiografía *f* echocardiography; echocardiogram
ecocardiograma *m* echocardiogram
ectópico -ca *adj* ectopic
ecuatoriano -na *adj & mf* Ecuadoran
eczema *See* **eccema**.
edad *f* age; —— **madura** *or* **mediana** middle age; —— **ósea** bone age
edema *m* edema; —— **pulmonar** pulmonary edema
educación *f* education
educar *vt* to educate
EEG *See* **electroencefalograma**.
efecto *m* effect; —— **adverso** adverse effect; —— **colateral** *or* **secundario** side effect; **hacer** —— to take effect, to have an effect; **No me hizo ningún efecto.**.It didn't do anything for me.
efedrina *f* ephedrine
eficaz *adj* (*pl* **-caces**) effective
eficiente *adj* efficient
ego *m* (*psych*) ego
egocéntrico -ca *adj* self-centered, egocentric
egoísmo *m* egoism
egoísta *adj* egoistic; *mf* egoist
egotismo *m* egotism

egotista *adj* egotistic; *mf* egotist
eje *m* axis
ejercicio *m* exercise; **hacer** —— to exercise
elástico -ca *adj & m* elastic
eléctrico -ca *adj* electric, electrical
electrocardiografía *f* electrocardiography; electrocardiogram (ECG *o* EKG)
electrocardiograma (ECG) *m* electrocardiogram (ECG *o* EKG)
electrocutar *vt* to electrocute
electrodo *m* electrode
electroencefalograma (EEG) *m* electroencephalogram (EEG)
electroforesis *f* electrophoresis
electrolítico -ca *adj* pertaining to electrolytes, electrolyte
electrólito, electrolito *m* electrolyte
electromiografía (EMG) *f* electromyography (EMG)
elefantiasis *f* elephantiasis
elegible *adj* eligible
elemento *m* element
elevación *f* elevation, rise
elevar *vt* to elevate, raise; *vi, vr* to rise
eliminar *vt* to eliminate, (*parásitos, una piedra, etc.*) to pass
elíxir, elixir *m* elixir
emaciado -da *adj* emaciated
emascular *vt* to emasculate
embarado -da *adj* (*fam*) bloated
embarazada *adj* pregnant
embarazo *m* pregnancy; **Tengo cuatro meses de embarazo.**.I'm four months pregnant; —— **ectópico** ectopic pregnancy; —— **tubárico** tubal pregnancy

embolectomía f embolectomy
embolia f embolism, (fam) stroke; —— **pulmonar** pulmonary embolism
embolio (Mex) See **embolia**.
émbolo m embolus; (de una jeringa) plunger
emborracharse vr to get drunk
embriagarse vr to get drunk
embriología f embryology
embrión m embryo
emergencia f emergency; **sala de** —— emergency room (ER)
emético -ca adj & m emetic
EMG See **electromiografía**.
emoción f emotion, feeling
emocional adj emotional
emotivo -va adj emotional (said of a person)
empacharse vr to develop indigestion, to get a stomachache. See **empacho**.
empacho m indigestion, folk illness manifest by abdominal bloating and other gastrointestinal complaints and believed due to food sticking to the sides of the intestine
empañado -da adj blurred; **vista empañada** blurred vision
empañarse vr (la vista) to blur, to become blurred; **Me empaña la vista**..My vision blurs..My vision gets blurred.
empastar vt (dent) to fill (a tooth)
empaste m (dent) filling
empatía f empathy
empeine m instep; groin; ringworm
empeoramiento m worsening
empeorar vt to make worse; vi, vr to get worse, deteriorate
empiema m empyema
emplasto m plaster (medicinal)
empleador -ra mf employer
empleo m employment, occupation, job
enalapril m enalapril
enanismo m dwarfism
enano -na mf dwarf, midget
encamado -da adj in bed, in a bed; mf patient in a bed
encefalitis f encephalitis
encefalomielitis f encephalomyelitis
encefalopatía f encephalopathy; —— **de Wernicke** Wernicke's encephalopathy
enchufe m electrical outlet

encía f (anat) gum
encinta adj pregnant
encoger vt (la pierna, el brazo) to bend; vi to get smaller; vr to get smaller; (fam) to get stiff, to cramp (up), to become contracted
enconarse vr to fester
encorvado -da adj stooped, bent over
encorvamiento m curvature (of the spine)
encorvarse vr to bend down, stoop
endarterectomía f endarterectomy
endémico -ca adj endemic
enderezar vt, vr (los dientes, un hueso, etc.) to straighten; **Enderece el brazo**..Straighten your arm.
endocardio m endocardium
endocarditis f endocarditis
endocrino -na adj endocrine
endocrinología f endocrinology
endocrinólogo -ga mf endocrinologist
endodoncia f root canal
endometrio m endometrium
endometriosis f endometriosis
endometritis f endometritis
endorfina f endorphin
endoscopia, endoscopía f endoscopy
endoscópico -ca adj endoscopic
endoscopio m endoscope
endotraqueal adj endotracheal
endovenoso -sa adj intravenous (IV)
endurecer vt to harden, make hard; vr to harden, become hard
endurecido -da adj hardened
endurecimiento m hardening
enema m&f enema; —— **de bario** barium enema
energía f energy
enérgico -ca adj energetic
enfermarse vr to get sick
enfermedad f disease, sickness, illness; —— **articular degenerativa** degenerative joint disease; —— **celiaca** celiac disease; —— **colágeno-vascular** or **del colágeno** collagen-vascular disease; —— **de Addison** Addison's disease; —— **de almacenamiento de glucógeno** glycogen storage disease; —— **de Alzheimer** Alzheimer's disease; —— **de células**

falciformes *or* drepanocíticas sickle cell disease; —— de Crohn Crohn's disease; —— de Cushing Cushing's disease; —— de Chagas Chagas' disease; —— de Gaucher Gaucher's disease; —— de Gilbert Gilbert's disease *o* syndrome; —— de Gilles de la Tourette Gilles de la Tourette syndrome; —— de Graves Graves' disease; —— de Hansen Hansen's disease; —— de Hirschsprung Hirschsprung's disease; —— de Hodgkin Hodgkin's disease; —— de Huntington Huntington's disease; —— de Kawasaki Kawasaki's disease; —— de lesiones mínimas minimal change disease; —— del injerto contra el huésped graft-versus-host disease; —— de los legionarios Legionnaire's disease; —— del sueño sleeping sickness; —— del suero serum sickness; —— del tejido conectivo *or* conjuntivo connective tissue disease; —— de Lyme Lyme disease; —— de mano, pie y boca hand-foot-and-mouth disease; —— de membrana hialina hyaline membrane disease; —— de Paget Paget's disease; —— de Parkinson Parkinson's disease; —— de Pott Pott's disease; —— de transmisión sexual sexually transmitted disease (STD); —— de Vincent Vincent's angina, trench mouth; —— de von Willebrand von Willebrand's disease *o* syndrome; —— de Whipple Whipple's disease; —— de Wilson Wilson's disease; —— fibroquística fibrocystic disease; —— inflamatoria pélvica pelvic inflammatory disease (PID); —— intersticial pulmonar interstitial lung disease; —— mamaria benigna benign breast disease; —— mental mental illness; —— ocupacional *or* profesional occupational illness; —— por arañazo de gato cat-scratch disease; —— por descompresión decompression sickness, the bends; —— pulmonar de los granjeros farmer's lung; —— pulmonar obstructiva crónica (EPOC) chronic obstructive pulmonary disease (COPD); —— vascular periférica peripheral vascular disease; —— venérea sexually transmitted disease (STD); quinta —— fifth disease

enfermera *f* nurse; —— **domiciliaria** home nurse; —— **visitadora** visiting nurse

enfermería *f* nursing; infirmary

enfermero *m* male nurse

enfermizo -za *adj* sickly

enfermo -ma *adj* sick, ill; *mf* sick person, patient

enfisema *m* emphysema

enflaquecerse *vr* to become thin

enfocar *vt* to focus

enfrentarse *vr* —— **a** to cope with

enfrente *adv* de —— front; **la parte de enfrente de..**the front of

engarrotado -da *adj* stiff

engarrotarse *vr* to become stiff

engarruñarse *vr* (*esp Mex*) to become stiff, contracted

engordar *vi* to get fat

enjuagar *vt* to rinse

enjuague *m* rinse; —— **bucal** mouthwash

enjugar *vt* to wipe

enlace *m* (*psych, obst*) bond

enlazamiento *m* (*psych, obst*) bonding

enloquecerse *vr* to go crazy

enmascarar *vt* (*signos, síntomas*) to mask

enojado -da *adj* angry, mad

enojarse *vr* to get angry *o* mad

enojo *m* rage, anger

enriquecido -da *adj* enriched

enrojecimiento *m* redness, reddening

ensalada *f* salad

ensayo *m* trial

enseñar *vt* to teach

ensimismado -da *adj* self-absorbed, lost in thought

ensuciar *vt* to soil, to get (*something*) dirty; *vr* to soil oneself, to get dirty

entablillar *vt* to splint

entérico -ca *adj* enteric; **con capa entérica** enteric-coated

enteritis *f* enteritis; —— **regional** regional enteritis

entero -ra *adj* whole

enterococo *m* enterococcus

enterocolitis *f* enterocolitis

enteropatía f enteropathy; —— **con pérdida de proteínas** protein-losing enteropathy
enterotoxina f enterotoxin
entrada f entrance
entrañas fpl entrails, bowels
entrecejo m space between eyebrows
entrecerrar vt —— **los ojos** to squint
entrenamiento m training
entrenar vt, vr to train
entrepiernas, entrepierna f crotch
entretenedor m pacifier
entristecerse vr to become sad
entuertos mpl postpartum cramps
entumecerse vr to become numb, to become numb and swollen
entumecido -da adj numb, numb and swollen
entumecimiento m numbness, numbness and swelling
entumido -da adj numb, numb and swollen
entumirse vr to become numb, to become numb and swollen
enuresis f (form) bed-wetting
envejecer vi, vr to grow old
envejecimiento m aging
envenenamiento m poisoning; —— **de la sangre** blood poisoning
envenenar vt to poison
enviciar vt to addict; vr to become addicted
envolver vt to wrap
enzima f enzyme
eosinófilo m eosinophil
epidemia f epidemic
epidémico -ca adj epidemic
epidemiología f epidemiology
epididimitis f epididymitis
epidídimo m epididymis
epidural adj epidural
epiglotis f epiglottis
epiglotitis f epiglottitis
epilepsia f epilepsy
epinefrina f epinephrine
episiotomía f episiotomy
episodio m episode
epispadias m epispadias
EPOC abbr **enfermedad pulmonar obstructiva crónica**. See **enfermedad**.
épulis m epulis

equilibrado -da adj balanced
equilibrio m equilibrium, balance
equinococosis f echinococcosis
equipo m (de profesionales de la salud) team; —— **de urgencia** first aid kit
equivalente adj & m equivalent
erección f erection
eréctil adj erectile
erecto -ta adj erect
ergocalciferol m ergocalciferol
ergotamina f ergotamine
erisipela f erysipelas
eritema m erythema; —— **infeccioso** erythema infectiosum; —— **multiforme** erythema multiforme; —— **nodoso** erythema nodosum
eritrocito m erythrocyte
eritromicina f erythromycin
erizarse vr —— **la piel** or **el pelo** to have goose pimples
erizo de mar m sea urchin
erógeno -na adj erogenous
erosión f erosion
erosionar vt, vr to erode
erótico -ca adj erotic
erradicar vt to eradicate
error m error
eructar vi to burp, belch; **hacer** —— (a un bebé) to burp (a baby)
erupción f eruption, rash
escala f scale (of measurement); —— **móvil** or **flexible** sliding scale
escaldadura f scald
escaldar vt to scald
escalofrío m chill
escalpelo m scalpel
escama f (de la piel) scale, flake
escamoso -sa adj squamous; flaky, scaly
escán m (Ang) scan
escape m (psych) outlet
escápula f scapula
escara f (form) scab, crust; —— **de presión** pressure sore
escaso -sa adj scarce, (el pelo) thin
Escherichia coli Escherichia coli
esclera f sclera
escleritis f scleritis
esclerodermia, escleroderma f scleroderma

esclerosis *f* sclerosis; —— **lateral amiotrófica** amyotrophic lateral sclerosis; —— **múltiple** multiple sclerosis; —— **sistémica progresiva** progressive systemic sclerosis; —— **tuberosa** tuberous sclerosis

escleroterapia *f* sclerotherapy

esclerótica *f* sclera

escocer *vi* to itch; to burn, sting, smart

escoliosis *f* scoliosis

escopolamina *f* scopolamine

escorbuto *m* scurvy

escorpión *m* scorpion

escozor *m* itching; smarting, stinging, burning

escritura *f* handwriting

escrófula *f* scrofula

escroto *m* scrotum

escuchar *vt* to listen to; *vi* to listen

escuela *f* school

escupidera *f* emesis basin

escupir *vt, vi* to spit

escupitajo *m* (*fam*) spit, gob of phlegm

escurrir *vi* **escurrirle la nariz** (*fam*) to have a runny nose

escutelaria *f* (*bot*) skullcap

esencial *adj* essential

esfigmomanómetro *m* blood pressure cuff

esfínter *m* sphincter

esforzarse *vr* to exert oneself; **No se esfuerce demasiado..**Don't overdo it.

esfuerzo *m* effort, exertion

esguince *m* (*form*) sprain, twist

esmalte *m* enamel; —— **para las uñas** nail polish

esmog *m* (*Ang*) smog

esofagitis *f* esophagitis; —— **por reflujo** reflux esophagitis

esófago *m* esophagus

espacio *m* space, gap

espalda *f* back; **parte baja de la** —— lower back

español -la *adj* Spanish; *mf* Spaniard

espárrago *m* asparagus

espasmo *m* spasm

espasmódico -ca *adj* spasmodic

espasticidad *f* spasticity

espástico -ca *adj* spastic

especia *f* spice

especialidad *f* specialty

especialista *mf* specialist

especie *f* species

específico -ca *adj* specific

espécimen *m* (*pl* **-címenes**) specimen

espectinomicina *f* spectinomycin

espectro *m* spectrum

espéculo *m* speculum

espejo *m* mirror

espejuelos *mpl* (*esp Carib*) eyeglasses, glasses

esperanza *f* hope; —— **de vida** life expectancy

esperar *vt* to hope for; to wait for; to expect; *vi* to hope; to wait

esperma *f* sperm, semen

espermaticida, espermicida *adj* spermicidal, spermatocidal; *m* spermicide, spermatocide

espermatocele *m* spermatocele

espermatozoide *m* sperm, spermatozoon

espeso -sa *adj* thick

espesor *m* thickness

espesura *f* thickness

espina *f* (*anat*) spine; (*bot*) thorn, spine, burr; (*de un pescado*) fish bone; —— **bífida** spina bifida; —— **dorsal** spinal column

espinacas *fpl* spinach

espinal *adj* spinal

espinarse *vr* to prick oneself (*with a thorn, etc.*)

espinazo *m* (*fam*) backbone, spine

espinilla *f* (*anat*) shin; (*derm*) blackhead, (*con pus*) pimple

espinillera *f* shin guard

espino *m* (*bot*) hawthorn

espirar *vt, vi* to expire, exhale

espirometría *f* spirometry

espirómetro *m* spirometer

espironolactona *f* spironolactone

espiroqueta *f* spirochete

esplenectomía *f* splenectomy

esplénico -ca *adj* splenic

espolón *m* (*ortho*) spur, bone spur

espondilitis *f* spondylitis; —— **anquilosante** ankylosing spondylitis

espondilosis *f* spondylosis

esponja *f* sponge

espontáneo -a *adj* spontaneous
espora *f* spore
esporádico -ca *adj* sporadic
esporotricosis *f* sporotrichosis
esposa *f* wife
esposo *m* husband
espray *m* (*Ang*) spray
esprue *m&f* sprue; —— **celiaco** *or* **no tropical** celiac *o* nontropical sprue; —— **tropical** tropical sprue
espuma *f* foam
espumarajo *m* foam, froth (*at the mouth*)
espumoso -sa *adj* foamy, frothy
esputo *m* sputum
esqueleto *m* skeleton
esquema *f* (*de vacunas, etc.*) schedule
esquistosomiasis *f* schistosomiasis
esquizofrenia *f* schizophrenia
esquizofrénico -ca *adj* & *mf* schizophrenic
esquizoide *adj* schizoid
estabilidad *f* stability
estabilización *f* stabilization
estabilizador *m* stabilizer
estabilizar *vt*, *vr* to stabilize
estable *adj* stable
estación *f* station; (*invierno, etc.*) season; —— **de enfermeras** nursing station
estadío, estadio *m* (*de una enfermedad, del cáncer, etc.*) stage
estadística *f* (*dato*) statistic
estado *m* status, state, condition; —— **de ánimo** mood; **en** —— (*fam*) pregnant
estadounidense *adj* American, of the United States
estafilococo *m* staphylococcus
estancarse *vr* (*la sangre*) to pool
estándar *adj* & *m* standard
estasis *f* stasis; —— **venosa** venous stasis
estenosis *f* stenosis (*form*), stricture
estenótico -ca *adj* stenotic
estéril *adj* sterile, infertile
esterilidad *f* sterility, infertility
esterilización *f* sterilization
esterilizar *vt* to sterilize
esternón *m* sternum, breastbone (*fam*)
esteroide *adj* & *m* steroid
estetoscopio *m* stethoscope
estilo de vida *m* lifestyle

estimulación *f* stimulation
estimulante *adj* stimulating; *m* stimulant
estimular *vt* to stimulate
estímulo *m* stimulus
estiramiento *m* (*form*) muscle pull
estirar *vt* to stretch; (*enderezar*) to straighten; *vi*, *vr* to stretch; **estirar(se) un músculo** to pull a muscle
estítico -ca *adj* (*esp ES*) constipated
estitiquez *f* (*esp ES*) constipation
estoico -ca *adj* stoic, stoical
estoma *m* (*Ang*) stoma
estomacal *adj* pertaining to the stomach
estómago *m* stomach; (*fam*) abdomen, belly; **boca del** —— pit of the stomach; **dolor** *m* **de** —— stomachache; **tener el** —— **revuelto** to have an upset stomach
estomaguito *m* (*ped*) tummy
estomatitis *f* stomatitis
estornudar *vi* to sneeze
estornudo *m* sneeze
estrabismo *m* strabismus
estradiol *m* estradiol
estrangulación *f* strangulation
estrangular *vt* to strangle, choke; (*una hernia*) to strangulate; *vr* to strangle, choke; to become strangulated
estrechez *f* stricture, narrowing
estrecho -cha *adj* narrow
estrella, estrellita *f* (*visual*) floater
estremecerse *vr* to shake, to shiver
estreñimiento *m* constipation
estreñir *vt* to constipate; *vr* to become constipated
estreptococo *m* streptococcus
estreptomicina *f* streptomycin
estreptoquinasa *f* streptokinase
estrés *m* (*pl* **estreses**) stress
estría *f* stretch mark
estribo *m* stirrup
estricnina *f* strychnine
estricto -ta *adj* strict
estriol *m* estriol
estrógeno *m* estrogen; **estrógenos conjugados** conjugated estrogens
estrongiloidiasis *f* strongyloidiasis
estuche *m* kit
estudiante *mf* student

estudio *m* study; —— **doble ciego** double-blind study

estupor *m* stupor

etambutol *m* ethambutol

etanol *m* ethanol

etapa *f* (*del sueño, etc.*) stage

éter *m* ether

ético -ca *adj* ethical

etilenglicol *m* ethylene glycol

etilo *m* ethyl

etionamida *f* ethionamide

etiqueta *f* label

étnico -ca *adj* ethnic

etodolaco *m* etodolac

etosuximida *f* ethosuximide

eucalipto *m* (*bot*) eucalyptus

euforia *f* euphoria

eufrasia *f* (*bot*) eyebright

eunuco *m* eunuch

eutanasia *f* euthanasia, mercy killing

evacuación *f* bowel movement

evacuar *vt* to evacuate; *vi* to have a bowel movement

evaluación *f* evaluation

evaluar *vt* to evaluate

evaporación *f* evaporation

evaporarse *vr* to evaporate

evitar *vt* to avoid, prevent; **Evite comer comidas grasosas.**.Avoid eating fatty foods.

evolución *f* evolution

exactitud *f* accuracy

exacto -ta *adj* exact, accurate

examen *m* examination, exam (*fam*), test; —— **de la vista** eye test; —— **de los senos** breast examination; —— **de Papanicolaou** *or* —— **del cáncer** (*fam*) Papanicolaou smear, Pap smear (*fam*); —— **físico** physical examination, physical (*fam*); —— **general de orina** urinalysis; —— **ginecológico** pelvic examination, pelvic (*fam*); —— **visual** eye examination, eye test

examinar *vt* to examine, to test

exantema súbito *m* exanthem subitum

excederse *vr* to overdo it; **Puede caminar, pero no se exceda.**.You can walk, but don't overdo it.

excesivo -va *adj* excessive

exceso *m* excess; **en** —— excessively

excitar *vt* to arouse, excite, stimulate; *vr* to become excited, to become aroused

excremento *m* stool

excusa *f* excuse

excusado *m* bathroom, toilet (*esp rural*)

exhalar *vt, vi* to exhale

exhausto -ta *adj* exhausted, run-down

expectativa de vida *f* life expectancy

expectorante *adj* & *m* expectorant

expectorar *vt* to cough up and spit (out)

expediente *m* chart, medical record, file

expeler *vt* to expel

experimental *adj* experimental

experimentar *vi* to experiment

experimento *m* experiment

experto -ta *adj* & *mf* expert

expirar *vi* to expire, die

explorador -ra *adj* (*surg*) exploratory

explorar *vt* (*form*) to examine; (*surg*) to explore

exploratorio -ria *adj* (*surg*) exploratory

exponer *vt* (*pp* **expuesto**) to expose; *vr* to be exposed, expose oneself

exposición *f* exposure

expuesto -ta (*pp of* **exponer**) *adj* exposed

expulsar *vt* to expel, (*parásitos, una piedra, etc.*) to pass; —— **el aire** to exhale, breathe out

expulsión *f* expulsion

extender *vt, vr* to extend, (*la pierna, el brazo*) to straighten

extensión *f* extension

extenso -sa *adj* extensive

extenuado -da *adj* debilitated, weak, exhausted

exterior *adj* outer, exterior, outside; *m* exterior, outside

externo -na *adj* external, outer, outside

extinguidor *m* fire extinguisher

extra *adj* extra

extracción *f* extraction, removal

extracto *m* (*pharm*) extract

extractor de leche *m* breast pump

extraer *vt* to extract, remove, take out

extrañar *vt* to miss; **¿Extraña a su hijo?**. Do you miss your son?

extraño -ña *adj* unusual
extremidad *f* extremity
extrovertido -da *adj* extroverted; *mf* extrovert

eyaculación *f* ejaculation; —— **nocturna** nocturnal emission; —— **precoz** premature ejaculation
eyacular *vi* to ejaculate

F

facciones *fpl* features
facial *adj* facial
factor *m* factor; —— **de protección solar (FPS)** solar protection factor (SPF); —— **de riesgo** risk factor; —— **intrínseco** intrinsic factor; —— **Rh** Rh factor
facultad *f* faculty, ability; *fpl* faculties
Fahrenheit *adj* Fahrenheit
faja *f* girdle, wide belt, (*para prevenir hernias*) truss, abdominal supporter
falda *f* skirt
fálico -ca *adj* phallic
falla *f* (*cardiaca, etc.*) failure
fallar *vi* to fail
fallecer *vi* to expire, die
fallo *See* **falla**.
falo *m* phallus
falsearse *vr* (*Mex*) to sprain, twist; **Me falseé la muñeca**..I sprained my wrist.
falseo *m* (*Mex*) sprain
falso -sa *adj* false
falta *f* lack, absence; —— **de(l) aire** shortness of breath
faltar *vi* to be low; **Le falta potasio**..Your potassium is low; —— **a** (*una cita, el trabajo*) to miss (*an appointment, work*); **faltarle (el) aire** to be short of breath; **¿Le falta el aire?**..Are you short of breath?
familia *f* family
familiar *adj* familial, family; *m* relative, family member; —— **consanguíneo** blood relative
famotidina *f* famotidine
fantasía *f* fantasy

farfallota *f* (*Carib*) mumps
faringe *f* pharynx
faringitis *f* pharyngitis
farmacéutico -ca *adj* pharmaceutical; *mf* pharmacist
farmacia *f* pharmacy, drugstore
fármaco *m* (*form*) medication
farmacodependencia *f* drug dependence, dependency
farmacodependiente *mf* person dependent on drugs, drug addict
farmacología *f* pharmacology
farmacológico -ca *adj* pharmacological, pharmacologic
farmacólogo -ga *mf* pharmacologist
farmacopea *f* pharmacopoeia
fascia *f* fascia
fascículo *m* tract
fascioliasis *f* fascioliasis
fasciotomía *f* fasciotomy
fascitis *f* fasciitis
fase *f* phase
fastidioso -sa *adj* annoying, irritating
fatal *adj* fatal
fatiga *f* fatigue, tiredness; (*fam*) asthma, shortness of breath
fatigante *See* **fatigoso -sa**.
fatigar *vt* to tire, tire out; *vr* to tire, get tired, tire out
fatigoso -sa *adj* tiring
febril *adj* febrile
fecha *f* date; —— **de caducidad** expiration date
fecundación *f* fertilization
fecundar *vt* to fertilize

felación _f_ fellatio
felicidad _f_ happiness; _(obst, etc.)_ **¡Felicidades!**..Congratulations!
feliz _(pl_ **felices)** _adj_ happy
felodipina _f_ felodipine
feminización _f_ feminization
femoral _adj_ femoral
fémur _m_ femur
fenacetina _f_ phenacetin
fenciclidina (PCP) _f_ phencyclidine (PCP)
fenilalanina _f_ phenylalanine
fenilbutazona _f_ phenylbutazone
fenilcetonuria _f_ phenylketonuria (PKU)
fenilefrina _f_ phenylephrine
fenilpropanolamina _f_ phenylpropanolamine
fenitoína _f_ phenytoin
fenobarbital _m_ phenobarbital
fenol _m_ phenol
fenómeno _m_ phenomenon; ——— **de Raynaud** Raynaud's phenomenon
fenotiacina _f_ phenothiazine
fenotipo _m_ phenotype
fentanil _m_ fentanyl
feo -a _adj_ ugly; bad, awful; **un dolor muy feo**..a really bad pain...**Sabe feo**..It tastes awful.
feocromocitoma _m_ pheochromocytoma
férrico -ca _adj_ ferric
fértil _adj_ fertile
fertilización _f_ fertilization
férula _f_ splint; _(sonda para mantener permeable un conducto)_ stent
fetal _adj_ fetal
fetiche _m_ fetish
fetichismo _m_ fetishism
feto _m_ fetus
fibra _f_ fiber; ——— **muscular** muscle fiber; ——— **nerviosa** nerve fiber; **de** ——— **óptica** fiberoptic
fibrilación _f_ fibrillation; ——— **auricular** atrial fibrillation; ——— **ventricular** ventricular fibrillation
fibrinógeno _m_ fibrinogen
fibroadenoma _m_ fibroadenoma
fibroma _m_ fibroma; ——— **pendular** skin tag
fibromioma _m_ fibromyoma; ——— **uterino** uterine fibromyoma, fibroid _(fam)_
fibroquístico -ca _adj_ fibrocystic

fibrosis _f_ fibrosis; ——— **quística** cystic fibrosis
fibrositis _f_ fibrositis
fibrótico -ca _adj_ fibrotic
fíbula _f_ fibula
fiebre _f_ fever, temperature _(fam)_; ——— **amarilla** yellow fever; ——— **de las trincheras** trench fever; ——— **del heno** hay fever; ——— **escarlatina** scarlet fever; ——— **manchada de las Montañas Rocosas** Rocky Mountain spotted fever; ——— **paratifoidea** paratyphoid fever; ——— **Q** Q fever; ——— **recurrente** relapsing fever; ——— **reumática** rheumatic fever; ——— **rompehuesos** breakbone fever, dengue; ——— **tifoidea** typhoid fever
figura _f (de una persona)_ figure
fijación _f_ fixation
fijar _vt (la vista)_ to stare; _vr_ to notice; **No me he fijado**..I haven't noticed.
fijo -ja _adj (mirada, etc.)_ steady
filariasis _f_ filariasis
filoso -sa _adj_ sharp
filtración _f_ filtration
filtrar _vt, vr_ to filter
filtro _m_ filter; ——— **solar** sunscreen
fin _m_ end; ——— **de semana** weekend
final _adj_ final
firma _f_ signature
firmar _vt, vi_ to sign
firme _adj_ firm, steady
firmeza _f_ firmness, stability, steadiness
fisiatra _mf_ physiatrist, specialist in physical medicine
fisiatría _f_ physiatry, physical medicine
físico -ca _adj_ physical; _m_ physique, build, physical appearance
fisicoculturista _mf_ bodybuilder
fisiología _f_ physiology
fisiológico -ca _adj_ physiological, physiologic
fisiólogo -ga _mf_ physiologist
fisioterapeuta _mf_ physical therapist, physiotherapist
fisioterapia _f_ physical therapy, physiotherapy
fisioterapista _mf_ physical therapist, physiotherapist
fisostigmina _f_ physostigmine
fístula _f_ fistula, sinus tract

fisura *f* fissure, crack, hairline fracture
fláccido -da, flácido -da *adj* flaccid, flabby
flaco -ca *adj* (*fam*) thin, lean
flanco *m* flank
flatulencia *f* flatulence
flatulento -ta *adj* flatulent
flebitis *f* phlebitis
flebografía *f* venography; venogram
flebograma *m* venogram
flebotomía *f* (*terapéutica*) phlebotomy; (*Ang, el sacar sangre*) phlebotomy, blood drawing
flema *f* mucus, phlegm
flemón *m* phlegmon
flexible *adj* flexible; (*persona*) supple, limber
flexionar *vt, vr* to flex
flojo -ja *adj* (*suelto*) loose; (*relajado*) relaxed, limp; (*fláccido*) flabby
flora *f* flora
fluconazol *m* fluconazole
fluctuar *vi* to fluctuate
flufenacina *f* fluphenazine
fluido *m* fluid
fluir *vi* to flow, to run; **fluirle la nariz** to have a runny nose; **Me fluye la nariz..I** have a runny nose.
flujo *m* flow, drainage; (*fam*) vaginal discharge; —— **menstrual** menstrual flow; —— **sanguíneo** blood flow
fluoración *f* fluoridation
fluorescente *adj* fluorescent
fluoridación *f* fluoridation
fluorización *f* fluoridation
fluoroscopia, fluoroscopía *f* fluoroscopy
fluorouracilo *m* fluorouracil
fluoruro *m* fluoride
fluoxetina *f* fluoxetine
flurazepam, fluracepam *m* flurazepam
fobia *f* phobia
focal *adj* focal
foco *m* focus
fogaje *m* (*Carib, fam*) hot flash, flush
fólico -ca *adj* folic
foliculitis *f* folliculitis
folículo *m* follicle; —— **ovárico** ovarian follicle; —— **piloso** hair follicle
folleto *m* booklet, pamphlet

fomento *m* compress; —— **caliente** hot compress
fondo *m* bottom; —— **de ojo** eyeground
fontanela *f* fontanel *o* fontanelle
fórceps *m* (*pl* **-ceps**) (*obst*) forceps
forense *adj* forensic
forma *f* form, shape; —— **de andar** gait; **en** —— **fit,** in shape
formación *f* formation
formaldehído *m* formaldehyde
formar *vt, vr* to form
fórmula *f* formula
formulario *m* formulary; (*papel*) form
fornido -da *adj* heavyset
fortalecer *vt* to strengthen, build up, to fortify; *vr* to become strong
fortificar *vt* to fortify
forzar *vt* —— **la vista** to strain one's eyes; —— **la voz** to strain one's voice
fosa *f* fossa; —— **nasal** nostril
fosfatasa alcalina *f* alkaline phosphatase
fosfato *m* phosphate
fósforo *m* phosphorus
fotocoagulación *f* photocoagulation
fotosensible *adj* photosensitive
fototerapia *f* phototherapy
FPS *abbr* factor *m* de protección solar. *See* **factor.**
fracasar *vi* to fail
fracaso *m* failure
fractura *f* fracture, break; —— **abierta** open fracture; —— **cerrada** closed fracture; —— **conminuta** comminuted fracture; —— **del cráneo** cranial *o* skull fracture; —— **en espiral** *or* **espiroidea** spiral fracture; —— **expuesta** open fracture; —— **por compresión** compression fracture; —— **por esfuerzo** stress fracture
fracturar *vt, vr* to fracture, break
frágil *adj* fragile, frail, delicate
fragmento *m* fragment
frambesia *f* frambesia, yaws
frambuesa *f* raspberry
frasco *m* bottle, pill bottle
fraterno -na *adj* fraternal
frazada *f* blanket; —— **eléctrica** electric blanket
frecuencia *f* frequency, rate; —— **cardiaca**

heart rate; —— **respiratoria** respiratory rate
freír *vt* to fry
frénico -ca *adj* phrenic
frenillos *mpl* bands, braces
frenos *mpl* bands, braces
frente *f* forehead, brow; **hacer** —— **a** to cope with
fresa *f* strawberry
fresco -ca *adj* fresh; cool
fricción *f* friction, rubbing; massage
frigidez *f* inability to respond sexually, frigidity (*ant*)
frígido -da *adj* unresponsive sexually, frigid (*ant*)
frijoles *mpl* beans
frío -a *adj* cold; *m* cold; **hacer** —— to be cold (*the weather*); **Me duele más cuando hace frío**..It hurts more when the weather is cold; **tener** *or* **sentir** —— to be *o* feel cold; **Tengo frío**..I'm cold.
friolento -ta *adj* sensitive to cold
frito -ta *adj* fried
friza *f* (*PR, SD*) blanket
frontal *adj* frontal
frotis *m* (*pl* **-tis**) (*micro*) smear; —— **de Papanicolaou** Papanicolaou smear
fructosa *f* fructose
fruncir *vt* —— **el entrecejo** *or* **el ceño** to frown; —— **los labios** to purse one's lips; —— **los ojos** *or* **la vista** to squint

fruta *f* fruit; —— **cítrica** *or* **ágria** citrus fruit; —— **seca** dried fruit
fuego *m* fire; (*úlcera en los labios*) cold sore, fever blister
fuente *f* source; (*obst*) bag of waters; —— **para beber** drinking fountain
fuera de, outside, outside of
fuerte *adj* strong, powerful; (*un resfriado, etc.*) bad; (*actividad*) strenuous
fuerza *f* strength, force; —— **de voluntad** will power; **de** —— **doble** double-strength; **de** —— **extra** extra-strength
fugaz *adj* (*pl* **fugaces**) (*dolor, etc.*) fleeting
fumador -ra *mf* smoker
fumar *vt, vi* to smoke; **No fumar**..No smoking
fumigar *vt* fumigate; —— **con avioneta** to crop-dust
función *f* function
funcionamiento *m* performance
funcionar *vi* to function
funda de almohada *f* pillowcase
funeraria *f* funeral home, mortuary
furia *f* rage
furoato de mometasona *f* mometasone
furosemida *f* furosemide
furúnculo *m* furuncle (*form*), boil
fusil *m* rifle, gun
fusión *f* fusion
fusionar *vi, vr* (*ortho*) to fuse
fútbol *m* soccer, football

G

gabinete *m* department, laboratory, office; —— **de fisioterapia, de rayos X, etc.** physical therapy department, x-ray department, etc.
gafas *fpl* spectacles, eyeglasses; —— **de sol** sunglasses
gago -ga *mf* (*esp Carib, fam*) stammerer,

stutterer
gaguear *vi* (*esp Carib, fam*) to stammer, stutter
galactosa *f* galactose
galactosemia *f* galactosemia
galio *m* gallium
galleta *f* cracker, cookie; —— **salada** saltine

galope *m* (*card*) gallop
gamma *f* gamma
gammagrafía *f* nuclear scanning; nuclear scan
gammagrama *m* nuclear scan; —— **de galio** gallium scan; —— **de talio** thallium scan
ganancia *f* gain
gancho *m* (*de pañal*) safety pin
ganciclovir *m* gancyclovir
ganglio *m* node; ganglion; **ganglios basales** basal ganglia; —— **linfático** lymph node
ganglioneuroma *m* ganglioneuroma
gangoso -sa *adj* (*la voz*) nasal
gangrena *f* gangrene; —— **gaseosa** gas gangrene; —— **seca** dry gangrene
Gardnerella vaginalis Gardnerella vaginalis
gargajear *vi* (*fam*) to cough up and spit out phlegm, to spit phlegm
gargajo *m* (*fam*) gob of phlegm
garganta *f* throat
gárgaras *fpl* **hacer** —— to gargle
garra *f* claw
garrapata *f* tick
garraspear *vi* to clear one's throat
garraspera *f* irritation of the throat
gas *m* (*pl* **gases**) gas; fumes; **gases arteriales** arterial blood gas; —— **hilarante** *or* **de la risa** laughing gas; —— **lacrimógeno** tear gas; —— **natural** natural gas; **pasar** —— to pass gas; **tener** —— to have gas; **tirar gases** to pass gas
gasa *f* gauze; —— *or* **gasita con alcohol** alcohol pad
gasolina *f* gasoline, gas (*fam*)
gasometría *f* arterial blood gas
gastrectomía *f* gastrectomy
gástrico -ca *adj* gastric
gastrina *f* gastrin
gastrinoma *m* gastrinoma
gastritis *f* gastritis
gastrocnemio *m* gastrocnemius
gastroenteritis *f* gastroenteritis
gastroenterología *f* gastroenterology
gastroenterólogo -ga *mf* gastroenterologist
gastrointestinal *adj* gastrointestinal (GI)
gatear *vi* (*ped*) to crawl
gato *m* cat

gaznate *m* (*fam*) windpipe
gel *m* gel
gelatina *f* gelatin
gemelo -la *adj* & *mf* twin; —— **dicigótico** *or* **fraterno** fraternal twin; —— **monocigótico** *or* **idéntico** identical twin; **gemelos siameses** conjoined twins, Siamese twins (*ant*)
gemfibrosilo, gemfibrozil *m* gemfibrozil
gemido *m* groan, moan
gemir *vi* to groan, moan
gen, gene *m* gene
genérico -ca *adj* generic
género *m* gender
genético -ca *adj* genetic; *f* genetics
genio *m* genius
genital *adj* genital; *m* **genitales** genitals, private parts (*fam*)
gentamicina *f* gentamicin
geriatra, geríatra *mf* geriatrician
geriatría *f* geriatrics
geriátrico -ca *adj* geriatric
germen *m* germ
germinoma *m* germinoma
gerontología *f* gerontology
gerontólogo -ga *mf* gerontologist
gestación *f* gestation
gestacional *adj* gestational
Giardia Giardia
giardiasis *f* giardiasis
gigantismo *m* gigantism
gimnasia *f* gymnastics
gimnasio *m* gymnasium
ginecología *f* gynecology
ginecólogo -ga *mf* gynecologist
gingiva *f* gingiva
gingivitis *f* gingivitis; —— **ulcerosa necrosante aguda** acute necrotizing ulcerative gingivitis
ginseng *m* (*bot*) ginseng
glande *m* glans
glándula *f* gland; —— **endocrina** endocrine gland; —— **paratiroides** parathyroid gland; —— **parótida** parotid gland; —— **pineal** pineal gland; —— **pituitaria** pituitary gland; —— **salival** salivary gland; —— **suprarrenal** adrenal gland; —— **tiroides** thyroid gland

glaucoma *m* glaucoma
glibenclamida *f* glyburide
gliburida *f* glyburide
glicerina *f* glycerin, glycerol
glicerol *m* glycerol
glicina *f* glycine
glioblastoma *m* glioblastoma
glioma *m* glioma
glipizida, glipicida *f* glipizide
globo *m* —— **ocular** *or* **del ojo** eyeball
globulina *f* globulin; —— **gamma** gamma
   globulin; —— **inmune** immune globulin
glóbulo *m* —— **blanco** white blood cell;
   —— **rojo** red blood cell
glomerulonefritis *f* glomerulonephritis
glositis *f* glossitis
glotis *f* glottis
glucagón *m* glucagon
glucagonoma *m* glucagonoma
gluconato *m* gluconate; —— **de calcio** calcium gluconate
glucosa *f* glucose
glutamato monosódico *m* monosodium glutamate (MSG)
glutámico -ca *adj* glutamic
glutamina *f* glutamine
gluten *m* gluten
glúteo -tea *adj* gluteal; *m* buttock
golf *m* golf
golpe *m* blow, stroke; —— **de calor** heatstroke; —— **precordial** *or* **torácico** precordial thump
golpear *vt* to hit, strike; **Me golpeé aquí..**
   It hit me here.
golpecito *m* pat; **dar golpecitos** to pat
goma *m* gumma; *f* rubber; gum; (*CA*)
   hangover; —— **de mascar** chewing gum;
   estar de —— (*CA*) to have a hangover
gónada *f* gonad
gonadotropina *f* gonadotropin; —— **coriónica humana** human chorionic gonadotropin (HCG)
gonce *m* (*CA, fam*) knuckle, joint
gonococo *m* gonococcus
gonorrea *f* gonorrhea
gordo -da *adj* fat
gordolobo *m* (*bot*) mullein
gorgotear *vi* to gurgle

gorgoteo *m* gurgle, gurgling
gorro *m* cap; —— **de baño** bathing *o*
   shower cap
gota *f* drop; (*enfermedad*) gout
gotear *vi* to drip
goteo *m* dripping, drip; —— **postnasal**
   postnasal drip
gotero *m* medicine dropper, eyedropper
gotoso -sa *adj* gouty
grado *m* degree; grade
gráfica *f* graph
gragea *f* coated pill
gramnegativo -va *adj* Gram-negative
gramo *m* gram
grampositivo -va *adj* Gram-positive
gran *See* **grande**.
grande *adj* (**gran** *before singular nouns*)
   big, large; **ponerse más** —— to get
   bigger; **¿Qué tan grande era?..**How big
   was it?
grandioso -sa *adj* grandiose
granito *m* small pimple; **granitos** rash, fine
   rash
granjero -ra *mf* farmer
grano *m* grain, cereal; (*pharm*) grain; (*derm*)
   pimple; —— **enterrado** deep pimple,
   boil; **de** —— **entero** whole-grain
granulación *f* granulation
granulocito *m* granulocyte
granuloma *m* granuloma; —— **piógeno**
   pyogenic granuloma
granulomatosis *f* granulomatosis; —— **de
   Wegener** Wegener's granulomatosis
grapa *f* (*surg*) staple
grasa *f* grease, fat; —— **de animal** animal
   fat
grasiento -ta *adj* greasy (*esp skin*)
grasoso -sa *adj* greasy, fatty
gratificación *f* gratification
grave *adj* serious, seriously ill, (*condición*)
   grave; (*tono*) low-pitched; **El está grave..**
   He is seriously ill.
gravedad *f* severity
greta *f* toxic Mexican folk remedy
grieta *f* crack
gripa *See* **gripe**.
gripe *f* influenza, flu; —— **asiática** Asian
   flu; —— **porcina** swine flu

gris *adj* gray
grisáceo -cea *adj* grayish
griseofulvina *f* griseofulvin
gritar *vi* to cry, to cry out
grito *m* cry
grosor *m* thickness
grueso -sa *adj* thick
gruñido *m* grunt
gruñir *vi* to grunt; (*esp Mex, las tripas*) to growl (*one's stomach*)
grupo *m* group; —— **de apoyo** support group; —— **sanguíneo** blood type
guabucho *m* (*PR, SD; fam*) lump, bump (*due to trauma*)
guaifenesina *f* guaifenesin

guante *m* glove
guapo -pa *adj* good-looking
guardar *vt* —— **cama** to stay in bed
guardería infantil *f* nursery, day care center
guardia, de on call
guatemalteco -ca *adj* & *mf* Guatemalan
güero -ra (*Mex*) *adj* blond; *m* blond; *f* blonde
guerra *f* war; —— **nuclear** nuclear war
guía *f* (*manual*) guide
guineo *m* (*variety of*) banana
guisante *m* pea
gusano *m* worm; maggot; —— **plano** flatworm; —— **redondo** roundworm
gusto *m* taste, flavor

H

habilidad *f* skill, ability
habitación *f* room, bedroom
hábito *m* habit
habituación *f* habituation
habituarse *vr* to become habituated, to get in the habit of
habla *f* speech; **desarrollo del** —— speech development
hablar *vt, vi* to speak; —— **con la lengua** *or* **voz pesada** to slur; —— **por señas** to sign
hacer *vi* **Hace tres años**..Three years ago... **¿Hace cuánto que tiene artritis?**..How long have you had arthritis? —— **del baño** (*Mex, fam*) to have a bowel movement; —— **del cuerpo** (*Carib, CA*) to have a bowel movement
hachís *m* hashish
Haemophilus Haemophilus
halitosis *f* halitosis
hallazgo *m* finding
hallus valgus, hallux valgus *m* hallux valgus
hallus varus, hallux varus *m* hallux varus

haloperidol *m* haloperidol
halotano *m* halothane
hamartoma *m* hamartoma
hambre *f* hunger; **tener** —— to be hungry; **¿Tiene hambre?**..Are you hungry?
harina *f* flour
haz *m* (*pl* **haces**) tract; —— **espinotalámico** spinothalamic tract
hebilla *f* buckle
heces *fpl* (*also* —— **fecales**) feces
helado *adj* frozen, cold; *m* ice cream
helio *m* helium
hemangioma *m* hemangioma; —— **cavernoso** cavernous hemangioma
hematocele *m* hematocele
hematócrito *m* hematocrit
hematología *f* hematology
hematólogo -ga *mf* hematologist
hematoma *m* hematoma; —— **subdural** subdural hematoma
hembra *adj* & *f* female
hemiplejía *f* hemiplegia
hemisferio *m* hemisphere
hemocromatosis *f* hemochromatosis

hemocultivo *m* blood culture
hemodiálisis *f* hemodialysis
hemofilia *f* hemophilia
hemoglobina *f* hemoglobin
hemofílico -ca *mf* hemophiliac
hemólisis *f* hemolysis
hemolítico -ca *adj* hemolytic
hemorragia *f* hemorrhage, bleeding; —— nasal nosebleed; —— **subaracnoidea** subarachnoid hemorrhage
hemorrágico -ca *adj* hemorrhagic
hemorroide *f* hemorrhoid
hemorroidectomía *f* hemorrhoidectomy
hemosiderosis *f* hemosiderosis
heno *m* hay
heparina *f* heparin
hepático -ca *adj* hepatic
hepatitis *f* hepatitis; —— **A, B, no A no B, etc.** hepatitis A; B; non-A, non-B; etc.
hepatoma *m* hepatoma
hepatorrenal *adj* hepatorenal
herbario -ria *adj* herbal
herbicida *m* herbicide
herbolario -ria *mf* herbalist, person who sells herbs; *m* herb shop
heredado -da *adj* inherited
heredar *vt* to inherit
hereditario -ria *adj* hereditary
herencia *f* heredity
herido -da *adj* injured, hurt, wounded; *mf* wounded person; *f* injury, wound, cut, incision; **herida de bala** gunshot wound; **herida punzante** *or* **por punción** puncture wound
herir *vt* to injure, hurt, wound
hermafrodita *adj* & *mf* hermaphrodite
hermafroditismo *m* hermaphroditism
hermanastra *f* stepsister
hermanastro *m* stepbrother
hermano -na *m* brother, sibling; *f* sister; **hermanos -nas siameses** Siamese twins
hernia *f* hernia; —— **estrangulada** strangulated hernia; —— **femoral** femoral hernia; —— **hiatal** hiatal hernia; —— **incarcerada** incarcerated hernia; —— **incisional** incisional hernia; —— **inguinal** inguinal hernia; —— **reducible** reducible hernia; —— **umbilical** umbilical hernia

heroína *f* heroin
herpangina *f* herpangina
herpes *m* herpes; —— **simple** herpes simplex; —— **zoster** herpes zoster, shingles
herpético -ca *adj* herpetic
hervido -da *adj* boiled; **agua hervida** boiled water
hervir *vt* (*also* hacer ——) to boil; *vi* to boil; **hervirle el pecho** (*fam*) to breathe noisily (*as with bronchitis or asthma*), to be congested in the chest, to wheeze
hervor *m* (*fam, del pecho*) congestion of the chest, wheezing
heterosexual *adj* & *mf* heterosexual
hidátide, hidatídico -ca *adj* hydatid
hidatiforme, hidatidiforme *adj* hydatidiform
hidradenitis supurativa *f* hidradenitis suppurativa
hidralacina *f* hydralazine
hidratante *adj* moisturizing
hidratar *vt* to hydrate
hidrato de cloral *m* chloral hydrate
hidrocarburo *m* hydrocarbon
hidrocefalia *f* hydrocephaly
hidrocéfalo *m* hydrocephalus
hidrocele *m* hydrocele
hidroclorotiazida *f* hydrochlorothiazide
hidrocortisona *f* hydrocortisone
hidrofobia *f* hydrophobia
hidrogenado -da *adj* hydrogenated
hidronefrosis *f* hydronephrosis
hidroquinona *f* hydroquinone
hidroterapia *f* hydrotherapy
hidroxicina *f* hydroxizine
hidróxido de sodio *m* sodium hydroxide
hiedra venenosa *f* poison ivy
hielo *m* ice; **bolsa con** —— ice pack
hierba *f* grass; herb
hierbería *f* herb shop
hierbero -ra *mf* herbalist
hierro *m* iron
hifema *See* **hipema**.
hígado *m* liver; **enfermedad** *f* **del** —— liver disease
higiene *f* hygiene
higiénico -ca *adj* hygienic
higienista *mf* hygienist
higo *m* fig

hijastro -tra *m* stepson, stepchild; *f* stepdaughter
hijo -ja *m* son, child; *f* daughter
hilo dental *m* dental floss
himen *m* hymen
hinchado -da *adj* swollen, puffy; —— del estómago bloated
hincharse *vr* to swell, swell up; —— el estómago to become bloated
hinchazón *f* swelling
hioides *m* hyoid bone
hipema *f* hyphema
hiperactividad *f* hyperactivity
hiperactivo -va *adj* hyperactive
hiperalimentación *f* hyperalimentation
hiperbárico -ca *adj* hyperbaric
hipercalcemia *f* hypercalcemia
hiperextensible *adj* double-jointed
hiperglucemia *f* hyperglycemia
hiperlipemia, hiperlipidemia *f* hyperlipidemia
hiperlipoproteinemia *f* hyperlipoproteinemia
hipermétrope *adj* farsighted
hipermetropía *f* farsightedness
hiperosmolar *adj* hyperosmolar
hiperparatiroideo -a *adj* hyperparathyroid
hiperparatiroidismo *m* hyperparathyroidism
hiperpigmentación *f* hyperpigmentation
hiperplasia *f* hyperplasia
hipersensibilidad *f* hypersensitivity
hipersensible *adj* hypersensitive
hipertensión *f* hypertension; —— maligna malignant hypertension; —— portal portal hypertension; —— pulmonar pulmonary hypertension
hipertermia *f* hyperthermia
hipertiroideo -a *adj* hyperthyroid
hipertiroidismo *m* hyperthyroidism
hipertrofia *f* hypertrophy; —— prostática benigna benign prostatic hypertrophy
hiperventilación *f* hyperventilation
hipnosis *f* hypnosis
hipnótico -ca *adj* & *m* hypnotic
hipnotismo *m* hypnotism
hipnotizador -ra *mf* hypnotist
hipnotizar *vt* to hypnotize
hipo *m* hiccup; tener —— to have the

hiccups, to hiccup
hipoalergénico -ca *adj* hypoallergenic
hipocondríaco -ca, hipocondriaco -ca *adj* & *mf* hypochondriac
hipodérmico -ca *adj* hypodermic
hipoglucemia *f* hypoglycemia
hipoglucemiante *m* hypoglycemic agent; —— oral oral hypoglycemic agent
hipoglucémico -ca *adj* hypoglycemic
hipoparatiroideo -a *adj* hypoparathyroid
hipoparatiroidismo *m* hypoparathyroidism
hipopituitarismo *m* hypopituitarism
hipospadias *m* hypospadias
hipotálamo *m* hypothalamus
hipotensión *f* hypotension
hipotermia *f* hypothermia
hipotiroideo -a *adj* hypothyroid
hipotiroidismo *m* hypothyroidism
hisopo *m* swab
histamina *f* histamine
histerectomía *f* hysterectomy; —— abdominal abdominal hysterectomy; —— vaginal vaginal hysterectomy
histeria *f* hysteria
histérico -ca *adj* hysterical
histidina *f* histidine
histiocitosis X *f* histiocytosis X
histología *f* histology
histoplasmosis *f* histoplasmosis
historia *f* history; —— clínica history, medical history; —— clínica previa past medical history
histriónico -ca *adj* histrionic
hogar *m* home; sin —— homeless
hoja *f* (*de cuchillo, etc.*) blade; —— de afeitar *or* rasurar razor blade
holístico -ca *adj* (*Ang*) holistic
hombre *m* man
hombro *m* shoulder
homeópata *mf* homeopath
homeopatía *f* homeopathy
homeopático -ca *adj* homeopathic
homofobia *f* homophobia
homofóbico -ca *adj* homophobic
homosexual *adj* & *mf* homosexual
hondo -da *adj* deep
hondureño -ña *adj* & *mf* Honduran
hongo *m* fungus, mushroom; hongos (*fam*)

yeast infection

honorarios *mpl* fee

hora *f* hour, time; **¿A qué hora comió?..** What time did you eat?..When did you eat? **horas de consulta** *or* **oficina** office hours; **horas de visita** visiting hours

horario *m* schedule

hormiga *f* ant

hormiguear *vi* to tingle

hormigueo *m* tingling

hormona *f* hormone; —— **adrenocorticotrópica** adrenocortical hormone (ACTH); —— **del crecimiento** growth hormone (GH); —— **estimulante del folículo** follicle-stimulating hormone (FSH); —— **estimulante del tiroides** thyroid-stimulating hormone (TSH); —— **liberadora de gonadotropinas** gonadotropin-releasing hormone (GnRH); —— **luteinizante** luteinizing hormone (LH); —— **paratiroidea** parathyroid hormone (PTH); —— **tiroidea** thyroid hormone; —— **tirotrópica** thyroid-stimulating hormone (TSH)

hormonal *adj* hormonal

horneado -da *adj* baked

hornear *vt* to bake

horno, al baked

hortensia *f* (*bot*) hydrangea

hospital *m* hospital; —— **de la comunidad** community hospital; —— **del condado** county hospital (*US*); —— **general** general hospital; —— **para veteranos** Veterans Administration (VA) hospital; —— **privado** private hospital; —— **psiquiátrico** mental hospital; —— **público** public hospital; **administración** *f* **del** —— hospital administration

hospitalario -ria *adj* pertaining to a hospital, hospital

hospitalizar *vt* to hospitalize

hostil *adj* hostile

hostilidad *f* hostility

hoy *adv* today

hoyo *m* hole; —— **de la nariz** (*fam*) nostril

hoyuelo *m* dimple

huata *f* (*ortho, surg*) padding

hueco -ca *adj* & *m* hollow; —— **de la rodilla** hollow of the knee

huelgo *m* breath; **tomar** *or* **agarrar** —— to catch one's breath

huellas *fpl* traces

huérfano -na *mf* orphan

huesecillo, huesillo *m* ossicle

hueso *m* bone; **huesos** (*esp Mex, CA; fam*) joints; **Se me hinchan los huesos**..My joints swell; —— **de la cadera** hipbone; —— **del pecho** breastbone; —— **del tobillo** anklebone; —— **iliaco** ilium

huevecillo *m* small egg (*of a parasite, etc.*)

huevo *m* egg; (*fam*) egg (*fam*), ovum; (*vulg, frec pl*) ball (*vulg, frec pl*), testicle

hule *m* rubber

humanitario -ria *adj* humanitarian

humano -na *adj* & *m* human; **ser humano** human being

humectante *adj* moisturizing

humedad *f* humidity, dampness, moisture

humedecedor *m* humidifier

humedecer *vt* to humidify, moisturize, moisten

húmedo -da *adj* damp, moist, humid

húmero *m* humerus

humo *m* smoke, fumes

humor *m* mood; (*anat*) humor; —— **acuoso** aqueous humor; —— **vítreo** vitreous humor; **estar de mal** —— to be in a bad mood

huracán *m* hurricane

I

ibuprofén, ibuprofeno *m* ibuprofen
id *m* (*psych*) id
ideal *adj* ideal
identidad *f* identity
identificación *f* identification
identificar *vt* to identify; *vr* (*psych*) identificarse con to identify with
idiopático -ca *adj* idiopathic
ido -da *adj* absent-minded, distracted
ilegal *adj* illegal
íleo *m* ileus
íleon *m* ileum
ileostomía *f* ileostomy
iliaco -ca *adj* iliac
ilusión *f* illusion
IM *See* intramuscular.
imagen *f* image; —— corporal body image; —— diagnóstica diagnostic imaging, X-ray, scan; imágenes por resonancia magnética magnetic resonance imaging (MRI)
imipenem *m* imipenem
imipramina *f* imipramine
impacción *f* impaction
impactación *f* impaction
impactado -da *adj* impacted
impacto *m* impact
imperdible *m* safety pin
imperforado -da *adj* imperforate
impétigo *m* impetigo
implantación *f* implantation
implantar *vt* to implant; *vr* to become implanted
implante *m* implant
impotencia *f* impotence
impotente *adj* impotent
impregnar *vt* to impregnate
impulsar *vt* (*sangre*) to pump
impulsivo -va *adj* impulsive

impureza *f* impurity
impuro -ra *adj* impure
inactividad *f* inactivity
inactivo -va *adj* inactive
inanición *f* starvation
inapropiado -da *adj* inappropriate
incansable *adj* tireless, untiring
incapacidad *f* disability; —— de trabajo (*Mex*) work excuse, certificate of disability
incapacitado -da *adj* disabled
incapacitante *adj* incapacitating
incapaz *adj* (*pl* -paces) incapable, unable
incendio *m* fire
incesto *m* incest
incestuoso -sa *adj* incestuous
incidencia *f* incidence
incisión *f* incision
inclinar *vt* to bend, bend down; **Incline la cabeza**..Bend your head down...**Incline la cabeza a la izquierda**..Bend your head to the left; *vr* to lean, lean forward, stoop; **Inclínese**..Lean forward.
incoherente *adj* incoherent
incomodidad *f* discomfort
incómodo -da *adj* uncomfortable
incompatible *adj* incompatible
incompetente *adj* incompetent
incompleto -ta *adj* incomplete
inconsciente *adj* unconscious
incontinencia *f* incontinence; —— de esfuerzo stress incontinence
incontinente *adj* incontinent
incordio *m* bubo, enlarged inguinal node
incrustación *f* (*dent*) inlay
incubadora *f* incubator
incurable *adj* incurable
indebido -da *adj* improper, inappropriate
independiente *adj* independent
indeseable *adj* undesirable

indicación f indication; (*en el expediente*) order; (*instrucción*) instruction; **poner indicaciones** to order

índice adj (*dedo*) index; m index; —— de Apgar Apgar score; —— de metabolismo basal basal metabolic rate; —— de mortalidad death rate; —— de mortalidad infantil infant mortality rate; —— de natalidad birth rate

indiferencia f indifference, apathy

indiferenciado -da adj undifferentiated

indigestión f indigestion

indisposición f indisposition, slight illness

indistinto -ta adj indistinct, dim

individuo m individual, person

indoloro -ra adj painless

indometacina f indomethacin

inducir vt to induce

ineficaz adj (*pl* -**caces**) ineffective

inelegible adj ineligible

inerte adj inert

inespecífico -ca adj nonspecific

inesperado -da adj unexpected

inestable adj unstable

inevitable adj unavoidable

infancia f infancy, childhood

infante m infant

infantil adj infantile

infarto m infarct, infarction; —— de miocardio myocardial infarction

infatigable adj tireless, untiring

infección f infection; —— del tracto urinario urinary tract infection (UTI); —— pélvica pelvic inflammatory disease (PID)

infeccioso -sa adj infectious

infectar vt to infect; vr to become infected

infeliz adj (*pl* -**lices**) unhappy

inferior adj (*anat*) inferior, lower

infertilidad f infertility

infestación f infestation

infestar vt to infest

infiltración f infiltration

infiltrar vt, vr to infiltrate

inflado -da adj (*del estómago*) bloated

inflamable adj flammable, inflammable; **no** —— nonflammable

inflamación f inflammation

inflamado -da adj inflamed

inflamarse vr to become inflamed

inflamatorio -ria adj inflammatory

inflarse vr —— el estómago to become bloated

influenza f influenza, flu

información f information, data

infrarrojo -ja adj infrared

infundir vt to infuse

infusión f infusion

ingeniería genética f genetic engineering

ingerir vt to ingest

ingle f groin

ingrediente m ingredient

ingresar vt to admit (*to the hospital*); vr to be admitted

ingreso m admission; **Ingresos** Admitting

inguinal adj inguinal

inhabilitado -da adj disabled

inhalación f inhalation

inhalador -ra adj inhalant; m inhaler

inhalante m inhalant

inhalar vt, vi to inhale, breathe in; (*cocaína, cemento, etc.*) to sniff (*cocaine, glue, etc.*)

inhibición f inhibition

inhibido -da adj inhibited

inhibir vt to inhibit

inicial adj initial; f initial

injertar vt (*pp* -**tado** or **injerto**) to graft

injerto (*pp of* **injertar**) m graft; —— cutáneo skin graft

inmaduro -ra adj immature; (*fruta*) green, not yet ripe

inmediatamente adv immediately

inmediato -ta adj immediate

inmersión f immersion

inmóvil adj immobile

inmovilización f immobilization

inmovilizador m immobilizer

inmovilizar vt to immobilize

inmune adj immune

inmunidad f immunity

inmunización f immunization

inmunizar vt to immunize

inmunocompetente adj immunocompetent

inmunocomprometido -da adj immunocompromised

inmunodeficiencia f immunodeficiency

inmunodepresión f immunodepression

inmunodeprimido -da *adj* immunodepressed
inmunoglobulina *f* immunoglobulin
inmunología *f* immunology
inmunológico -ca *adj* immunological
inmunólogo -ga *mf* immunologist
inmunosupresor -ra *adj* immunosuppressive; *m* immunosuppressant
inmunoterapia *f* immunotherapy
inoculación *f* inoculation
inocular *vt* to inoculate
inodoro *m* toilet; **taza del —— toilet bowl**
inofensivo -va *adj* harmless
inoperable *adj* inoperable
inorgánico -ca *adj* inorganic
inquieto -ta *adj* restless, uneasy
insaturado -da *adj* unsaturated
insecticida *m* insecticide
insecto *m* insect
inseguridad *f* insecurity
inseguro -ra *adj* insecure
inseminación *f* insemination; **—— artificial** artificial insemination
inseminar *vt* to inseminate
insolación *f* sunstroke, heatstroke
insomnio *m* insomnia
insoportable *adj* unbearable
inspirar *vt, vi* to inspire, inhale
instinto *m* drive, instinct
instrucción *f* instruction
instructivo *m* package insert
instrumento *m* instrument
insuficiencia *f* insufficiency, failure; **—— aórtica, mitral, etc.** aortic insufficiency, mitral insufficiency, etc.; **—— cardiaca congestiva** congestive heart failure; **—— hepática** hepatic insufficiency, liver failure; **—— renal** renal insufficiency *o* failure; **—— respiratoria** respiratory failure; **—— venosa** venous insufficiency
insulina *f* insulin; **—— de acción rápida** regular insulin; **—— lenta** lente insulin; **—— NPH** *or* **de acción intermedia** NPH insulin; **—— semilenta** semilente insulin; **—— ultralenta** ultralente insulin
intacto -ta *adj* intact
intelecto *m* intellect
intelectual *adj* intellectual
intelectualizar *vi* to intellectualize

inteligencia *f* intelligence; **cociente de —— (CI)** intelligence quotient (IQ)
intensidad *f* intensity
intensificar *vt* to intensify
intensivo -va *adj* intensive
intenso -sa *adj* intense
interacción *f* interaction
interactuar *vi* to interact
interferón *m* interferon; **—— alfa** alpha interferon; **—— beta** beta interferon; **—— gamma** gamma interferon
interior *adj & m* interior
intermedio -dia *adj* intermediate
intermitente *adj* intermittent
internar *vt* to admit (*to the hospital*), to hospitalize; *vr* to be admitted *o* hospitalized; **¿Ha estado internado aquí antes?**..Have you been hospitalized here before?
internista *mf* internist
interno -na *adj* internal, inner, inside; (*anat*) medial; *mf* intern
interpersonal *adj* interpersonal
interpretar *vt, vi* to interpret
intérprete *mf* interpreter
intersticial *adj* interstitial
intervalo *m* interval
intervención *f* intervention
interventricular *adj* interventricular
intestinal *adj* intestinal
intestino *m* intestine, bowel, gut; **—— delgado** small intestine *o* bowel; **—— grueso** large intestine *o* bowel
intimidad *f* intimacy
intolerable *adj* intolerable, unbearable
intolerancia *f* intolerance
intolerante *adj* intolerant
intoxicación *f* poisoning, intoxication; **—— alimenticia** *or* **alimentaria** food poisoning
intraarticular *adj* intraarticular
intracraneal *adj* intracranial
intracutáneo -nea *adj* intradermal
intradérmico -ca *adj* intradermal
intramuscular (IM) *adj* intramuscular
intranquilo -la *adj* restless
intraocular *adj* intraocular
intravenoso -sa (IV) *adj* intravenous (IV)
introducir *vt* to insert

introvertido -da *adj* introverted; *mf* introvert
intubación *f* intubation
intubar *vt* to intubate
intususcepción *f* intussusception
inundación *f* flood
inútil *adj* useless
inválido -da *adj* disabled; *mf* disabled person
invasivo -va *adj* invasive; **no —** non-invasive
invasor -ra *adj* invasive; **no —** non-invasive
investigación *f* research; **en —** (*medicamento, etc.*) investigational
invierno *m* winter
invisible *adj* invisible
involuntario -ria *adj* involuntary
inyección *f* injection, shot (*fam*); **¿Me van a poner una inyección?**..Are you going to give me an injection?
inyectable *adj* injectable
inyectar *vt* to inject, to give (*someone*) an injection; **¿Me va a inyectar?**..Are you going to give me an injection? *vr* to inject oneself, give oneself an injection
iontoforesis *f* iontophoresis
ipecacuana *f* ipecac
ir *vi* **— y venir** to come and go; **El dolor me va y me viene**..The pain comes and goes.

ira *f* anger, rage
iris *m* (*pl* **iris**) iris
iritis *f* iritis
irradiación *f* irradiation
irradiar *vt* to irradiate
irregular *adj* irregular
irreversible *adj* irreversible
irrigación *f* irrigation
irrigar *vt* to irrigate
irritabilidad *f* irritability
irritable *adj* irritable
irritación *f* irritation
irritante *adj* irritating; *m* irritant
irritar *vt* to irritate; *vr* to become irritated
irrompible *adj* unbreakable
isoetarina *f* isoetharine
isoleucina *f* isoleucine
isométrico -ca *adj* isometric
isoniacida *f* isoniazid (INH)
isótopo *m* isotope
isotretinoína *f* isotretinoin
isquemia *f* ischemia; **— cerebral transitoria** transient ischemic attack
isquémico -ca *adj* ischemic
isradipina *f* isradipine
itraconazol *m* itraconazole
IV *See* **intravenoso**.
izquierdo -da *adj* left; left-handed; *f* left, left-hand side

J

jabón *m* soap
jadear *vi* to pant
jalar *vt* **— aire** to gasp
jalea *f* jelly
jamón *m* ham
jaqueca *f* migraine, severe headache
jarabe *m* syrup; **— para la tos** cough syrup
jardinero -ra *mf* gardener

jarra *f* pitcher
jefe -fa *mf* employer; **— de enfermeras** head nurse; **— de turno** charge nurse
jején *m* gnat, no-see-um, sandfly
jengibre *m* (*bot*) ginger
jeringa *f* syringe
jeringuilla *f* (*esp Carib*) syringe
jimagua *mf* (*Cub*) twin
jiricua *f* (*Mex, fam*) vitiligo

joroba *f* hump
jorobado -da *adj* humpbacked; *mf* humpback
joven *adj* young; *m* young man, young
person; *f* young woman
juanete *m* bunion
judo *m* judo

jugo *m* juice; —— **de fruta, naranja,
tomate, etc.** fruit juice, orange juice,
tomato juice, etc.
juntar *vt, vr* (*dos objetos*) to join
juramento hipocrático *m* Hippocratic Oath
juvenil *adj* juvenile
juventud *f* youth

K

karate *m* karate
ketoconazol *m* ketoconazole
ketorolaco *m* ketorolac
kilo *See* **kilogramo**.

kilogramo *m* kilogram
Klebsiella Klebsiella
kwashiorkor *m* kwashiorkor

L

laberintitis *f* labyrinthitis
laberinto *m* labyrinth
labetolol *m* labetolol
labial *adj* labial
labio *m* lip; (*genital*) labium (*form*), lip
(*fam*); —— **inferior** lower lip; ——
superior upper lip
laboratorio *m* laboratory
laceración *f* laceration
lacerar *vt* to lacerate
lacrimal, lagrimal *adj* lacrimal *o* lachrymal
lacrimógeno *m* tear gas
lactancia *f* lactation; —— **materna** breast-
feeding
lactante *mf* nursing infant, breast-fed infant
lactar *vi* to lactate
lactasa *f* lactase
lácteo -tea *adj* milk, pertaining to milk;
producto —— milk product

láctico -ca *adj* lactic
Lactobacillus Lactobacillus
lactosa *f* lactose; **intolerancia a la** ——
lactose intolerance
lactulosa *f* lactulose
ladilla *f* crab louse, crab (*fam*)
lado *m* side; **por el lado de mi madre**..on
my mother's side
lagaña *f* sleep (*eye secretions*)
lagartija *f* push-up
lágrima *f* tear
laguna mental *f* blackout, lapse of memory
lamentar *vt, vr* to mourn
lamer *vt* to lick
laminectomía *f* laminectomy
lámpara *f* lamp; —— **de hendidura**
slitlamp; —— **solar** *or* **bronceadora**
sunlamp
lana *f* wool

lanceta *f* lancet

lanolina *f* lanolin

lanugo *m* lanugo

laparoscopia, laparoscopía *f* laparoscopy

laparascópico -ca *adj* laparoscopic

laparoscopio *m* laparoscope

laparotomía *f* laparotomy

lapso *m* lapse

largo -ga *adj* long; a —— plazo long-term; hacer más —— to lengthen; *m* length

laringe *f* larynx

laringectomía *f* laryngectomy

laríngeo -a *adj* laryngeal

laringitis *f* laryngitis

laringoscopia, laringoscopía *f* laryngoscopy

laringoscopio *m* laryngoscope

larva *f* larva; —— migrans larva migrans

láser *m* laser

lastimadura *f* sprain, dislocation, muscle pull, bruise, minor injury (*in which skin remains intact*)

lastimar *vt* to hurt, injure; *vr* to get hurt, to hurt oneself; ¿Se lastimó?..Did you hurt yourself?...¿Se lástimo la cabeza?..Did you hurt your head?

lata *f* can

latente *adj* latent

lateral *adj* lateral

látex *m* latex

latido *m* beat; —— del corazón heartbeat

latir *vi* (*el corazón*) to beat; (*un dolor*) to throb

lavable *adj* washable

lavado *m* lavage; (*intestinal*) enema; —— broncoalveolar bronchoalveolar lavage; —— gástrico gastric lavage; —— peritoneal peritoneal lavage

lavar *vt* to wash; *vr* lavarse la cabeza *or* el pelo to wash one's hair; lavarse las manos, la cara, etc. to wash one's hands, one's face, etc.

lavativa *f* enema

lavatorio *m* lavatory

laxante *adj & m* laxative

lazo *m* loop

lb. *See* libra.

leche *f* milk; —— baja en grasas low fat milk; —— bronca (*Mex*) raw milk; —— condensada condensed milk; —— de cabra goat's milk; —— descremada *or* desnatada skim milk; —— de vaca cow's milk; (*fam*) raw milk; —— en polvo powdered milk; —— entera whole milk; —— evaporizada evaporated milk; —— materna breast milk; —— pasteurizada pasteurized milk; —— sin procesar raw milk; producto de —— milk *o* dairy product

leche de magnesia *f* milk of magnesia

lecho *m* bed, sickbed, deathbed; —— vascular vascular bed

lecitina *f* lecithin

lectura *f* (*de un instrumento*) reading

leer *vt, vi* to read; —— los labios to lipread

legaña *f* sleep (*eye secretions*)

lego -ga *adj* lay (*opinion, etc.*)

legrado *m* (*fam*) curettage

legumbre *f* legume; (*vegetal*) vegetable

leiomiofibroma *m* leiomyofibroma

leiomioma *m* leiomyoma

leiomiosarcoma *m* leiomyosarcoma

leishmaniasis *f* leishmaniasis; —— mucocutánea americana American *o* mucocutaneous leishmaniasis

lejía *f* lye

lengua *f* tongue; —— saburral coated tongue; sacar la —— to stick out one's tongue; Saque la lengua..Stick out your tongue.

lenguaje *m* language (*structure and development*); —— corporal body language

lente *m&f* lens; —— de aumento magnifying glass; —— de contacto (*duro, blando*) contact lens (*hard, soft*)

lentes *mpl* eyeglasses, glasses; —— para el sol *or* oscuros sunglasses; —— protectores protective eyewear, goggles

lepra *f* leprosy

leptospirosis *f* leptospirosis

lesbiana *f* lesbian

lesión *f* lesion, injury; —— por latigazo whiplash

lesionar *vt* to hurt, injure; *vr* to hurt oneself, to get injured

letal *adj* lethal

letárgico -ca *adj* lethargic

letargo *m* lethargy
letra *f* handwriting
letrina *f* latrine
leucemia *f* leukemia; —— **granulocítica** granulocytic leukemia; —— **linfoblástica** lymphoblastic leukemia; —— **linfocítica aguda** acute lymphocytic leukemia; —— **mielógena crónica** chronic myelogenous leukemia; —— **mieloide** myeloid leukemia
leucina *f* leucine
leucocito *m* leukocyte
leucoencefalopatía multifocal progresiva *f* progressive multifocal leukoencephalopathy
levantar *vt* to raise, to lift; **Levante la pierna..**Raise your leg; —— **pesas** to lift weights, to work out; *vr* to get up, to stand (up)
leve *adj* slight, light, mild
liberación *f* release; **de —— prolongada** slow-release; **de —— sostenida** sustained-release
liberador -ra *adj* releasing; —— **de cobre,** —— **de hormona, etc.** copper-releasing, hormone-releasing, etc.
liberar *vt* to release; (*virus, etc.*) to shed
libido *f* libido
libra (lb.) *f* pound (lb.)
libre *adj* free, loose
licor *m* liquor
lidocaína *f* lidocaine
liendre *f* nit
lienzo *m* cloth, towel
ligado -da *adj* —— **al cromosoma X** *or* —— **al X** X-linked; —— **al sexo** sex-linked
ligadura *f* ligation; —— **de las trompas** *or* **tubárica** tubal ligation
ligamento *m* ligament
ligar *vt* to join (*two objects*)
ligero -ra *adj* light, slight; gentle
lima *f* lime; file; —— **para uñas** nail file
limar *vt* to file
limitar *vt* to limit
límite *m* limit; —— **inferior normal** lower limit of normal; —— **superior normal** upper limit of normal

limón *m* lemon; —— **verde** lime
limpia *f* (*Mex, CA; fam*) healing ritual
limpiador -ra de casa *mf* housecleaner
limpiar *vt* to clean; *vr* (*después de defecar*) to wipe (*oneself*)
limpieza *f* cleaning; cleanliness; (*fam*) healing ritual
limpio -pia *adj* clean
lindano *m* lindane
línea *f* line, streak
linfa *f* lymph
linfadenitis *f* lymphadenitis
linfangitis *f* lymphangitis
linfático -ca *adj* lymphatic
linfocito *m* lymphocyte; —— **B** B lymphocyte; —— **T ayudante** helper T lymphocyte; —— **T supresor** suppressor T lymphocyte
linfogranuloma venéreo *or* **inguinal** *m* lymphogranuloma venereum (LGV)
linfoide *adj* lymphoid
linfoma *m* lymphoma; —— **linfocítico** *or* **no Hodgkin** lymphocytic *o* non-Hodgkin's lymphoma
linimento *m* liniment
linoleico -ca *adj* linoleic
liofilizado-da *adj* lyophilized
liomioma *m* leiomyoma
liomiosarcoma *m* leiomyosarcoma
lipasa *f* lipase
lípido *m* lipid
lipoma *m* lipoma
lipoproteína *f* lipoprotein; —— **de alta densidad (LAD)** high density lipoprotein (HDL); —— **de baja densidad (LBD)** low density lipoprotein (LDL); —— **de muy baja densidad (LMBD)** very low density lipoprotein (VLDL)
liposarcoma *m* liposarcoma
liposucción *f* liposuction
liquen plano *m* lichen planus
líquido -da *adj* liquid, runny; *m* liquid, fluid; —— **amniótico** amniotic fluid; —— **cefalorraquídeo (LCR)** cerebrospinal fluid (CSF); —— **pleural** pleural fluid; —— **seminal** seminal fluid; —— **sinovial** synovial fluid
lisiado -da *adj* crippled; *mf* crippled person

lisiar *vt* to cripple
lisina *f* lysine
lisinopril *m* lisinopril
liso -sa *adj* smooth, even
lista de espera *f* waiting list
listeriosis *f* listeriosis
litio *m* lithium
litotripsia *f* lithotripsy
litro *m* liter
liviano -na *adj* light (*weight*)
llaga *f* ulcer, sore
llamada *f* page; —— **por el bíper** page by beeper; —— **por vocina** overhead page
llamar *vt* (*por vocina, por bíper*) to page
llanto *m* cry, crying
llenar *vt* to fill
lleno -na *adj* full; **¿Está lleno?**..Are you full?
llenura *f* fullness
llevar *vt* (*ropa, etc.*) to wear
llorar *vt* to mourn; *vi* to cry
lobar *adj* lobar
lobectomía *f* lobectomy
lobelia *f* (*bot*) lobelia
lobotomía *f* lobotomy
lóbulo *m* lobe; (*del oído*) earlobe
local *adj* local
loción *f* lotion; —— **bronceadora** suntan lotion
loco -ca *adj* crazy, insane; **volver** —— (*a alguien*) to drive (*someone*) crazy; **volverse** —— to go crazy, lose one's mind; *mf* crazy person
locura *f* insanity, craziness

lombriz *f* (*pl* -**brices**) worm, intestinal worm
lomo *m* (*fam*) loin, lower back
lonche *m* (*Ang*) lunch
longevidad *f* longevity
longitud *f* length; —— **de onda** wavelength
loperamida *f* loperamide
loracarbef *m* loracarbef
loracepam *m* lorazepam
loratidina *f* loratidine
lordosis *f* lordosis
lordótico -ca *adj* lordotic
lote *m* (*pharm*) lot
lovastatina *f* lovastatin
LSD *See* **dietilamida del ácido lisérgico.**
lubricación *f* lubrication
lubricante *adj* & *m* lubricant
lubricar *vt* to lubricate
lucecita *f* (*visual*) floater
lumbar *adj* lumbar
lumpectomía *f* (*Ang*) lumpectomy
lunar *m* mole, birthmark
lupa *f* magnifying glass, hand lens
lúpulo *m* (*bot*) hops
lupus *m* lupus; —— **eritematoso generalizado** *or* **sistémico** systemic lupus erythematosus (SLE)
luteínico -ca *adj* luteal
lúteo -a *adj* luteal
luxación *f* dislocation
luxar *vt, vr* to dislocate, to become dislocated; **Me luxé el hombro**..I dislocated my shoulder...**Se me luxó el hombro**..My shoulder became dislocated.
luz *f* (*pl* **luces**) light; —— **del sol** sunlight

M

macerar *vt* to macerate
machucadura *f* mash, mild crush injury
machucar *vt* to mash, crush
machucón *m* mash, mild crush injury

macrobiótico -ca *adj* macrobiotic
madrastra *f* stepmother
madre *f* mother; —— **subrogada** surrogate mother

madrugada *f* early morning (*before dawn*)

madurar *vi* to mature; (*un absceso*) to come to a head, to secrete pus

madurez *f* maturity

maduro -ra *adj* mature; (*absceso, fruta*) ripe

maestro -tra *mf* teacher

magnesio *m* magnesium

magro -gra *adj* (*persona*) lean, thin; (*carne*) lean

magullado -da *adj* bruised, sore

magulladura *f* bruise

magullar *vt* to bruise; *vr* to bruise, get bruised

maicena *f* cornstarch

maíz *m* corn

mal *adj See* **malo**; *adv* **estar** —— to be sick, to feel ill; **Estoy mal de los pulmones.**.I have a problem with my lungs; **sentirse** —— to feel sick; *m* illness, sickness, ailment, disease; —— **del pinto** pinta, mal del pinto; —— **de montaña** mountain sickness; —— **de ojo** (*fam*) eye infection, conjunctivitis; evil eye, pediatric folk illness believed to occur when a person with magical powers eyes an infant with ill intent; —— **de orín** (*fam*) urinary tract infection

malabsorción *f* malabsorption

malaria *f* malaria

malatión *m* malathion

malestar *m* malaise

maletín *m* (*del médico*) doctor's bag

malformación *f* malformation

malignidad *f* malignancy

maligno -na *adj* malignant

malla *f* mesh

mallugar *See* **magullar**.

malo -la *adj* (**mal** *before masculine singular nouns*) bad; sick, ill; **¿Está mala ella?**.Is she sick?

malparir *vi* to have a miscarriage

malparto *m* miscarriage

mama *f* breast

mamá *f* (*pl* **mamás**) mom

mamadera *f* nursing bottle, baby's bottle; nipple of nursing bottle

mamar *vi* to nurse, suck (*at mother's breast*); (*vulg*) to perform fellatio

mamario -ria *adj* mammary

mamila *f* nipple (*of a nursing bottle*)

mamografía *f* mammography; mammogram

mamograma *m* mammogram

mamoplastia, mamoplastía *f* mammoplasty

mancha *f* spot, stain; —— **de vino oporto** port-wine stain

manco -ca *adj* one-handed, one-armed

mandíbula *f* jaw, lower jaw, jawbone

manejar *vt* to manage; (*un vehículo*) to drive

manejo *m* management

manguera *f* hose, tube

maní *m* peanut

manía *f* mania

maniaco -ca, maníaco -ca *adj* manic

maniacodepresivo -va *adj* manic-depressive

manicomio *m* insane asylum

manicura *f* manicure

manifestación *f* manifestation

maniobra *f* maneuver; —— **de Heimlich** Heimlich maneuver

maniobrar *vt, vi* to maneuver

manipular *vt* to manipulate

mano *f* hand; —— **péndula** wrist drop

manometría *f* manometry

manta *f* blanket, light blanket; —— **eléctrica** electric blanket

manteca *f* lard, fat, cooking grease; —— **de cacao** cocoa butter

mantener *vt* to maintain; —— **la respiración** *or* **el resuello** to hold one's breath; **Mantenga la respiración.**.Hold your breath.

mantenimiento *m* maintenance

mantequilla *f* butter; —— **de cacahuate** peanut butter

manual *adj* manual, hand-held; *m* manual, booklet

manubrio *m* manubrium

manzana *f* apple; —— **de Adán** Adam's apple

manzanilla *f* (*bot*) chamomile

mañana *adv* tomorrow; **pasado** —— the day after tomorrow; *f* morning; **inyección de la mañana.**.morning injection

mapache *m* raccoon

maquillaje *m* make-up, cosmetics

máquina de afeitar *f* electric razor, shaver

marca *f* mark; brand; **marcas** (*de los drogadictos*) tracks; —— **de nacimiento** birthmark

marcapaso *m* pacemaker

marcha *f* gait

mareado -da *adj* dizzy, lightheaded, faint

mareo *m* dizziness, lightheadedness, (*en avión*) airsickness, (*en un barco*) seasickness, (*en un vehículo*) carsickness, (*debido al movimiento en general*) motion sickness; **dar** —— to make dizzy; **tener** —— to feel dizzy, to feel lightheaded

margarina *f* margarine

margen *m* margin, border, edge

marido *m* husband

marihuana, marijuana *f* marijuana, grass (*fam*), pot (*fam*)

marisco *m* (*frec pl*) shellfish, seafood

marital *adj* marital

martillo *m* hammer

masa *f* mass, lump; —— **muscular** muscle mass

masaje *m* massage; —— **cardiaco externo (MCE)** chest compressions; **dar** —— to massage

masajear *vt* to massage

masajista *m* masseur; *f* masseuse

mascar *vt, vi* to chew

máscara, mascarilla *f* (*para oxígeno, etc.*) mask, face mask

mascota *f* pet

masculino -na *adj* masculine, male

masivo -va *adj* massive

masoquismo *m* masochism

masoquista *mf* masochist

mastectomía *f* mastectomy; —— **radical modificada** modified radical mastectomy

masticable *adj* chewable

masticar *vt, vi* to chew

mastitis *f* mastitis

mastoideo -a *adj* mastoid

masturbarse *vr* to masturbate

matar *vt* to kill

matasanos *m* quack

material *m* material

maternal *adj* maternal, motherly

maternidad *f* maternity

materno -na *adj* maternal

matrimonio *m* married couple

matriz *f* (*pl* **-trices**) uterus, womb

matutino -na *adj* (*form*) pertaining to morning, morning

maxilar *adj* maxillary; *m* jaw, jawbone; —— **inferior** lower jaw; —— **superior** maxilla, upper jaw

maxilofacial *adj* maxillofacial

máximo -ma *adj* & *m* maximum

mayonesa *f* mayonnaise

mayor *adj* (*comp of* **grande**) bigger, larger; older; (*anat, surg*) major

MCE *abbr* **masaje cardiaco externo**. *See* **masaje**.

mear *vi* (*vulg*) to piss (*vulg*), to urinate

meato *m* meatus

mebendazol *m* mebendazole

mecanismo *m* mechanism; —— **de defensa** defense mechanism

mecha *f* wick, packing

meconio *m* meconium

media *f* hose, stocking

mediano -na *adj* medium; (*anat*) median

mediastino *m* mediastinum

medicamento *m* medication, medicine, drug; —— **a base de sulfas** sulfa drug

medicar *vt* to medicate

medicastro *m* quack

medicina *f* medicine; —— **alternativa** alternative medicine; —— **del primer nivel** primary care; —— **del tercer nivel** tertiary care; —— **deportiva** sports medicine; —— **familiar** family medicine, family practice; —— **interna** internal medicine; —— **nuclear** nuclear medicine; —— **ocupacional** occupational medicine; —— **podiátrica** podiatric medicine; —— **preventiva** preventive medicine; —— **socializada** socialized medicine

medicinal *adj* medicinal

médico -ca *adj* medical; *m* doctor, physician; —— **adscrito** attending physician; —— **clínico** clinician, practitioner; —— **de cabecera** *or* **de la familia** family doctor, family physician; —— **forense** coroner; —— **general** general practitioner; —— **interno** intern; —— **privado** private doctor, private physician; —— **residente** resident (*physician*)

medicolegal *adj* medicolegal

medicucho *m* quack

medida *f* measurement, size; measure; **medidas sanitarias** sanitation, sanitary measures

medidor *m* meter, measuring device

medio -dia *adj* half, half a, a half; middle; —— **dormido** half asleep; **media hermana** half sister; —— **hermano** half brother; **media pastilla** half a pill; *m* middle; medium; —— **ambiente** environment; —— **de contraste** contrast medium

mediodía *m* noon

mediquillo *m* quack

medir *vt* to measure

meditar *vi* to meditate

medroxiprogesterona *f* medroxyprogesterone

médula *f* medulla; marrow; —— **espinal** spinal cord; —— **ósea** bone marrow

medusa *f* jellyfish

megacolon *m* megacolon

megadosis *f* megadose

mejilla *f* cheek

mejor *adj & adv* (*comp of* **bueno** *and* **bien**) better

mejorar *vt* to improve; *vr* to improve, get better

mejoría *f* improvement

melancolía *f* melancholy

melancólico -ca *adj* melancholic

melanina *f* melanin

melanoma *m* melanoma

melatonina *f* melatonin

mellizo -za *adj & mf* twin

membrana *f* membrane, web; —— **esofágica** esophageal web; —— **mucosa** mucous membrane; —— **timpánica** tympanic membrane

memoria *f* memory; —— **reciente** short-term memory; —— **remota** long-term memory

meninge *f* meninx (*en inglés se emplea casi siempre la forma plural*: meninges)

meningioma *m* meningioma

meningitis *f* meningitis

meningocele *m* meningocele

meningococo *m* meningococcus

menisco *m* meniscus

menopausia *f* menopause

menor *adj* (*comp of* **pequeño**) smaller; younger; (*anat, surg*) minor; *m* (*de edad*) minor

menstruación *f* menstruation

menstrual *adj* menstrual

menstruar *vi* to menstruate

menta *f* (*bot*) mint; —— **verde** spearmint

mental *adj* mental

mente *f* mind

mentol *m* menthol

mentón *m* chin

menudo, a often

meperedina *f* meperedine

mercurio *m* mercury

mes *m* (*pl* **meses**) month

mesa *f* table; —— **de cirugía** operating table; —— **de exploración** (*form*) *or* **de exámenes** examining table; —— **de operaciones** operating table

mescalina *f* mescaline

mesencéfalo *m* midbrain

mesentérico -ca *adj* mesenteric

mesenterio *m* mesentery

mesotelioma *m* mesothelioma

meta *f* goal

metabólico -ca *adj* metabolic

metabolismo *m* metabolism

metacarpiano -na *adj & m* metacarpal

metadona *f* methadone

metal *m* metal; —— **pesado** heavy metal

metálico -ca *adj* metallic

metanfetamina *f* methamphetamine

metano *m* methane

metanol *m* methanol

metaproterenol *m* metaproterenol

metaqualona *f* methaqualone

metastásico -ca *adj* metastatic

metástasis *f* (*pl* **-sis**) metastasis; **dar —— to** metastasize

metastatizar *vi* to metastasize

metatarsiano -na *adj & m* metatarsal

meter *vt* to insert; —— **aire** (*Mex, fam*) to breathe in, inhale

meticilina *f* methicillin
metilcelulosa *f* methylcellulose
metildopa *f* methyldopa
metilfenidato *m* methylphenidate
metilprednisolona *f* methylprednisolone
metionina *f* methionine
metoclopramida *f* metoclopramide
método *m* method, technique; —— **del ritmo** rhythm method
metoprolol *m* metoprolol
metotrexato *m* methotrexate
metro *m* meter; —— **cuadrado** meter squared *o* square meter
metronidazol *m* metronidazole
mexicano -na *adj* & *mf* Mexican
mezcal *m* mescal
mezcalina *f* mescaline
mezcla *f* mixture
mezclar *vt* to mix
mezquino *m* (*Mex, CA*) wart
mialgia *f* myalgia
miastenia grave *or* **gravis** *f* myasthenia gravis
miconazol *m* miconazole
microbiano -na *adj* microbial
microbio *m* microbe
microbiología *f* microbiology
microcirugía *f* microsurgery
microgramo *m* microgram
microonda *f* microwave
microorganismo *m* microorganism
microscópico -ca *adj* microscopic
microscopio *m* microscope; —— **electrónico** electron microscope
miedo *m* fear; **tener** —— to be afraid *o* scared
miel *f* (*de abeja*) honey
mielina *f* myelin
mielograma *m* myelogram
mieloma múltiple *m* multiple myeloma
mielomeningocele *m* myelomeningocele
miembro *m* member; (*brazo o pierna*) limb; (*fam*) penis, member (*fam*)
migraña *f* migraine headache, migraine
milagro *m* miracle
milenrama *f* (*bot*) yarrow
miliar *adj* miliary
miligramo *m* milligram

mililitro *m* milliliter
milímetro *m* millimeter
mimar *vt* to pamper, coddle
mineral *adj* & *m* mineral
minero *m* miner
mínimo -ma *adj* & *m* minimum
minoxidil *m* minoxidil
minuto *m* minute
miocárdico -ca *adj* myocardial
miocardio *m* myocardium
miocarditis *f* myocarditis
mioglobina *f* myoglobin
mioma *m* myoma; —— **uterino** uterine leiomyoma, fibroid (*fam*)
miopatía *f* myopathy
miope *adj* myopic, nearsighted
miopía *f* myopia
miositis *f* myositis
mirada *f* gaze
mirar *vi* to look; **Mire arriba**..Look upward.
mitad *f* half; middle; **Tome la mitad de una pastilla**..Take half a pill.
mitral *adj* mitral
mixedema *m* myxedema
mixoma *m* myxoma
mochar *vt* (*vulg*) to cut off
moco *m* mucus
mocosidad *f* (*fam*) mucus; **tener** —— to have a runny nose, to have the sniffles
mocoso -sa *adj* **estar** —— (*vulg*) to have a runny nose
modelo *mf* (*a seguir*) role model
moderación *f* moderation
moderado -da *adj* moderate
modificación *f* modification, adjustment
modificar *vt* to modify, adjust
modo de vida *m* lifestyle
moho *m* mold, mildew
moisés *m* cradle, bassinet
mojado -da *adj* wet, damp
mojar *vt* to wet; *vr* to get wet
mola *f* (*obst*) mole; —— **hidatiforme** hydatidiform mole
molar *adj* (*obst, dent*) molar; *m* (*dent*) molar
molde *m* (*dent, etc.*) mold
moldear *vt* to mold
molécula *f* molecule

moler *vt* to grind, crush

molestar *vt* to bother; (*sexualmente*) to fondle, to molest; **Me molesta el brazo.**. My arm is bothering me...**¿Ha sido molestada?**..Has she been molested?

molestia *f* discomfort, trouble; **Tengo una molestia en la espalda.**.My back is bothering me.

molesto -ta *adj* annoying, irritating

mollera *f* fontanel *o* fontanelle

molusco contagioso *m* molluscum contagiosum

momentáneo -a *adj* fleeting, momentary

mometasona *f* mometasone

monitor *m* monitor; —— **cardiaco** cardiac monitor; —— **cardiaco fetal** *or* —— **cardiotocográfico** fetal heart monitor; —— **cardiaco ambulatorio** *or* **Holter** Holter monitor

monitoreo *m* monitoring

monitorización *f* monitoring

monitorizar *vt* to monitor

monoclonal *adj* monoclonal

monogamia *f* monogamy

monógamo -ma *adj* monogamous

monoinsaturado -da *adj* monounsaturated

mononucleosis *f* mononucleosis

monóxido de carbono *m* carbon monoxide

monstruo *m* monster; —— **de Gila** Gila monster

moquear *vi* (*fam*) to run (*one's nose*); **Me moquea la nariz.**.My nose is running..I have a runny nose.

moquera *f* (*fam*) nasal secretions, mucus; **tener** —— to have a runny nose, to have the sniffles

morado -da *adj* purple; cyanotic; bruised; *m* (*esp Carib*) bruise

morbilidad *f* morbidity

morboso -sa *adj* morbid

mordedura *f* bite

morder *vt*, *vi* to bite

mordida *f* bite

moreno -na *adj* dark-skinned; *mf* dark-skinned person, black, black person

morete *m* (*Mex, CA*) bruise; **hacerse** *or* **salirle moretes** to bruise, get bruises, get bruised

moreteado -da *adj* bruised (*all over*), black-and-blue

moretón *m* bruise; **hacerse** *or* **salirle moretones** to bruise, get bruises, get bruised

morfina *f* morphine

morfología *f* morphology

morgue *f* morgue

morir *vi*, *vr* (*pp* **muerto**) to die, expire; —— **de hambre** to starve

mormado -da *adj* (*Mex, fam*) congested, having nasal congestion

mortal *adj* fatal

mortalidad, mortandad *f* mortality

mosca *f* fly; —— **doméstica** housefly

mosquito *m* mosquito, gnat; —— **simúlido** sandfly

mota *f* (*Mex*) grass, pot, marijuana

motivación *f* motivation

moto *See* **motocicleta**.

motocicleta *f* motorcycle

motor -ra *adj* motor

mover *vi*, *vr* to move, to wiggle; **No se mueva.**.Don't move...**Mueva los dedos del pie.**.Wiggle your toes.

móvil *adj* mobile

movilidad *f* mobility

movilizar *vt* to mobilize

movimiento *m* movement; **movimientos oculares rápidos (MOR)** *or* **movimientos rápidos de los ojos** rapid eye movements (REM)

muchacho -cha *m* boy, child; *f* girl

mucho -cha *adj* a lot of, much; **mucho vómito.**.a lot of vomiting...**no mucho dolor.**.not much pain; **muchos -chas** a lot of, many; **muchos granos.**.a lot of pimples..many pimples; *adv* much, a lot; **mucho peor.**.much worse..a lot worse

mucinoso -sa *adj* mucinous

mucocele *m* mucocele

mucocutáneo -nea *adj* mucocutaneous

mucolítico -ca *adj* & *m* mucolytic

mucosidad *f* mucus; **tener** —— to have a runny nose, to have the sniffles

mucoso -sa *adj* mucous

mudez *f* mutism

mudo -da *adj* & *mf* mute

muela *f* molar, back tooth (*fam*); —— **del**

juicio or **cordal** wisdom tooth
muerte f death; —— **cerebral** brain death; —— **piadosa** mercy killing
muerto -ta (pp of **morir**) adj dead, deceased; mf dead person, corpse
muestra f sample, specimen
mujer f woman, wife
muleta f crutch
múltiple adj multiple
multiplicarse vr to multiply
multivitamina f multivitamin
multivitamínico -ca adj pertaining to multivitamins, multivitamin
muñeca f wrist

muñón m (anat) stump
mupirocin m mupirocin
murciélago m (zool) bat
murmullo m (card) murmur
muscular adj muscular
músculo m muscle
musculoso -sa adj muscular
músico -ca mf musician
muslo m thigh
mutación f mutation
mutante adj & m mutant
mutilar vt to mutilate, to cripple
mutismo m mutism (esp elective)
Mycoplasma Mycoplasma

N

nabumetone m nabumetone
nacer vi to be born
nacido -da adj born; —— **muerto** stillborn; **recién** —— newborn; m (esp Carib) boil
nacimiento m birth
nadar vi to swim
nalga f (fam) buttock; fpl bottom
nalidíxico -ca adj nalidixic
naloxona f naloxone
napalm m napalm
naproxén m naproxen
naranja adj orange; f (fruta) orange
narcisismo m narcissism
narcisista adj narcissistic; mf narcissist
narcolepsia f narcolepsy
narcótico -ca adj & m narcotic
nariz f (pl **narices**) nose; nostril
nasal adj nasal
nasofaringe f nasopharynx
nasogástrico -ca adj nasogastric
natación f swimming
natural adj natural
naturaleza f nature
naturismo m naturopathy

naturista adj naturopathic; mf naturopath
naturópata mf naturopath
naturopatía f naturopathy
naturopático -ca adj naturopathic
náusea f (frec pl) nausea; **náuseas del embarazo** morning sickness; **dar** —— to make nauseated, to make gag; **sentir** or **tener** —— to feel o be nauseated, to gag
nauseabundo -da adj nauseating
navaja f (de afeitar or rasurar) razor blade
nebulizador m nebulizer, inhaler
necrofilia f necrophilia
necrofobia f necrophobia
necrólisis tóxica epidérmica f toxic epidermal necrolysis
necrosis f necrosis
necrótico -ca adj necrotic
nefrectomía f nephrectomy
nefritis f nephritis
nefrología f nephrology
nefrólogo -ga mf nephrologist
nefropatía f nephropathy
nefrosis f nephrosis
nefrótico -ca adj nephrotic

negación *f* denial
negativismo *m* negativism
negativo -va *adj* negative
negligencia *f* neglect; —— **médica** malpractice
negligente *adj* negligent
negro -gra *adj* black; *mf* (*persona*) black, black person
Neisseria Neisseria
nene -na *mf* (*fam*) baby
neomicina *f* neomycin
neonatal *adj* neonatal
neonatología *f* neonatology
neonatólogo -ga *mf* neonatologist
neoplasia *f* neoplasm
neoplásico -ca *adj* neoplastic
neostigmina *f* neostigmine
nervio *m* nerve; —— **atrapado** pinched nerve; —— **auditivo** *or* **acústico** acoustic nerve; —— **ciático** sciatic nerve; —— **comprimido** entrapped nerve, pinched nerve (*fam*); —— **craneal** cranial nerve; —— **cubital** ulnar nerve; —— **espinal** spinal nerve; —— **facial** facial nerve; ——**femoral** femoral nerve; —— **frénico** phrenic nerve; —— **laríngeo recurrente** recurrent laryngeal nerve; —— **mediano** median nerve; —— **motor** motor nerve; —— **óptico** optic nerve; —— **parasimpático** parasympathetic nerve; —— **peroneo** *or* **peroneal** peroneal nerve; —— **pudendo** pudendal nerve; —— **radial** radial nerve; —— **raquídeo** spinal nerve; —— **sensitivo** sensory nerve; —— **simpático** sympathetic nerve; —— **trigémino** trigeminal nerve; —— **vago** vagus nerve
nervios *mpl* (*esp Mex, CA*) nerves, anxiety
nerviosidad *f* nervousness
nerviosismo *m* nervousness
nervioso -sa *adj* nervous
neumococo *m* pneumococcus
neumoconiosis *f* pneumoconiosis
neumología *f* pulmonology
neumólogo -ga *mf* pulmonologist
neumonía *f* pneumonia; —— **por aspiración** aspiration pneumonia
neumonitis *f* pneumonitis

neumotórax *m* pneumothorax
neural *adj* neural
neuralgia *f* neuralgia; —— **del trigémino** trigeminal neuralgia; —— **postherpética** postherpetic neuralgia
neurinoma *m* neurinoma
neuritis *f* neuritis
neuroblastoma *m* neuroblastoma
neurocirugía *f* neurosurgery
neurocirujano -na *mf* neurosurgeon
neurofibroma *m* neurofibroma
neurofibromatosis *f* neurofibromatosis
neurogénico -ca, neurógeno -na *adj* neurogenic
neuroléptico -ca *adj* & *m* neuroleptic
neurología *f* neurology
neurológico -ca *adj* neurological, neurologic
neurólogo -ga *mf* neurologist
neuroma *m* neuroma; —— **del acústico** acoustic neuroma
neuromuscular *adj* neuromuscular
neuropatía *f* neuropathy; —— **diabética** diabetic neuropathy; —— **periférica** peripheral neuropathy
neurosífilis *f* neurosyphilis
neurosis *f* (*pl* **-sis**) neurosis; —— **de guerra** shell shock; —— **postraumática** posttraumatic stress disorder
neurótico -ca *adj* & *mf* neurotic
neutral *adj* neutral
neutralizar *vt* to neutralize
neutrófilo *m* neutrophil
nevo *m* nevus, birthmark; —— **en araña** spider angioma
niacina *f* niacin
nica *f* (*Mex, CA*) bedpan, chamber pot, portable commode
nicaragüense *adj* & *mf* Nicaraguan
niclosamida *f* niclosamide
nicotina *f* nicotine
nicotínico -ca *adj* nicotinic
nieto -ta *m* grandson, grandchild; *f* granddaughter
nieve *f* snow
nifedipina *f* nifedipine
nigua *f* chigger, redbug, harvest mite
nilón *m* nylon
niña *f* (*del ojo*) pupil

niñera *f* baby-sitter
niñez *f* childhood
niño -ña *m* boy, child; *f* girl
níquel *m* nickel
nistagmo *m* nystagmus
nistatina *f* nystatin
nitrato *m* nitrate; —— **de plata** silver nitrate
nitrito *m* nitrite
nitrofurantoína *f* nitrofurantoin
nitrógeno *m* nitrogen
nitroglicerina *f* nitroglycerin
nivel *m* level; **del primer** —— primary; **del tercer** —— tertiary
nizatidina *f* nizatidine
nocardiosis *f* nocardiosis
noche *f* night, late evening
nocivo -va *adj* harmful; —— **para la salud** bad for one's health
nocturno -na *adj* nocturnal
nodo *m* (*card*) node; —— **auriculoventricular** atrioventricular node; —— **sinoauricular** sinoatrial node
nodriza *f* wet nurse
nodular *adj* nodular
nódulo *m* nodule
nombre *m* name, first name
norepinefrina *f* norepinephrine
norfloxacina *f* norfloxacin
norma *f* norm, standard
normal *adj* normal
normalizar *vt* to normalize

norteamericano -na *adj & mf* North American, American
nortriptilina *f* nortriptyline
nostalgia *f* homesickness; **sentir** —— to be homesick
notar *vt* to notice; **¿Ha notado sangre en el excremento?**..Have you noticed blood in your stool?
notificar *vt* to notify
novacaína *f* novacaine
novia *f* fiancée, girl friend
novio *m* fiancé, boy friend
nube *f* (*del ojo*) cataract, opacity, cloudy spot
nublado -da *adj* blurred, cloudy
nublarse *vr* (*la vista, etc.*) to cloud (up), become blurred
nubosidad *f* (*en el ojo*) cloudy spot, cataract
nuca *f* back of the neck
nuclear *adj* nuclear
nudillo *m* knuckle
nuera *f* daughter-in-law
nuez *f* (*pl* **nueces**) nut; —— **de Adán** Adam's apple
número dos *m* (*el defecar*) number two
número uno *m* (*el orinar*) number one
nutrición *f* nutrition; —— **parenteral total** total parenteral nutrition (TPN)
nutricional *adj* nutritional
nutriólogo -ga *mf* nutritionist
nutrir *vt* to nourish, to feed
nutritivo -va *adj* nutritious, nourishing

O

obesidad *f* obesity
obeso -sa *adj* obese
obrar *vi* (*Mex, CA*) to have a bowel movement
obrero -ra *mf* worker
obsesión *f* obsession
obsesivo-compulsivo -va *adj* obsessive-compulsive
obstetra *mf* obstetrician
obstetricia *f* obstetrics
obstétrico -ca *adj* obstetrical, obstetric
obstrucción *f* obstruction, blockage
obstructivo -va *adj* obstructive
obstruído -da *adj* obstructed

obstruir *vt* to obstruct, block; *vr* to become obstructed *o* blocked
occipital *adj* occipital
oclusión *f* occlusion
oclusivo -va *adj* occlusive
octogenario -ria *mf* octogenarian
ocular *adj* ocular
oculista *mf* ophthalmologist, eye doctor
ocupación *f* occupation
ocupacional *adj* occupational
odiar *vt* to hate
odio *m* hate, hatred
odontología *f* dentistry
odontólogo -ga *mf* dentist, oral surgeon
oficina *f* office
ofloxacina *f* ofloxacin
oftálmico -ca *adj* ophthalmic
oftalmología *f* ophthalmology
oftalmólogo -ga *mf* ophthalmologist
oftalmoscopio *m* ophthalmoscope
oído *m* ear; hearing, sense of hearing; —— **externo** external ear; —— **interno** internal *o* inner ear; —— **medio** middle ear; **oídos, nariz, y garganta** ear, nose, and throat (ENT)
oír *vt, vi* to hear; **¿Cómo oye Ud.?**..How is your hearing?
ojera *f* dark circle under one's eye
ojeroso -sa *adj* having rings under one's eyes
ojo *m* eye; —— **de pescado** (*fam*) wart, plantar wart; —— **morado** black eye; —— **rojo** *or* **enrojecido** pinkeye, conjunctivitis
oleada *f* wave; —— **de calor** hot flash
oler *vt, vi* to smell; (*cocaína, cemento, etc.*) to sniff (*cocaine, glue, etc.*) ; —— **a** to smell like; —— **mal** to smell bad
olfatorio -ria *adj* olfactory
oligoelemento *m* trace element
olor *m* odor, smell
olvidadizo -za *adj* forgetful, absent-minded
olvidar *vt* to forget
ombligo *m* umbilicus (*form*), navel, belly-button (*fam*)
omeprazol *m* omeprazole
omóplato *m* scapula, shoulder blade (*fam*)
oncocerciasis *f* onchocerciasis

oncocercosis *f* onchocerciasis
oncología *f* oncology
oncólogo -ga *mf* oncologist
onda *f* wave; —— **cerebral** brain wave
onza (onz.) *f* ounce (oz.)
opacidad *f* opacity
opaco -ca *adj* opaque
operable *adj* operable
operación *f* operation; —— **cesárea** cesarean section; **sala de operaciones** operating room (OR)
operar *vt* to operate on; **Tenemos que operarle la pierna.**.We need to operate on your leg; *vi* to operate; *vr* to have an operation; **Ud. tiene que operarse.**.You need to have an operation.
opiáceo -a *adj & m* opiate
opinión *f* opinion; **segunda** —— second opinion
opio *m* opium
oportunista *adj* opportunistic
opresivo -va *adj* (*dolor*) crushing
óptico -ca *adj* optical, optic; *m* optician; *f* optics
optometrista *mf* optometrist
oral *adj* oral
órbita *f* (*anat*) orbit
orciprenalina *f* metaproterenol
orden *f* (*en el expediente*) order
ordenar *vt* to order
oreja *f* ear
orfanatorio *m* orphanage
orfelinato *m* orphanage
orgánico -ca *adj* organic
organismo *m* body, organism; **No descuide su organismo.**.Don't neglect your body.
órgano *m* organ
organofosforado *m* organophosphate
orgasmo *m* orgasm, climax
orificio *m* orifice
origen *m* source
orín *m* (*frec pl*) urine
orina *f* urine
orinadera *f* (*esp Mex, fam*) bout of frequent urination
orinal *m* urinal
orinar *vi* to urinate; *vr* **orinarse en la cama** to wet the bed

oro *m* gold
orofaringe *f* oropharynx
orquiectomía, orquidectomía *f* orchiectomy
orquitis *f* orchitis
ortiga *f* (*bot*) nettle
ortodoncia *f* orthodontia, orthodontics
ortodoncista, ortodontista *mf* orthodontist
ortopedia *f* orthopedics *o* orthopaedics
ortopédico -ca *adj* orthopedic *o* orthopaedic
ortopedista *mf* orthopedist
ortosis *f* orthosis
oruga *f* caterpillar
orzuelo *m* sty *o* stye
oscuro -ra *adj* dark, dim
óseo -a *adj* osseous, pertaining to bone, bone; **médula ósea** bone marrow
osteítis *f* osteitis; —— **fibroquística** osteitis fibrosa cystica
osteoartritis *f* osteoarthritis
osteofito *m* osteophyte
osteogénesis *or* **osteogenia imperfecta** *f* osteogenesis imperfecta
osteoma *m* osteoma
osteomalacia *f* osteomalacia
osteomielitis *f* osteomyelitis
osteópata *mf* osteopath
osteopatía *f* osteopathy
osteoporosis *f* osteoporosis
osteosarcoma *m* osteosarcoma

ótico -ca *adj* otic
otitis *f* otitis; —— **externa** otitis externa; —— **interna** otitis interna; —— **media** otitis media
otolaringología *f* otolaryngology
otolaringólogo -ga *mf* otolaryngologist
otoño *m* fall, autumn
otorrinolaringología *f* otolaryngology
otorrinolaringólogo -ga *mf* otolaryngologist
otosclerosis *f* otosclerosis
otoscopio *m* otoscope
ovárico -ca *adj* ovarian
ovario *m* ovary; —— **poliquístico** polycystic ovary
ovulación *f* ovulation
ovular *vi* to ovulate
óvulo *m* ovum, egg (*fam*); vaginal suppository
oxacepam *m* oxazepam
oxacilina *f* oxacillin
oxalato *m* oxalate
oxicodona *f* oxycodone
oxidado -da *adj* rusty; **clavo** —— rusty nail
óxido *m* oxide; —— **de cinc** zinc oxide; —— **nitroso** nitrous oxide
oxígeno *m* oxygen
oxitocina *f* oxytocin
oxiuro *m* pinworm
ozono *m* ozone

P

pabellón *m* (*de un hospital*) ward
pacha *f* (*CA*) nursing bottle, baby's bottle
paciente *adj* patient; *mf* patient; —— **externo** *or* **ambulatorio** outpatient
padecer *vi* to suffer, to have (*a disease, symptom, etc.*); **Padezco dolores de la espalda**..I have back pains..I suffer from back pains; —— **de** to suffer from; **Padezco de artritis**..I suffer from arthritis.
padecimiento *m* ailment

padrastro *m* stepfather; hangnail
padre *m* father, parent; priest
país *m* (*pl* **países**) country
pájaro *m* bird
paladar *m* palate; —— **blando** soft palate; —— **duro** hard palate; —— **hendido** cleft palate
palangana *f* basin
paleta *f* shoulder blade; (*fam*) tongue blade
paliativo -va *adj* & *m* palliative

palidez *f* paleness, pallor
pálido -da *adj* pale
palma *f* (*anat, bot*) palm
palmada, palmadita *f* pat
palmar *adj* palmar
palomita *f* (*ped*) penis
palpar *vt* to palpate
palpitación *f* palpitation
palpitante *adj* throbbing
palpitar *vi* to palpitate; to beat
paludismo *m* malaria
pamplina *f* (*bot*) chickweed
pan *m* bread; —— **integral** whole-grain
  bread; —— **tostado** toast
panadero -ra *mf* baker
panadizo *m* felon, whitlow
panameño -ña *adj & mf* Panamanian
páncreas *m* (*pl* **-as**) pancreas
pancreatectomía *f* pancreatectomy
pancreático -ca *adj* pancreatic
pancreatitis *f* pancreatitis
pánico *m* panic; **ataque** *m* **de** —— panic
  attack
pantaletas *fpl* (*Mex*) panties, (*women's*)
  underpants
pantalón *m* (*frec pl*) pants, trousers; **pantalones antichoque** military antishock
  trousers (MAST)
panties *mpl* (*esp Carib*) panties, (*women's*)
  underpants
pantimedias *fpl* pantyhose
pantorilla *f* (*anat*) calf
pantoténico -ca *adj* pantothenic
panza *f* paunch, belly
panzón -na *adj* (*fam*) potbellied
pañal *m* diaper
pañalitis *f* (*fam*) diaper rash
paño *m* cloth, towel, compress; mask of
  pregnancy
pañuelo *m* handkerchief; —— **de papel**
  tissue
papa *f* potato
papá *m* (*pl* **papás**) dad
papada *f* double chin
Papanicolaou *m* (*fam*) Pap smear
papel *m* role; paper; —— **sanitario,
  higiénico,** *or* **de baño** toilet paper
paperas *fpl* mumps

papila *f* papilla; —— **gustativa** taste bud
papilar *adj* papillary
papilomavirus *m* papillomavirus
paracetamol *m* acetaminophen
paracoccidioidomicosis *f* paracoccidioidomycosis
parado -da *adj* (*de pie*) standing
paradójico -ca *adj* paradoxical
paraespinal *adj* paraspinal *o* paraspinous
paragonimiasis *f* paragonimiasis
paraguayo -ya *adj & mf* Paraguayan
parálisis *f* paralysis; —— **cerebral** cerebral
  palsy; —— **de Bell** *or* **facial** Bell's palsy
paralizador -ra, paralizante *adj* paralyzing;
  m paralyzing agent
paralizar *vt* to paralyze
paramédico -ca *adj & m* paramedic
paranasal *adj* paranasal
paranoia *f* paranoia
paranoico -ca *adj* paranoid
paranoide *adj* paranoid
parapléjico -ca *adj & mf* paraplegic
paraquat *m* paraquat
parar *vi* to quit; *vr* to stand, to stand up
parasitario -ria *adj* parasitic
parásito *m* parasite
paratión *m* parathion
paratiroideo -a *adj* parathyroid
parche *m* patch
parcial *adj* partial
pared *f* (*anat*) wall
paregórico *m* paregoric
parejo -ja *adj* even; *f* partner; couple
parenteral *adj* parenteral
parentérico -ca *adj* parenteral
paresia, paresis *f* paresis
pariente *mf* relative; —— **consanguíneo**
  blood relative
parietal *adj* parietal
parir *vt* (*esp Carib, fam*) to bear (*a child*)
paro *m* arrest; —— **cardiaco** cardiac arrest;
  —— **respiratorio** respiratory arrest
paroniquia *f* paronychia
parotiditis *f* parotiditis, parotitis
parótido -da *adj* parotid; *f* parotid gland
paroxetina *f* paroxetine
paroxismal, paroxístico -ca *adj* paroxysmal
paroxismo *m* paroxysm

parpadear *vi* to blink
parpadeo *m* blinking, blink
párpado *m* eyelid
partera *f* midwife
partero *m* general practitioner who attends deliveries; male midwife
partes *fpl* private parts, genitals (*esp female*); —— **privadas** *or* **íntimas** private parts, genitals (*esp female*)
partícula *f* particle
partida *f* certificate
partido -da *adj* cracked, split, chapped
partidura *f* (*Cub*) fracture, break
partir *vt, vr* to split, (*los labios*) to chap; (*Cub, un hueso*) to break
parto *m* birth, childbirth; delivery; —— **natural** natural childbirth; **dolor** *m* **del** —— labor pain, contraction; **estar de trabajo de** —— to be in labor; **sala de partos** delivery room; **trabajo de** —— labor
pasado -da de peso *adj* overweight
pasaje *m* passage; **pasajes nasales** nasal passages
pasajero -ra *adj* fleeting, transient
pasar *vt* to pass; (*esp Mex*) to swallow; —— **gas** to pass gas; —— **saliva** (*esp Mex*) to swallow (*dry swallow*); **Pase saliva, por favor**..Swallow, please; *vr* to wear off; (*a disease*) to spread; **El dolor se le va a pasar**..The pain will wear off...**¿Se pasa a los demás?**..Is it contagious?
pasatiempo *m* pastime, hobby
paseo *m* walk; **dar un** —— to go for a walk
pasillo *m* hall, hallway
pasionaria *f* (*bot*) passionflower
pasivo-agresivo -va *adj* passive-aggressive
pasivo -va *adj* passive
paso *m* step, pace; pass; **dar un** —— to step, take a step
pasta *f* paste; —— **dental** *or* **dentífrica** toothpaste
pastilla *f* pill; —— **para dormir** sleeping pill
patada *f* kick
patela *f* patella, kneecap
paternidad *f* paternity
paterno -na *adj* paternal

patizambo -ba *adj* knock-kneed
pato *m* urinal (*hand-held*); bedpan
patología *f* pathology
patológico -ca *adj* pathological, pathologic
patólogo -ga *mf* pathologist
patrón -na *mf* employer; *m* pattern
pauta *f* guideline
pavo *m* turkey
PCP *See* **fenciclidina**.
peca *f* freckle
pecho *m* chest, breast
pecoso -sa *adj* freckled
pectoral *adj* pectoral
pediatra, pedíatra *mf* pediatrician
pediatría *f* pediatrics
pediátrico -ca *adj* pediatric
pediculosis *f* pediculosis
pedicure *m* pedicure
pedicuro -ra *mf* podiatrist
pegadizo -za *adj* (*Mex, fam*) catching
pegajoso -sa *adj* sticky
pegar *vt* to strike, to hit; **pegarle** (*una enfermedad*) to catch, get; to give; **Me pegó la gripe**..I caught the flu...**¡Ud. me la pegó!**..You gave it to me!
peinar *vt* to comb; *vr* to comb one's hair
peine *m* comb
pelado -da *adj* (*la piel*) raw, peeling, chapped
pelagra *f* pellagra
pelarse *vr* to peel
peligro *m* danger, hazard
peligroso -sa *adj* dangerous, hazardous
pellejo *m* (*fam*) skin
pelo *m* hair
pelota *f* (*fam*) bump, lump
peluca *f* wig
peluquero -ra *mf* haircutter; *m* barber
pélvico -ca *adj* pelvic
pelvis *f* pelvis
pena *f* grief; embarrassment
pendiente *adj* pending
pene *m* penis
penetración *f* penetration
penetrante *adj* penetrating; (*herida*) deep; (*frío, dolor*) piercing
penetrar *vt* to penetrate, pierce, to puncture
pénfigo *m* pemphigus

penfigoide *adj & m* pemphigoid
penicilamina *f* penicillamine
penicilina *f* penicillin
pensamiento *m* thought
pensar *vt, vi* to think
pentamidina *f* pentamidine
pentazocina *f* pentazocine
pentoxifilina *f* pentoxifylline
peor *adj & adv* (*comp of* **malo** *and* **mal**) worse; **ponerse** —— to get worse
pepe *m* (*Guat*) pacifier
pepino *m* cucumber
pepsina *f* pepsin
péptico -ca *adj* peptic
pequeño -ña *adj* small, little
pera *f* pear
percepción *f* perception; —— **de la profundidad** depth perception
perceptible *adj* detectable
percutáneo -a *adj* percutaneous
perder *vt* to lose; (*una cita*) to miss; (*un hábito*) to outgrow, grow out of; —— **el conocimiento** *or* **la conciencia** to lose consciousness, to black out; —— **peso** to lose weight
pérdida *f* loss; —— **de la audición** hearing loss
perejil *m* parsley
perfeccionismo *m* perfectionism
perfeccionista *adj & mf* perfectionist
perfil *m* profile
perforación *f* perforation
perforar *vt* to perforate
perfume *m* perfume
periarteritis nodosa *f* polyarteritis nodosa
pericárdico -ca, pericardiaco -ca *adj* pericardial
pericardio *m* pericardium
pericarditis *f* pericarditis; —— **constrictiva** constrictive pericarditis
periferia *f* periphery
periférico -ca *adj* peripheral
perilla *f* bulb syringe
perinatología *f* neonatology, study of human development and disease at or near the time of birth
perineal *adj* perineal
periodo, período *m* period; —— **de incubación** incubation period
periodoncista *mf* periodontist
periodontal *adj* periodontal
peristalsis *f* peristalsis
peritoneal *adj* peritoneal
peritoneo *m* peritoneum
peritonitis *f* peritonitis
perjudicar *vt* to impair
perjudicial *adj* harmful
permanente *adj* permanent
permetrina *f* permethrin
permiso *m* permission, consent
peroné *m* fibula
peroneal *adj* peroneal
peroneo -a *adj* peroneal
peróxido *m* peroxide; —— **de benzoílo** benzoyl peroxide; —— **de hidrógeno** hydrogen peroxide
perrilla *f* (*Mex, fam*) sty *o* stye
perro *m* dog; —— **guía** guide dog, Seeing Eye dog
persistir *vi* to persist
persona *f* person
personal *adj* personal
personalidad *f* personality; —— **antisocial** antisocial personality; —— **ciclotímica** cyclothymic personality; —— **esquizoide** schizoid personality; —— **histriónica** histrionic personality; —— **limítrofe** borderline personality; —— **narcisista** narcissistic personality; —— **obsesivo-compulsiva** obsessive-compulsive personality; —— **paranoide** paranoid personality; —— **pasivo-agresiva** passive-aggressive personality
perspectiva *f* outlook
pertussis *f* pertussis
peruano -na *adj & mf* Peruvian
pesadez *f* heaviness
pesadilla *f* nightmare
pesado -da *adj* heavy
pesar *m* grief; *vt, vi* to weigh; ¿**Cuánto pesa Ud.?**..How much do you weigh?...**Tenemos que pesarlo**..We have to weigh you.
pesario *m* pessary
pescado *m* fish
pescador -ra *mf* fisherman
pescar *vt* (*fam, una enfermedad*) to catch

pesimismo *m* pessimism
peso *m* weight; —— **al nacer** *or* **al nacimiento** birthweight; **bajar de** —— to lose weight; **ganar** —— to gain weight; **perder** —— to lose weight; **tener** —— **excesivo** to be overweight
pesquisa *f* inquest
pestaña *f* eyelash
peste *f* pest, plague; —— **bubónica** bubonic plague
pesticida *m* pesticide
pestilencia *f* pestilence
petrolato *m* petroleum jelly
petróleo *m* petroleum; **destilado del** —— petroleum distillate
peyote *m* peyote
pez *m* (*pl* **peces**) fish
pezón *m* nipple (*female*)
pezonera *f* nipple shield
pH *m* pH
pián *m* yaws
picada *f* (*de insecto*) sting, bite
picadura *f* prick, stick, puncture; (*de insecto*) bite, sting
picante *adj* hot, spicy; **salsa** —— hot sauce
picar *vt* (*insecto*) to bite, to sting; (*esp Mex*) to stick, prick; *vi* to itch; **¿Le pica el brazo?**..Does your arm itch?
picazón *f* itch, itching; **tener** —— to itch
pico *m* peak; **alcanzar el** —— to peak
pie *m* foot; —— **caído** foot drop; —— **de atleta** athlete's foot; —— **deforme congénito** clubfoot; —— **péndulo** foot drop; —— **plano** flatfoot; **de** —— standing
piedra *f* stone; —— **de la vesícula** gallstone; —— **del riñón** kidney stone; —— **pómez** pumice stone
piel *f* skin; —— **de gallina** goose pimples; —— **de oveja** sheepskin
pielografía *f* pyelography; pyelogram
pielograma *m* pyelogram
pielonefritis *f* pyelonephritis
pierna *f* leg
pigmentación *f* pigmentation
pigmento *m* pigment
píldora *f* pill; —— **anticonceptiva** birth control pill
pilonidal *adj* pilonidal

pilórico -ca *adj* pyloric
píloro *m* pylorus
piloroplastia *f* pyloroplasty
pinchar *vt* to puncture, prick, stick
pinchazo *m* puncture, prick, stick; —— **del dedo** fingerstick
pindolol *m* pindolol
pineal *adj* pineal
pinta *f* pint; pinta, mal del pinto
pintarse *vr* —— **la cara** to put on makeup; —— **las uñas** to put on fingernail polish, to paint one's nails; —— **los labios** to put on lipstick
pintura *f* paint
pinza *f* clamp, clip; *fpl* tweezers, clamp, forceps
pinzar *vt* to clamp, to clip
piña *f* pineapple
piodermia, pioderma *m&f* pyoderma
piógeno -na *adj* pyogenic
piojo *m* louse
piorrea *f* pyorrhea
pipa *f* pipe (*for smoking*)
piperacilina *f* piperacillin
pipí *m* (*esp ped*) pee; penis; **hacer** —— to pee
pique *m* chigger, harvest mite, redbug
piquetazo *m* (*esp Mex, CA; fam*) strong sharp pain, jab
piquete *m* (*dolor*) stabbing pain, sharp pain; (*de insecto*) bite, sting; (*esp Mex, de aguja o espina*) prick, stick; —— **del dedo** fingerstick
pirazinamida *f* pyrazinamide
piridoxina *f* pyridoxine
pirosis *f* pyrosis, heartburn
pispelo *m* (*ES*) sty *o* stye
pistola *f* gun
pitar *vi* pitarle el pecho (*esp PR*) to wheeze
pitiriasis *f* pityriasis; —— **versicolor** pityriasis versicolor
pituitario -ria *adj* pituitary
placa *f* (*dent, bacteriana*) plaque; (*dent, surg*) plate; (*rayos X*) film, x-ray; —— **de Hawley** (*orthodontia*) retainer
placebo *m* placebo
placenta *f* placenta, afterbirth (*fam*); —— **previa** placenta previa; **desprendimiento**

prematuro de —— placenta abruptio
placer *m* pleasure
plaga *f* plague
planificación familiar *f* family planning, planned parenthood
plano -na *adj* even, flat
planta *f* (*del pie*) sole; (*bot*) plant
plantar *adj* plantar
plantilla *f* insole, footpad (*fam*)
plaqueta *f* platelet
plasma *m* plasma
plasmaféresis *f* plasmapheresis
plástico -ca *adj* & *m* plastic
plata *f* silver
plátano *m* banana
platelminto *m* flatworm
platino *m* platinum
plazo *m* **a corto** —— short-term; **a largo** —— long-term
pleito *m* suit, lawsuit; **poner** —— to sue
plenitud *f* fullness
pletismografía *f* plethysmography
pleura *f* pleura
pleural *adj* pleural
pleuresía *f* pleurisy
pleurítico -ca *adj* pleuritic
pleuritis *f* pleuritis
plexo *m* plexus; —— **solar** solar plexus
pliegue *m* fold; —— **cutáneo** skin fold
plomo *m* lead
Pneumocystis carinii Pneumocystis carinii
pócima *f* potion
poción *f* potion
poco -ca *adj* little, not much; **poca náusea**.. little nausea..not much nausea; **pocos -cas** few, not many; **unas pocas veces**..a few times...**Quedan pocas manchas**..Not many spots are left; *adv* little, not much; **Come poco**...He doesn't eat much; *m* little; —— **a** —— little by little, gradually
poder *m* power; —— **legal** power of attorney
poderoso -sa *adj* powerful
podíatra, podiatra *mf* podiatrist
podiatría *f* podiatry
podiatrista *mf* podiatrist
podofilina *f* podophyllin
podrido -da (*pp of* **pudrir**) *adj* rotten

polen *m* pollen
poliarteritis nudosa *f* polyarteritis nodosa
policitemia *f* polycythemia; —— **vera** polycythemia vera
poliinsaturado -da *adj* polyunsaturated
polimialgia reumática *f* polymyalgia rheumatica
polimiositis *f* polymyositis
polimixina *f* polymyxin
polio *f* polio
poliomielitis *f* poliomyelitis
polipectomía *f* polypectomy
pólipo *m* polyp; —— **adenomatoso** adenomatous polyp; **pólipos juveniles** juvenile polyps; —— **nasal** nasal polyp
poliposis *f* polyposis
poliquístico -ca *adj* polycystic
polivitamínico -ca *adj* & *m* multivitamin
pollo *m* chicken
polución *f* pollution; —— **nocturna** nocturnal emission
polvo *m* dust, powder; —— **de ángel** (*Ang*) angel dust, PCP; **polvos de talco** talcum powder; **en** —— powdered
pomada *f* ointment, salve
pomo *m* small bottle
pomposo -sa *adj* grandiose
pómulo *m* cheekbone
ponerse *vr* (*pp* **puesto**) (*ropa, etc.*) to put on; **Póngase esta bata**..Put on this gown; —— **azul, dormido, pálido, etc.** to turn *o* become blue, numb, pale, etc. **¿Se le ponen blancos los dedos cuando hace frío?**..Do your fingers turn white when it gets cold? —— **de pie** to stand (up)
ponzoña *f* poison, venom
poplíteo -a *adj* popliteal
popó (*fam*) *m* stool, (*ped*) poopoo; **hacer** —— to have a bowel movement
por *prep* per; **respiraciones por minuto**..respirations per minute; —— **ciento** percent; —— **día** per day
porcelana *f* porcelain
porcentaje *m* percentage
porcino -na *adj* porcine
porción *f* portion
porfiria *f* porphyria
poro *m* pore

portador -ra *mf* carrier
portal *adj* portal
portar *vt* (*una enfermedad*) to carry
portátil *adj* portable
posición *f* position
positivo -va *adj* positive
posos del café *m* coffee grounds
posponer *vt* (*pp* **-puesto**) to postpone
pospuesto *pp of* **posponer**
postemilla *f* (*Mex, CA; fam, dent*) abscess
post mortem *adj & adv* postmortem
posterior *adj* posterior
postizo -za *adj* prosthetic (*form*), artificial, false
postnasal *adj* postnasal
postnatal *adj* postnatal
postoperatorio -ria *adj* postoperative
postparto *adj* postpartum
postrado -da *adj* prostrate (*form*), exhausted, debilitated
postre *m* dessert
postura *f* posture, stance
postural *adj* postural
potable *adj* potable
potasio *m* potassium
potencia *f* potency, strength
potencial *adj & m* potential; —— **evocado** evoked potential
potente *adj* potent, strong, powerful
PPD *abbr* **proteína purificada derivada de la tuberculina.** *See* **proteína.**
práctica *f* practice
practicar *vt* to practice; (*un estudio, etc.*) to perform
pravastatina *f* pravastatin
praziquantel *m* praziquantel
prazosina *f* prazosin
precaución *f* precaution; **por** —— just in case
precisión *f* precision, accuracy
preciso -sa *adj* precise, exact
precoz *adj* (*pl* **-coces**) precocious; premature
predecir *vt* (*pp* **-dicho**) to predict
predicho *pp of* **predecir**
predisponer *vt* (*pp* **-puesto**) to predispose
predisposición *f* predisposition
predispuesto -ta (*pp of* **predisponer**) *adj* predisposed

prednisona *f* prednisone
preeclampsia *f* preeclampsia
preliminar *adj* preliminary
prematuro -ra *adj* premature; *mf* premature newborn, preemie (*fam*)
premedicación *f* premedication
premolar *adj & m* premolar
prenatal *adj* prenatal
prendido -da *adj* (*esp Mex*) hooked (*on drugs, etc.*)
prensión *f* grip, grasp
preñada *adj* (*fam*) pregnant
preñez *f* (*fam*) pregnancy
preocuparse *vr* to worry; **¿Está preocupado?..**Are you worried?...**No se preocupe..**Don't worry.
preoperatorio -ria *adj* preoperative
preparación *f* preparation
preparado *m* (*pharm*) preparation
preparar *vt* (*una prescripción*) to prepare, to fill
prepucio *m* foreskin
presbiacusia *f* presbycusis
presbicia *f* presbyopia, farsightedness
presbiopía *f* presbyopia, farsightedness
prescribir *vt* (*pp* **-scrito**) to prescribe, order
prescripción *f* prescription
prescrito *pp of* **prescribir**
presentación *f* presentation; —— **pélvica** *or* **de nalgas** breech presentation
preservar *vt* to preserve
preservativo *m* preservative; condom, rubber (*fam*)
presión *f* pressure; (*fam*) blood pressure; —— **alta** (*fam*) high blood pressure; —— **arterial** *or* **sanguínea** blood pressure; —— **diastólica** diastolic pressure; —— **sistólica** systolic pressure
presionado -da *adj* stressed, under stress
presionar *vt* to press
pretérmino *adj* preterm
prevalencia *f* prevalence
prevención *f* prevention
prevenible *adj* preventible
prevenir *vt* to prevent
preventivo -va *adj* preventive
previo -via *adj* previous
primario -ria *adj* primary

primavera *f* spring, springtime
primer *See* **primero.**
primero -ra *adj* (**primer** *before masculine singular nouns*) first; **primeros auxilios** first aid
primo -ma *mf* cousin
principio *m* beginning, onset
prisión *f* prison
privacía *f* privacy
privacidad *f* privacy
privado -da *adj* private
probabilidad *f* probability
probablemente *adv* probably
probar *vt* to test; (*comida, etc.*) to taste
problema *m* problem
probucol *m* probucol
procaína *f* procaine
procainamida *f* procainamide
procedimiento *m* procedure
proceso *m* process
proctitis *f* proctitis
pródromo *m* prodrome
producir *vt* to produce
producto *m* product; —— **lácteo** *or* **de leche** milk *o* dairy product
profesional *adj* professional
profiláctico -ca *adj & m* prophylactic
profilaxis *f* prophylaxis
profundidad *f* depth
profundo -da *adj* deep
progeria *f* progeria
progesterona *f* progesterone
programa *m* program
progresar *vi* to progress
progresión *f* progression
progresivo -va *adj* progressive
progreso *m* progress
prolactina *f* prolactin
prolactinoma *m* prolactinoma
prolapso *m* prolapse; —— **del cordón umbilical, del útero, de la vejiga, etc.** prolapsed umbilical cord, uterus, bladder, etc.; —— **valvular mitral** mitral-valve prolapse
prolina *f* proline
prolongación *f* extension
prolongar *vt* to prolong, extend
promedio *m* average; **como** —— on aver-

age; **el** —— **de altura** the average height
prono -na *adj* prone
pronosticar *vt* to predict, to make a prognosis
pronóstico *m* prognosis
propagación *f* spread
propagar *vt, vr* to spread
propensión *f* predisposition, susceptibility
propiltiouracilo *m* propylthiouracil
propioceptivo -va *adj* proprioceptive
proporción *f* proportion
proporcionar *vt* to provide, supply
propoxifeno *m* propoxyphene
propranolol *m* propranolol
proptosis *f* proptosis
prostaglandina *f* prostaglandin
próstata *f* prostate
prostatectomía *f* prostatectomy
prostatitis *f* prostatitis
prostituto -ta *mf* prostitute
protección *f* protection
protector -ra *adj* protective; *m* guard, (*para una aguja*) cap, needle cap; —— **solar** sunscreen
proteger *vt* to protect; *vr* to protect oneself
proteína *f* protein; —— **purificada derivada de la tuberculina (PPD)** purified protein derivative of tuberculin (PPD)
protésico -ca, protético -ca *adj* prosthetic
prótesis *f* (*pl* **-sis**) prosthesis
Proteus Proteus
protocolo *m* protocol
protozoario -ria *adj & m* protozoan
protuberancia *f* protuberance, bump
provocar *vt* to bring on, trigger, provoke; **¿Hay algo en particular que le provoca los dolores?**..Is there anything in particular that brings on the pains?
próximo -ma *adj* next
proyección *f* projection
proyectil *m* projectile
prueba *f* test, trial; proof; —— **cruzada** crossmatch; —— **cutánea** skin test; —— **de cáncer** (*fam*) Pap smear; —— **de embarazo** pregnancy test; —— **de esfuerzo** exercise stress test; —— **de función pulmonar** pulmonary function test; —— **de la audición** hearing test;

—— de la orina urine test, urinalysis; —— de la tuberculosis TB test; —— del parche patch test; —— de sangre blood test; —— de tolerancia a la glucosa glucose tolerance test; —— VDRL VDRL; a —— de agua, a —— de niños, etc. waterproof, childproof, etc.

prurito *m* pruritis

Pseudomonas Pseudomonas

psicoactivo -va *adj* psychoactive

psicoanálisis *m* psychoanalysis

psicoanalista *mf* psychoanalyst, analyst (*fam*)

psicoanalizar *vt* to psychoanalyze

psicodélico -ca *adj* psychedelic

psicología *f* psychology

psicológico -ca *adj* psychological

psicólogo -ga *mf* psychologist

psicópata *mf* psychopath

psicosis *f* psychosis

psicosomático -ca *adj* psychosomatic

psicoterapeuta *mf* psychotherapist, therapist (*fam*)

psicoterapia *f* psychotherapy

psicoterapista *mf* psychotherapist, therapist (*fam*)

psicótico -ca *adj & mf* psychotic

psicotrópico -ca *adj & m* psychotropic

psilocibina *f* psilocybin

psique *f* psyche

psiquiatra, psiquíatra *mf* psychiatrist

psiquiatría *f* psychiatry

psiquiátrico -ca *adj* psychiatric

psitacosis *f* psittacosis

psoas *m* (*pl* -as) psoas

psoriasis *f* psoriasis

pterigión *m* pterygium

ptosis *f* ptosis

pubertad *f* puberty

pubiano -na *adj* pubic

púbico -ca *adj* pubic

pubis *m* (*form*) pubic area

público -ca *adj* public

pudendo -da *adj* pudendal

pudrir *vt, vr* (*pp* **podrido**) to rot

puente *m* (*dent*) bridge; (*anat*) pons; (*card*) bypass; —— **coronario** coronary bypass

puerco *m* pork

puerperal *adj* puerperal

puerperio *m* puerperium

puertorriqueño -ña *adj & mf* Puerto Rican

puesto *pp of* **poner**

pujar *vi* to bear down, to strain (*at stool*); (*obst*) to push; **¿Tiene que pujar para defecar?**..Do you have to strain to have a bowel movement?...**Respire profundo y puje**..Take a deep breath and push.

pujo *m* straining, straining at stool

pulga *f* flea

pulgada *f* inch

pulgar *m* thumb

pulir *vt* (*los dientes, etc.*) to polish

pulmón *m* lung

pulmonar *adj* pulmonary, pulmonic

pulmonía *f* pneumonia; —— **por aspiración** aspiration pneumonia

pulpejo *m* soft flesh; (*del dedo*) finger pad; (*del oído*) earlobe

pulsación *f* pulsation

pulsante *adj* throbbing

pulsar *vi* (*un dolor*) to throb

pulsátil *adj* throbbing

pulso *m* pulse; **Quisiera tomarle el pulso**..I would like to take your pulse.

punción *f* puncture, tap; —— **digital** fingerstick; —— **lumbar** lumbar puncture, spinal tap; **herida por** —— puncture wound

puncionar *vt* (*form*) to puncture, tap

punta *f* tip; —— **del dedo** fingertip

puntada *f* stitch, suture

punteagudo -da *adj* pointed, sharp

punto *m* point; (*de sutura*) stitch; —— **doloroso** trigger point; —— **máximo** peak; **alcanzar el** —— **máximo** to peak; **poner puntos** to suture, stitch

punzada *f* prick, stick; (*de dolor*) shooting pain, pang, twinge; **dar punzadas** to give sudden, sharp pains

punzante *adj* (*dolor*) sharp, stabbing, shooting, throbbing

punzar *vt* to prick, stick; *vi* to give sudden sharp pains

puñalada *f* stab wound

puño *m* fist; **apretar** *or* **cerrar el** —— to make a fist

pupila *f* pupil (*of the eye*)

pupú *m* (*fam*) stool, (*ped*) poopoo; **hacer** —— to have a bowel movement
puré *m* purée; —— **de manzana** applesauce
purgación *f* purge; (*fam*) gonorrhea, the clap (*vulg*)
purgante *adj* & *m* purgative
purgativo -va *adj* & *m* purgative
purificador *m* purifier
purificar *vt* to purify
purina *f* purine

puro -ra *adj* pure; *m* cigar
púrpura *f* purpura; —— **de Henoch-Schönlein** Henoch-Schönlein purpura; —— **trombocitopénica idiopática** idiopathic thrombocytopenic purpura (ITP); —— **trombocitopénica trombótica** thrombotic thrombocytopenic purpura (TTP)
pus *m* pus
pústula *f* pustule

Q

quebradizo -za *adj* fragile
quebrado -da *adj* broken, chipped, split
quebradura *f* break, split
quebrar *vt, vr* to break, fracture, chip, split; **¿Cuándo se quebró la pierna?**..When did you break your leg?
quedarse *vr* —— **en cama** to stay in bed
queja *f* complaint
quejarse *vr* to complain
quelado -da *adj* chelated
queloide *m* keloid
quemadura *f* burn; —— **de sol** sunburn
quemante *adj* burning
quemar *vt* to burn; *vr* to burn oneself, to get burned; **¿Se quemó?**..Did you burn yourself?...**¿Se quemó la mano?**..Did you burn your hand? **quemarse por el sol** to get sunburned
quemazón *f* burning, burn
queratina *f* keratin
queratotomía *f* keratotomy
querer *vt, vi* to love
queso *m* cheese
quieto -ta *adj* quiet, calm
quijada *f* jawbone, jaw
quilate *m* carat; **oro de 24 quilates** 24 carat gold

químico -ca *adj* chemical; *f* chemistry
quimioterapia *f* chemotherapy
quinacrina *f* quinacrine
quinaprilo *m* quinapril
quinidina *f* quinidine
quinina *f* quinine
quinta enfermedad *f* fifth disease
quintillizo -za *mf* quintuplet
quintupleto -ta *mf* quintuplet
quíntuplo -pla, **quíntuple** *mf* quintuplet
quirófano *m* operating room (OR)
quiropodista *mf* podiatrist
quiropráctico -ca *mf* chiropractor; *f* chiropractic
quirúrgico -ca *adj* surgical
quiste *m* cyst; —— **de Baker** Baker's cyst; —— **de Bartholin** Bartholin's cyst; —— **del conducto tirogloso** thyroglossal duct cyst; —— **dermoide** dermoid cyst; —— **hidátide** hydatid cyst; —— **ovárico** ovarian cyst; —— **pilonidal** pilonidal cyst; —— **poplíteo** popliteal cyst; —— **sebáceo** sebaceous cyst; —— **tirogloso** thyroglossal duct cyst
quístico -ca *adj* cystic
quitar *vt* to remove; (*arith*) to subtract; **Quítele siete a cien**..Subtract seven from

one hundred; *vr* (*ropa*) to take off; (*dolor, hábito, etc.*) to go away; **Quítese la camisa**..Take off your shirt...**No se me quita el dolor**..The pain won't go away.

R

rabadilla *f* tailbone, area around tailbone
rabdomiólisis *f* rhabdomyolysis
rabdomioma *m* rhabdomyoma
rabdomiosarcoma *m* rhabdomyosarcoma
rabdosarcoma *m* rhabdosarcoma
rabia *f* rabies; rage
rabioso -sa *adj* rabid
racionalización *f* rationalization
racionalizar *vi* to rationalize
radiación *f* radiation
radiactividad *f* radioactivity
radiactivo -va *adj* radioactive
radial *adj* radial
radiarse *vr* (*dolor, calor*) to radiate
radical *adj* radical
radiculopatía *f* radiculopathy
radio *m* (*anat*) radius; (*chem*) radium
radioactividad *f* radioactivity
radioactivo -va *adj* radioactive
radiografía *f* x-ray (*film*); radiography
radioisótopo *m* radioisotope
radiología *f* radiology
radiólogo -ga *mf* radiologist
radionúclido *m* radionuclide
radioterapia *f* radiotherapy, radiation therapy
rádium *m* radium
radón *m* radon
raíz *f* (*pl* **raíces**) root; —— **nerviosa** nerve root
rajado -da *adj* (*piel, labios*) chapped, cracked, split
rajar *vt* (*fam*) to cut, to split, (*la cabeza*) to crack
ralo -la *adj* thin (*hair*)
rama *f* branch
ramipril *m* ramipril

rango *m* range; —— **de movimiento** range of motion; —— **de valores** range of values
ranitidina *f* ranitidine
ranurado -da *adj* (*tableta*) scored
rapé *m* (*tabaco*) snuff
raquídeo -a *adj* spinal
raquitismo *m* rickets
raro -ra *adj* rare, unusual
rascacio *m* stonefish
rascar *vt* to scratch; *vr* to scratch (*oneself*); **Procure no rascarse**..Try not to scratch (*yourself*).
rasgos *mpl* features
rasguñar *vt* to scratch
rasguño *m* scratch
rash *m* rash
raspadita *f* small scrape, abrasion
raspado *m* (*fam*) curettage
raspadura *f* scrape, abrasion
raspar *vt* to scrape, to scratch
raspón *m* scrape, abrasion
rasquera *f* (*fam*) itching
rasquiña *f* (*esp Carib, fam*) itching
rastrillo *m* razor
rasuradora *f* electric razor, shaver
rasurar *vt, vr* to shave
rata *f* rat
raticida *m* rat poison
rato *m* short time
ratón *m* mouse
raya *f* streak; (*zool*) stingray
rayo *m* ray, beam; —— **láser** laser, laser beam; —— **X** x-ray; **los rayos solares** *or* **del sol** the sun's rays; **el departamento de rayos X**..the x-ray department...**los rayos X del señor Smith**..Mr. Smith's

x-ray.

raza *f* race (*of people*)

razón *f* **perder la** —— to lose one's mind, go crazy

RCP *abbr* **resucitación cardiopulmonar.** *See* **resucitación.**

reabsorber *vt, vi* to resorb

reacción *f* reaction; —— **adversa** adverse reaction; —— **alérgica** allergic reaction; —— **conversiva** conversion reaction; —— **cruzada** cross reaction; —— **del injerto contra el huésped** graft-versus-host reaction *o* disease; —— **tardía** delayed reaction

reaccionar *vi* to react

reactivación *f* reactivation

reactivar *vt* to reactivate

reactivo -va *adj* reactive

realidad *f* reality

reanimación *f* resuscitation; —— **cardio-pulmonar (RCP)** cardiopulmonary resuscitation (CPR)

reanimar *vt, vr* to revive

rebaba *f* burr (*metal*)

rebajar *vi* to reduce, lose weight

rebote *m* rebound

recaer *vi* to relapse

recaída *f* relapse

recámara *f* bedroom

recesivo -va *adj* recessive

receta *f* (*médica*) prescription, order

recetar *vt* to prescribe, to order

rechazar *vt* to reject

rechazo *m* rejection

rechinar *vi* (*los dientes*) to grind (*one's teeth*)

recién nacido -da *mf* newborn

recientemente *adv* recently

recipiente *m* container

recobrar *vt, vr* to recover

recombinante *adj* recombinant

recomendación *f* recommendation

recomendar *vt* to recommend

reconstruir *vt* to reconstruct

récord *m* (*Ang*) record, chart

recordar *vt* to remember

recostado -da *adj* lying down, recumbent

recostarse *vi* to lie down

recreación *f* recreation

recreo *m* recreation

recrudecer *vi* (*una enfermedad*) to flare, to get worse

rectal *adj* rectal

recto -ta *adj* straight; *m* rectum

rectocele *m* rectocele

recubrimiento *m* coating, lining

recubrir *vt* (*el estómago, etc.*) to coat

recuento *m* count; —— **de glóbulos blancos** white blood cell count; —— **sanguíneo** blood count

recuperación *f* recuperation, recovery; **sala de** —— recovery room

recuperar *vt* to regain, recover; —— **el aire** to catch one's breath; *vr* to recuperate, recover

recurrencia *f* recurrence

recurso *m* recourse

red *f* mesh, network

redondo -da *adj* round

reducción *f* reduction

reducible *adj* reducible

reducir *vt* to reduce; (*ortho*) to reduce, set; *vr* to get smaller, shrink

reemplazar *vt* to replace

reemplazo *m* replacement; —— **total de cadera** total hip replacement

reevaluar *vt* to reevaluate

referencia *f* reference

refinado -da *adj* refined

reflejo *m* reflex; —— **condicionado** conditioned reflex; —— **nauseoso** gag reflex; —— **patelar** *or* **rotuliano** patellar reflex, knee jerk (*fam*)

reflexología *f* (*Ang*) reflexology

reflujo *m* reflux; —— **esofágico** esophageal reflux

reforzar *vt* to reinforce, strengthen

refracción *f* refraction

refractivo -va *adj* refractive

refrescante *adj* refreshing

refrescar *vt* to refresh; *vr* to refresh oneself, to get some fresh air

refresco *m* soft drink

refrigeración *f* refrigeration; **en** —— refrigerated

refrigerador *m* refrigerator

refrigerio *m* snack
refuerzo *m* reinforcement; **dosis** *f* **de** —— booster dose
refugio *m* shelter; —— **para mujeres, para personas sin hogar, etc.** women's shelter, homeless shelter, etc.
regaderazo *m* (*Mex, fam*) shower
regaliz *m* (*bot*) licorice
regarse *vr* (*fam, dolor*) to spread; **El dolor se me riega por todo el brazo**..The pain spreads through my whole arm.
regazo *m* lap (*of a person*)
regeneración *f* regeneration
regenerarse *vr* to regenerate
régimen *m* (*pl* **regímenes**) regimen; diet
registro *m* (*de un monitor, ECG, etc.*) tracing; (*de signos vitales, etc.*) record; (*de nacimientos, etc.*) register
regla *f* (*periodo menstrual*) period; **bajarle la** —— (*fam*) to have one's period
reglar *vi* to menstruate
regresión *f* regression
regulador *m* regulator
regular *adj* regular; *vt* to regulate
regurgitación *f* regurgitation; —— **aórtica, mitral, etc.** aortic regurgitation, mitral regurgitation, etc.
regurgitar *vt* to regurgitate
rehabilitación *f* rehabilitation
rehabilitar *vt* to rehabilitate; *vr* to become rehabilitated
rehidratación *f* rehydration
rehidratar *vt* to rehydrate
reinfección *f* reinfection
reinfestación *f* reinfestation
reír *vi, vr* to laugh
rejuvenecer *vt* to rejuvenate; *vr* to become rejuvenated
relación *f* relation; —— **sexual** sexual intercourse; **¿Cuándo fue la última vez que tuvo relación sexual?**..When was the last time you had sexual intercourse?
relajación *f* relaxation
relajante *adj* relaxing; *m* relaxant
relajar *vt, vr* to relax; **Relaje la pierna**.. Relax your leg...**Relájese**..Relax.
relámpago *m* lightning
rellenar *vt* (*un diente*) to fill (*a tooth*)

relleno *m* (*Mex, CA; dent*) filling
remedio *m* remedy, cure; —— **casero** home remedy
remisión *f* remission
remojar *vt* to soak
remordimiento *m* remorse
renal *adj* renal
rendimiento *m* performance
renovar *vt* to renew
renovascular *adj* renovascular
renquear *vi* to limp
reparación *f* repair
reparar *vt* to repair, fix
repelente *m* repellant; —— **de insectos** insect repellant
repente, de suddenly
repentino -na *adj* sudden
repetir *vt* to repeat; *vi* (*Mex, fam*) to burp
repetitivo -va *adj* repetitive
reponer *vt* to replace, restore, replenish
reportable *adj* reportable
reportar *vt* to report
reposar *vi* to rest, take a rest
reposo *m* rest; **en** —— at rest
represión *f* repression
reprimir *vt* to repress
reproducción *f* reproduction
reproducir *vt, vr* to reproduce
reproductivo -va *adj* reproductive
reproductor -ra *adj* reproductive
requesón *m* cottage cheese
res *f* beef
resaca *f* hangover; **tener una** —— to have a hangover, to be hungover
resbalar *vi, vr* to slip
resbalón *m* slip
rescatar *vt* to rescue
rescate *m* rescue
resecarse *vi* to become dry, dry out
resección *f* resection
reseco -ca *adj* dry, dried, dried out
resequedad *f* dryness; —— **de boca** dry mouth
reserpina *f* reserpine
reserva *f* reserve, store
reservorio *m* reservoir
resfriado *m* cold
resfriarse *vr* to catch a cold

residente *mf* (*médico*) resident
residuo *m* residue
resina *f* resin
resistencia *f* resistance; stamina
resistente *adj* resistant
resistir *vt, vr* to resist
resollar *vi* to breathe; to breathe hard, pant
resolverse *vr* (*pp* **resuelto**) to resolve, clear up
resonancia magnética nuclear *f* (*ant*) nuclear magnetic resonance (*ant*), magnetic resonance imaging (MRI)
resorber *vt, vi* to resorb
respaldo *m* backup
respeto *m* respect; —— **de sí mismo** self-esteem
respiración *f* respiration, breath; **Tome una respiración profunda.**.Take a deep breath; —— **boca-a-boca** mouth-to-mouth respiration *o* resuscitation; **falta de la** —— shortness of breath; **faltarle la** —— to be short of breath; **¿Le faltaba la respiración?**..Were you short of breath?
respirador *m* respirator
respirar *vt, vi* to breathe; **Respire profundo.**.Breathe deeply..Take a deep breath.
respiratorio -ria *adj* respiratory
responder *vi* to respond
respuesta *f* response; —— **acondicionada** conditioned response; —— **inmune** immune response
restablecer *vt* to restore; *vr* (*de una enfermedad*) to recover
restablecimiento *m* recovery
restañar *vt* to stanch
restar *vt, vi* (*arith*) to subtract; **Réstele siete a cien.**.Subtract seven from one hundred.
restauración *f* restoration
restaurar *vt* to restore
restricción *f* restriction
restringir *vt* to restrict
resucitación *f* resuscitation; —— **boca-a-boca** mouth-to-mouth resuscitation; —— **cardiopulmonar (RCP)** cardiopulmonary resuscitation (CPR)
resucitar *vt* to resuscitate
resuelto *pp* of **resolver**
resultado *m* result, outcome

resultar *vi* to turn out; **¿Y si resulta positivo?**..And if it turns out positive?
retardado -da *adj* retarded, delayed; —— **mental** mentally retarded
retardar *vt* to delay
retardo *m* retardation; delay; —— **mental** mental retardation
retención *f* retention
retenedor *m* (*orthodontia*) retainer
retener *vt* to retain; —— **agua** to retain water
retículo *m* network
reticulocito *m* reticulocyte
retina *f* retina; —— **desprendida** detached retina
retinopatía *f* retinopathy
retorcerse *vr* to writhe; (*el estómago*) to cramp; **Se me retuerce el estómago.**.My stomach is cramping..I have stomach cramps.
retorcijón, retortijón *m* abdominal cramp
retrasado -da *adj* retarded, delayed; —— **mental** mentally retarded
retrasar *vt* (*desarrollo, etc.*) to delay; *vr* to lag
retraso *m* retardation; delay, lag; —— **mental** mental retardation
retroalimentación *f* feedback
retrógrado -da *adj* retrograde
reúma, reuma *f* rheumatism, joint pain; watery discharge
reumático -ca *adj* rheumatic
reumatoide *adj* rheumatoid
reumatología *f* rheumatology
reumatólogo -ga *mf* rheumatologist
reusable *adj* reusable
revacunación *f* booster shot, revaccination
revalorar *vt* to reevaluate
reventar *vt, vr* to rupture, burst
reversible *adj* reversible
revestido -da *adj* lined, coated
revestimiento *m* (*del estómago, etc.*) lining, coating
revestir *vt* to line, to coat; **Células mucosas revisten el intestino.**.Mucous cells line the intestine...**Este medicamento reviste la pared interna de su estómago.**.This medicine coats the walls of your stomach.

revisar *vt* to examine, to check

revisión *f* examination

revitalizador -ra *adj* revitalizing

revitalizar *vt* to revitalize

revivir *vt, vi* to revive

riboflavina *f* riboflavin

Rickettsia Rickettsia

rico -ca *adj* rich

riesgo *m* risk; **alto —** high risk; **correr el — de** to run the risk of; **factor de —** risk factor

rifampicina *f* rifampin

rigidez *f* stiffness

rígido -da *adj* rigid, stiff

rigor mortis *m* rigor mortis

rinitis *f* rhinitis; **— alérgica** allergic rhinitis

rinoplastia *f* rhinoplasty

riñón *m* kidney; emesis basin; **— poliquístico** polycystic kidney

riñonera *f* emesis basin

risa *f* laugh

rítmico -ca *adj* rhythmic

ritmo *m* rhythm; **— biológico** biorhythm; **método del —** rhythm method

ritual *m* ritual

rivalidad *f* rivalry; **— entre hermanos** sibling rivalry

robusto -ta *adj* heavyset

roca *f* (*fam*) crack, crack cocaine

rociada *f* spray

rociador *m* sprayer

rociar *vt* to spray

rodilla *f* knee

rodillera *f* kneepad

roedor -ra *adj & m* rodent

rojizo -za *adj* reddish

rojo -ja *adj* red

romper *vt, vr* (*pp* **roto**) to break

rompimiento *m* break

ron *m* rum

roncar *vi* to snore; **roncarle el pecho** to breathe noisily (*as with asthma or bronchitis*), to wheeze

roncha *f* wheal; *fpl* hives, (*fam*) rash

ronchitas *fpl* (*fam*) fine rash

ronco -ca *adj* hoarse

rondas *fpl* (*Ang, de los médicos*) rounds; **hacer —** to make rounds

ronquera *f* hoarseness

roña *f* (*esp Mex, fam*) scabies

ropa *f* clothes, clothing; **— de cama** bedclothes, bedding; **— interior** underwear

rosado -da *adj* pink

roséola *or* **roseola infantil** *f* roseola infantum

roto -ta (*pp of* **romper**) *adj* broken

rótula *f* patella, kneecap

rotura *f* rupture; (*muscular*) tear

rozadura *f* chafe, scrape

rozar *vt, vi* to graze, chafe, rub; **¿Le roza el pañal?**..Does the diaper chafe him? *vr* to graze (*oneself*); **Me rocé el brazo**..I grazed my arm.

rozón *m* graze

rubeola, rubéola *f* rubella, German measles (*fam*), three-day measles (*fam*)

rubio -bia *adj* blond; *m* blond; *f* blonde

rubor *m* (*physio*) flush, redness

ruborizarse *vr* (*physio*) to flush

ruibarbo *m* rhubarb

ruido *m* noise

ruptura *f* rupture; **— prematura de membranas** premature rupture of membranes

rural *adj* rural

rutina *f* routine

rutinario -ria *adj* routine

S

SA *See* **sinoauricular.**
sábana *f* sheet, bedsheet
saber *vi* to taste; —— **a** to taste like; —— **mal** to taste bad
sabor *m* flavor, taste; **con** —— **a cereza, con** —— **a plátano, etc.** cherry-flavored, banana-flavored, etc.
sacaleche *m* breast pump
sacar *vt* to remove, take out; (*sangre*) to draw; **¿Me van a sacar sangre?**..Are you going to draw blood? —— **aire** (*esp Mex, CA*) to breathe out; —— **la lengua** to stick out one's tongue; **Saque la lengua**..Stick out your tongue; **sacarle el aire** *or* **los gases** (*a un bebé*) to burp (*a baby*); **Debe sacarle el aire**..You should burp him.
sacarina *f* saccharin
sacerdote *m* priest
sacro -cra *adj* sacral; *m* sacrum
sacroiliaco -ca *adj* sacroiliac
sacudida eléctrica *f* electric shock
sacudirse *vr* —— **la nariz** (*esp Carib*) to blow one's nose
sádico -ca *adj* sadistic; *mf* sadist
sadismo *m* sadism
safeno -na *adj* saphenous
sal *f* salt; **sales aromáticas** smelling salts; —— **de Epsom** Epsom salt; **substituto de** —— salt substitute
sala *f* room, ward; —— **de cuneros** newborn nursery; —— **de emergencia** emergency room (ER); —— **de espera** waiting room; —— **de operaciones** operating room (OR); —— **de partos** delivery room; —— **de recuperación** recovery room; —— **de urgencias** emergency room (ER)
salado -da *adj* salted, salty

salazosulfapiridina *f* sulfasalazine
salbutamol *m* salbutamol
salicilato *m* salicylate
salicílico -ca *adj* salicylic
salida *f* exit
salino -na *adj* saline; **solución salina isotónica** normal saline solution
salir *vi* to turn out; to drain; **El estudio salió positivo**..The test turned out positive...**¿Le sale pus?**..Is it draining pus? **salirle agua de la nariz** (*Carib*) to have a runny nose; **salirle granos** to break out (*one's skin*); **Le están saliendo granos**..He's breaking out..His skin is breaking out; **salirle leche** to lactate (*form*), to produce milk; **salirle los dientes** to teethe, to come in (*one's teeth*); **¿Le están saliendo los dientes?**..Is he teething?..Are his teeth coming in? **salirle sangre** to bleed; **¿Le salió sangre?** ..Did you bleed? **salirle una piedra** (*al orinar*) to pass a stone
saliva *f* saliva, spit
salivación *f* salivation
salival *adj* salivary
Salmonella Salmonella
salmonelosis *f* salmonellosis
salpingitis *f* salpingitis
salpullido *m* rash (*esp due to heat or chafing*), diaper rash
salsa *f* sauce; —— **picante** hot sauce
saltar *vi* to hop
salto *m* hop
salubridad *f* health
salud *f* health; —— **mental** mental health; —— **pública** public health
saludable *adj* healthy
salvado *m* bran
salvadoreño -ña *adj & mf* Salvadoran, Salvadorian

salvamento *m* rescue

salvar *vt* to save, rescue, to salvage

sanar *vt* to heal, cure; *vi* to heal, become cured; (*Mex, fam*) to give birth

sanatorio *m* sanatorium

saneamiento *m* (*ambiental*) sanitation

sangrado *m* bleeding; —— menstrual menstrual bleeding, menstrual flow; —— por la nariz nosebleed

sangrante *adj* bleeding; úlcera —— bleeding ulcer

sangrar *vi* to bleed

sangre *f* blood; poner —— to give a transfusion, to transfuse; ¿Me van a poner sangre?..Are you going to give me a transfusion?

sangría *f* phlebotomy (*therapeutic*); hacer —— to phlebotomize, remove blood from

sangriento -ta *adj* bloody

sanguijuela *f* leech

sanguíneo -nea *adj* blood, pertaining to blood; tipo —— blood type

sanidad *f* health, healthiness; sanitation

sanitario -ria *adj* sanitary; *m* rest room

sano -na *adj* healthy

santero -ra *mf* (*Carib*) faith healer, witch doctor

santos óleos *mpl* last rites, extreme unction, anointing of the sick

sarampión *m* measles; —— alemán German measles, rubella

sarcoidosis *f* sarcoidosis

sarcoma *m* sarcoma; —— de Ewing Ewing's sarcoma; —— de Kaposi Kaposi's sarcoma

sarna *f* scabies

sarpullido *m* rash (*esp due to heat or chafing*), diaper rash

sarro dental *m* tartar

sasafrás *m* (*bot*) sassafras

satélite *adj* (*clínica, lesión*) satellite

saturado -da *adj* saturated; no —— unsaturated

sauna *m* sauna

sebáceo -a *adj* sebaceous

sebo *m* sebum

seborrea *f* seborrhea

seca *f* enlarged lymph node

secante *adj* drying

secar *vt* to dry; *vr* to dry, to dry out

sección *f* section

seco -ca *adj* dry, dried

secreción *f* secretion, discharge; —— nasal posterior postnasal drip

secretar *vt* to secrete

secretario -ria *mf* secretary; —— de sala ward clerk

secretorio -ria *adj* secretory

secundario -ria *adj* secondary

secundinas *fpl* afterbirth

sed *f* thirst; tener —— to be thirsty; ¿Tiene sed?..Are you thirsty?

seda *f* silk

sedante *adj & m* sedative

sedar *vt* to sedate

sedentario -ria *adj* sedentary

sedimento *m* sediment, deposit

seguido *adv* often; ¿Qué tan seguido le dan los dolores (del parto)?..How often are the contractions coming?

seguimiento *m* follow-up

segundo -da *adj* second; *m* second

seguridad *f* safety

seguro -ra *adj* safe, sure; para estar —— just in case, to be sure; *m* (*Mex*) safety pin; *mpl* insurance

selenio *m* selenium

semana *f* week

semen *m* semen

seminoma *m* seminoma

sen *m* (*bot*) senna

sena *See* sen.

senil *adj* senile

seno *m* sinus; (*pecho*) breast

sensación *f* sensation, feeling

sensibilidad *f* sensitivity

sensibilizar *vt* to sensitize; *vr* to become sensitized

sensible *adj* sensitive, susceptible

sensitivo -va *adj* sensitive, susceptible; (*nervio*) sensory

sensorio -ria *adj* sensory

sentaderas *fpl* bottom, buttocks (*form*)

sentarse *vr* to sit, sit down, (*cuando está acostado*) to sit up

sentido *m* sense; —— de la vista sense of

sight; —— **del gusto** sense of taste; ——
del oído sense of hearing; —— **del olfato**
sense of smell; —— **del tacto** sense of
touch

sentimiento *m* feeling, emotion

sentir *vt* to feel; to be sorry; **Va a sentir
algo de dolor**..You're going to feel some
pain...**Lə siento**..I'm sorry; *vr* to feel;
¿Cómo se siente?..How do you feel?...**¿Se
siente cansado?**..Do you feel tired?...**¿Se
siente mal?**..Do you feel sick?

seña *f* sign; **hablar por señas** (*comunicar
con sordomudos*) to sign

señal *f* sign; —— **de advertencia** *or* **alarma**
warning sign

señora *f* wife

sepsis *f* sepsis

séptico -ca *adj* septic

sequedad *f* dryness; —— **de boca** dry
mouth

ser *m* —— **amado** loved one; —— **humano**
human being

seriado -da *adj* serial

sérico -ca *adj* pertaining to serum, serum

serie *f* series; —— **ósea** bone scan

serina *f* serine

serio -ria *adj* serious

seroconversión *f* seroconversion

serología *f* serology

seronegativo -va *adj* seronegative

seropositivo -va *adj* seropositive

serpiente *f* snake; —— **de cascabel** rattlesnake

sertralina *f* sertraline

servicio *m* service; (*frec pl*) restroom; ——
social social service

seudoefedrina *f* pseudoephedrine

seudogota *f* pseudogout

seudohipoparatiroidismo *m* pseudohypoparathyroidism

seudoquiste *m* pseudocyst —— **pancreático**
pancreatic pseudocyst

seudosuicidio *m* staged suicide; suicide gesture

severo -ra *adj* severe

sexo *m* sex; —— **oral** oral sex; —— **seguro**
(*Ang*) safe sex, sex without risk of infection; **cambio de** —— sex change; **ligado**

al —— sex-linked

sexual *adj* sexual

sexualidad *f* sexuality

Shigella Shigella

shigelosis *f* shigellosis

shock *m* (*Ang*) shock

sibilancia *f* (*form*) wheeze

SIDA *abbr* **síndrome de inmunodeficiencia
adquirida**. *See* **síndrome**.

sidatorio *m* (*Cub*) AIDS sanatorium

siempre *adv* **como** —— as usual

sien *f* (*anat*) temple

sierra *f* saw

siesta *f* nap; **tomar una** —— to take a nap

sietemesino -na *mf* baby born at seven
months

sífilis *f* syphilis

sifilítico -ca *adj* syphilitic

sigmoideo -a *adj* sigmoid

sigmoidoscopia, sigmoidoscopía *f* sigmoidoscopy; —— **flexible** flexible sigmoidoscopy

sigmoidoscopio *m* sigmoidoscope

signo *m* (*de una enfermedad*) sign; —— **de
advertencia** *or* **alarma** warning sign;
signos vitales vital signs

siguiente *adj* next

silbar *vi* **silbarle el pecho** to wheeze

silbido *m* wheeze; **tener silbidos** to have
wheezing, to wheeze; **Tengo silbidos**..I
have wheezing.

sílice *f* silica

silicona *f* silicone

silicosis *f* silicosis

silla *f* chair; —— **de ruedas** wheelchair

simeticona *f* simethicone

simetría *f* symmetry

simétrico -ca *adj* symmetrical, symmetric

simpatectomía *f* sympathectomy

simpático -ca *adj* friendly, kind; (*neuro*)
sympathetic

simvastatina *f* simvastatin

sinapsis *f* synapse

síncope *m* syncope (*form*), faint

sincronizar *vt* to synchronize

síndrome *m* syndrome; —— **alcohólico
fetal** fetal alcohol syndrome; ——
carcinoide carcinoid syndrome; ——

cerebral orgánico organic brain syndrome; —— de abstinencia withdrawal; —— de Asherman Asherman's syndrome; —— de cefalea postraumática postconcussional syndrome; —— de Cushing Cushing's syndrome; —— de DiGeorge DiGeorge syndrome; —— de Down Down's syndrome; —— de Ehlers-Danlos Ehlers-Danlos syndrome; —— de Felty Felty's syndrome; —— de Gilles de la Tourette Gilles de la Tourette syndrome; —— de Guillain-Barré Guillain-Barré syndrome; —— de inmunodeficiencia adquirida (SIDA) acquired immune deficiency syndrome (AIDS); —— de insuficiencia respiratoria del adulto adult respiratory distress syndrome (ARDS); —— de Kawasaki Kawasaki's syndrome; —— de Klinefelter Klinefelter's syndrome; —— de Korsakoff Korsakoff's syndrome; —— del choque tóxico toxic shock syndrome; —— del intestino irritable irritable bowel syndrome; —— del niño hiperactivo attention deficit syndrome; —— del niño maltratado battered child syndrome; —— del seno enfermo sick sinus syndrome; —— del túnel carpiano carpal tunnel syndrome; —— de malabsorción malabsorption syndrome; —— de Mallory-Weiss Mallory-Weiss syndrome; —— de Marfan Marfan's syndrome; —— de Ménière Ménière's syndrome; —— de muerte súbita infantil sudden infant death syndrome (SIDS); —— de Osler-Rendu-Weber Osler-Rendu-Weber syndrome; —— de Peutz-Jeghers Peutz-Jeghers syndrome; —— de Pickwick Pickwickian syndrome; —— de piernas inquietas restless legs syndrome; —— de Reiter Reiter's syndrome; —— de Reye Reye's syndrome; —— de Sheehan Sheehan's syndrome; —— de Sjögren Sjögren's syndrome; —— de Stevens-Johnson Stevens-Johnson syndrome; —— de Turner Turner's syndrome; —— estafilococo de piel escaldada staphylococcal scalded skin syndrome; ——

hemolítico-urémico hemolytic-uremic syndrome; —— hepatorrenal hepatorenal syndrome; —— nefrótico nephrotic syndrome; —— posconmocional postconcussional syndrome; —— premenstrual premenstrual syndrome;
sinergia f synergy
sínfisis f symphysis
sinoauricular, sinoatrial (SA) adj sinoatrial (S-A)
sinovial adj synovial
sinovitis f synovitis
sintético -ca adj synthetic
sintetizar vt to synthesize
síntoma m symptom
sinusitis f sinusitis
siringomielia f syringomyelia
sirviente -ta mf housecleaner
sismo m earthquake
sistema m system; —— **cardiovascular** cardiovascular system; —— **digestivo** digestive system; —— **endocrino** endocrine system; —— **esquelético** skeletal system; —— **inmunitario** immune system; —— **métrico** metric system; —— **musculoesquelético** musculoskeletal system; —— **nervioso autónomo** autonomic nervous system; —— **nervioso central (SNC)** central nervous system (CNS); —— **nervioso parasimpático** parasympathetic nervous system; —— **nervioso periférico** peripheral nervous system; —— **nervioso simpático** sympathetic nervous system; —— **reproductor** reproductive system; —— **respiratorio** respiratory system
sistémico -ca adj systemic
sistólico -ca adj systolic
SNC abbr **sistema nerviosa central**. See **sistema**.
sobaco m (fam) armpit
sobador -ra mf folk healer who uses massage
sobar vt to rub, massage; (fam, los huesos) to reduce (a dislocation or fracture)
sobrecargar vt to overload
sobrecompensar vi to overcompensate
sobredosis f (pl -sis) overdose
sobreexcitar vt to overexcite; vr to become

overexcited
sobrepeso *m* excess weight
sobreviviente *mf* survivor
sobrevivir *vt, vi* to survive
sobrina *f* niece
sobrino *m* nephew
sobrio -ria *adj* sober
socio -cia *mf* partner, associate
socorrista *mf* rescuer
socorro *interj* Help! *m* help
soda *f* soda
sodio *m* sodium
sofocación *f* suffocation
sofocamiento *m* feeling of suffocation, hot flash
sofocar *vt, vr* to suffocate, smother
sol *m* sun
solar *adj* solar; **los rayos solares** the sun's rays
soldado *m* soldier
soldar *vi* (*ortho*) to fuse, knit
sóleo *m* soleus
sólido -da *adj & m* solid
solitaria *f* tapeworm
soltar *vt* (*pp* **suelto**) to loosen, free, (*fam*) to relax; **Suelte el cinturón..**Loosen your belt...**Suelte la pierna..**Relax your leg.
soltero -ra *adj* unmarried, single
soltura *f* (*Mex, fam*) diarrhea, loose bowels
soluble *adj* soluble
solución *f* solution; —— **amortiguadora** buffer solution; —— **salina isotónica** normal saline solution
solvente *m* solvent
somático -ca *adj* somatic
sombrero *m* hat
somnífero *m* sleeping pill
somnoliento -ta *adj* sleepy, drowsy
sonambulismo *m* sleepwalking
sonar *vi* (*las tripas*) to growl (*one's stomach*); *vr* **sonarse la nariz** to blow one's nose
sonda *f* catheter, tube; probe; —— **Foley** Foley catheter; —— **nasogástrica** nasogastric tube; —— **para alimentación** feeding tube
sondear, sondar *vt* to probe
sonido *m* sound

sonograma *m* sonogram
sonreír *vi, vr* to smile
sonrisa *f* smile
sonrojamiento *m* (*physio*) flush, flushing
sonrojarse *vr* (*physio*) to flush
soñar *vt, vi* to dream; —— **con** to dream of *o* about; —— **despierto** to daydream
soñoliento -ta *adj* sleepy, drowsy
sopa *f* soup
soplar *vi* to blow; **Sople lo más fuerte que pueda..**Blow as hard as you can; *vr* **soplarse la nariz** (*Carib*) to blow one's nose
soplo *m* (*cardiaco*) murmur, heart murmur
soportable *adj* bearable
soportar *vt* to bear, endure, stand; **No lo soporto..**I can't bear it.
soporte *m* support (*physical*); —— **para el arco del pie** arch support
sorber *vt* to sip; —— **los mocos** (*fam*) to sniffle
sorbitol *m* sorbitol
sorbo *m* sip
sordera *f* deafness
sordo -da *adj* deaf; (*dolor*) dull; **medio** —— hard of hearing; *mf* deaf person
sordomudez *f* deafmutism
sordomudo -da *adj* deaf and mute; *mf* deaf-mute
soroche *m* (*SA*) mountain sickness
sostén *m* brassiere, bra
sostener *vt* —— **la respiración** *or* **el resuello** to hold one's breath; **Sostenga la respiración..**Hold your breath.
soya, soja *f* soybean
Staphylococcus Staphylococcus
status *m* status; —— **asthmaticus** status asthmaticus; —— **epilepticus** status epilepticus
Streptococcus Streptococcus
Strongyloides Strongyloides
suave *adj* soft, smooth, gentle, mild
suavizador -ra *adj* (*una loción*) softening
suavizante *adj* (*una loción*) softening
suavizar *vt* (*la piel*) to soften
subagudo -da *adj* subacute
subalimentación *f* undernourishment
subaracnoideo -a *adj* subarachnoid

subclavio -via *adj* subclavian

subclínico -ca *adj* subclinical

subconciencia *f* subconscious, subconsciousness

subconsciente *adj* subconscious

subcutáneo -a *adj* subcutaneous

subdural *adj* subdural

subespecialidad *f* subspecialty

subida *f* rise

subir *vi* to rise, go up; **Le subió el azúcar..** Your sugar rose.

súbito -ta *adj* sudden

sublimación *f* (*psych*) sublimation

sublingual *adj* sublingual

subluxación *f* subluxation

substancia *f* substance; —— **blanca** white matter; —— **gris** gray matter; —— **química** chemical

substituir *vt* to substitute; **Ud. puede substituir huevos por pescado..**You can substitute fish for eggs (*Observe que los dos objetos* huevos y pescado *se invierten al traducir al inglés. Note that the two objects* fish *and* eggs *are inverted on translating to Spanish.*)

substituto *m* substitute

succión *f* suction

suciedad *f* dirt

sucio -cia *adj* dirty

sucralfato *m* sucralfate

sudamericano -na *adj & mf* South American

sudar *vi* to sweat, perspire

sudor *m* sweat, perspiration

sudoroso -sa *adj* sweaty

suegra *f* mother-in-law

suegro *m* father-in-law

suela *f* sole (*of a shoe*)

suelto -ta (*pp* of **soltar**) *adj* loose, free, relaxed; **estar** —— **del estómago** (*fam*) to have diarrhea

sueño *m* sleep; dream; —— **húmedo** *or* **mojado** wet dream; **dar** —— to make sleepy; **tener** —— to be sleepy

suero *m* serum; IV fluid, electrolyte solution (*IV or oral*); **¿Me van a poner suero?..** Are you going to give me IV fluids?

suéter *m* sweater

suficiente *adj* sufficient

sufrimiento *m* suffering

sufrir *vt, vi* to suffer

suicida *adj* suicidal

suicidarse *vr* to commit suicide

suicidio *m* suicide; **intento de** —— suicide attempt

sujetadores *mpl* restraints

sujetar *vt* to restrain

sulfacetamida *f* sulfacetamide

sulfadiacina *f* sulfadiazine

sulfametoxazol *m* sulfamethoxazole

sulfas *fpl* sulfa drugs

sulfato *m* sulfate; —— **de cobre** copper sulfate; —— **de magnesio** magnesium sulfate; —— **ferroso** ferrous sulfate

sulfisoxazol *m* sulfisoxazole

sulfito *m* sulfite

sulfonamida *f* sulfonamide

sulfonilurea *f* sulfonylurea

sulindaco *m* sulindac

sumar *vt* (*arith*) to add; **¿Cuánto es ocho y nueve?..**How much is eight and nine?

sumatriptan *m* sumatriptan

suministrar *vt* to supply, provide

suministro *m* supply

superar *vt* to overcome

superego *m* superego

superficial *adj* superficial

superficie *f* surface

superior *adj* (*anat*) superior, upper

supervivencia *f* survival

superviviente *mf* survivor

supino -na *adj* supine

suplementario -ria *adj* supplementary, supplemental

suplemento *m* supplement

supositorio *m* suppository

supresión *f* suppression

supresor *m* suppressant; —— **del apetito** appetite suppressant

suprimir *vt* to suppress; (*una medicina, etc.*) to eliminate, quit taking

supuración *f* discharge

supurar *vi* to form pus, to drain pus

suramericano -na *See* **sudamericano -na**.

surfactante *m* surfactant

surtir *vt* (*una prescripción*) to fill; —— **de**

nuevo to refill
susceptibilidad *f* susceptibility
susceptible *adj* susceptible
suspender *vt* to suspend
suspensión *f* suspension
suspensorio *m* athletic supporter, jockstrap (*fam*)
suspirar *vi* to sigh

suspiro *m* sigh
sustitución *See* **substitución.**
sustituir *See* **substituir.**
susto *m* fright, scare; folk illness manifest by anxiety and other symptoms and believed to be caused by a sudden fright
sutura *f* suture
suturar *vt* to suture, to stitch (up)

T

tabaco *m* tobacco
tábano *m* horsefly
tabaquismo *m* tobacco use
tabardillo *m* form of typhus; typhoid fever; (*fam*) sunstroke
tabique *m* septum; —— **desviado** deviated septum; —— **interventricular** interventricular septum; —— **nasal** nasal septum
tabla *f* (*de datos*) chart
tableta *f* tablet
tablilla *f* splint
tabú *m* (*pl* **-búes**) taboo
TAC *m* CAT scan. *See* **tomografía.**
tacón *m* heel (*of a shoe*); **de** —— **alto** high-heeled
tacrina *f* tacrine
tacto *m* touch, sense of touch; —— **rectal** rectal examination
tajo *m* cut, gash
taladrar *vt* (*dent*) to drill
taladro *m* (*dent*) drill
tálamo *m* thalamus
talasemia, talasanemia *f* thalassemia
talco *m* talcum powder, talc
talio *m* thallium
talla *f* height, size
tallo cerebral *m* brainstem
talón *m* (*anat*) heel
tamaño *m* size
tambalear *vi, vr* to stagger

tamoxifén, tamoxifeno *m* tamoxifen
tampón *m* tampon; (*chem*) buffer
tanino *m* tannin
tanque *m* tank; —— **de oxígeno** oxygen tank
tapa *f* (*de una botella*) cap; —— **de seguridad** safety cap
tapado -da *adj* (*nariz*) congested; (*esp Mex*) constipated, obstructed
tapar *vt* to cover; (*anat, surg*) to block; (*dent*) to fill; *vr* to become blocked; **taparse el ojo** to cover one's eye; **taparse la nariz** to hold one's nose
tapón *m* plug, stopper; —— **para el oído** earplug
taponamiento *m* tamponade; —— **cardiaco** cardiac tamponade
taquicardia *f* tachycardia
taranta *f* dizziness, lightheadedness, dizzy spell
tarántula *f* tarantula
tarde *f* afternoon, early evening
tardío -a *adj* late, delayed
tarjeta *f* (*del hospital, del negocio*) card
tarsal *adj* tarsal
tartamudear *vi* to stutter, stammer
tartárico -ca *adj* tartaric
tártaro *m* tartar
tasa *f* rate; —— **de metabolismo basal** basal metabolic rate; —— **de mortalidad**

death rate; —— **de mortalidad infantil** infant mortality rate; —— **de natalidad** birth rate

tatuaje *m* tattoo

taza *f* cup, cupful

TC *abbr* **tomografía computada**. *See* **tomografía**.

té *m* (*pl* **tes**) tea

TEC *abbr* **terapia electrochoque** *or* **electroconvulsiva**. *See* **terapia**.

tecato -ta *mf* (*PR*) junkie, person who injects drugs

techo *m* —— **de la boca** roof of the mouth

técnico -ca *mf* technician; *f* technique

tecnología *f* technology

tejido *m* tissue; —— **blando** soft tissue; —— **conectivo** *or* **conjuntivo** connective tissue; —— **de granulación** granulation tissue

tela *f* tape; film; —— **adhesiva** adhesive tape

telangiectasia *f* telangiectasia; —— **aracniforme** spider angioma

telefonear *vt, vi* to call (*by telephone*)

teléfono *m* telephone

telemetría *f* telemetry

tembladera *f* shaking spell, the shakes (*fam*)

temblar *vi* to tremble, shake; **¿Le tiemblan las manos?**..Do your hands shake?

temblor *m* earthquake; (*frec pl*) tremor, shiver, shaking spell; —— **familiar** familial tremor

tembloroso -sa *adj* tremulous

temor *m* fear

temperamento *m* temperament

temperatura *f* temperature; (*fam*) fever; —— **ambiente** room temperature; **tomarse la** —— to take one's temperature

temporada *f* season, time of year; **temporada de la gripe**..flu season

temporal *adj* temporary; (*anat*) temporal; **Este vendaje es solo temporal**..This bandage is only temporary.

temporomandibular *adj* temporomandibular

tendencia *f* tendency; trend

tendón *m* tendon; —— **de Aquiles** Achilles tendon; —— **de la corva** hamstring

tendonitis *f* tendinitis

tenia *f* taenia *o* tenia, tapeworm

tenis *m* tennis

tenosinovitis *f* tenosynovitis

tensiómetro *m* blood pressure cuff

tensión *f* tension, stress, strain; —— **nerviosa** nervous tension; **bajo** —— stressed, under stress

tenso -sa *adj* tense; **poner** —— (*el brazo, etc.*) to tense; **ponerse** —— to tense up; **Procure de no ponerse tenso**..Try not to tense up.

teofilina *f* theophylline

teoría *f* theory

TEP *abbr* **tomografía por emisión de positrones**. *See* **tomografía**.

terapeuta *mf* therapist

terapéutico -ca *adj* therapeutic; *f* therapy

terapia *f* therapy; —— **de grupo** group therapy; —— **del habla** speech therapy; —— **electrochoque** *or* **electroconvulsiva (TEC)** electroconvulsive therapy (ECT); —— **física** physical therapy; —— **intensiva** intensive care; —— **ocupacional** occupational therapy; —— **respiratoria** respiratory therapy

terapista *mf* therapist; —— **del habla** speech therapist; —— **físico** physical therapist; —— **ocupacional** occupational therapist

teratoma *m* teratoma

terazosina *f* terazosin

terbutalina *f* terbutaline

terfenadina *f* terfenadine

termal *adj* thermal

terminal *adj* terminal

término *m* term; **a** —— at term

termómetro *m* thermometer; —— **oral** *or* **bucal** oral thermometer; —— **rectal** rectal thermometer

terremoto *m* earthquake (*severe*)

terrores nocturnos *mpl* night-terrors

testículo *m* testicle; —— **no descendido** undescended testicle

Testigos de Jehová *mpl* Jehovah's Witnesses

testosterona *f* testosterone

tétanos *m* tetanus

tetera *f* nipple (*of nursing bottle*)

tetilla *f* nipple (*of a male*)

tetraciclina *f* tetracycline

tetracloruro de carbono *m* carbon tetrachloride

tetrahidrocanabinol *m* tetrahydrocannabinol (THC)

tetralogía de Fallot *f* tetralogy of Fallot

textura *f* texture

tez *f* complexion

tía *f* aunt

tiabendazol *m* thiabendazole

tiamina *f* thiamine

tibia *f* tibia, shinbone (*fam*)

tibio -bia *adj* lukewarm, tepid

tiburón *m* shark

tic *m* tic; —— **doloroso** tic douloureux

tiempo *m* time; weather; ¿**Cuánto tiempo estuvo inconsciente?**..How long were you unconscious? —— **de protrombina (TP)** prothrombin time (PT); —— **parcial de tromboplastina (TPT)** partial thromboplastin time (PTT); **con el** —— eventually, in time; **mucho** —— a long time; **poco** —— a short time; **todo el** —— all the time

tienda *f* tent; —— **de oxígeno** oxygen tent

tieso -sa *adj* stiff, rigid

tifo *m* typhus

tifus *m* typhus

tijeras *fpl* scissors

timectomía *f* thymectomy

timidez *f* shyness

tímido -da *adj* timid, shy, bashful

timo *m* thymus

timolol *m* timolol

timoma *m* thymoma

timpanectomía *f* tympanectomy

timpánico -ca *adj* tympanic

tímpano *m* eardrum

timpanoplastia *f* tympanoplasty

tina *f* (*de baño*) bathtub

tiner *m* thinner

tintura *f* tincture

tiña, tinea *f* tinea; —— **corporal** *or* **del cuerpo** tinea corporis, ringworm (*fam*) ; —— **crural** *or* **inguinal** tinea cruris; —— **de la cabeza** tinea capitis; —— **del pie** tinea pedis, athlete's foot (*fam*)

tío *m* uncle

tioridacina *f* thioridazine

típico -ca *adj* typical

tipo *m* type; —— **de sangre** blood type

tira *f* strap, strip; —— **reactiva** test strip, dipstick

tiraleche *m* breast pump

tiramina *f* tyramine

tirantes *mpl* suspenders

tirar *vt* (*esp Mex*) *vt* to pass, to shed; —— **gases** *or* **vientos** to pass gas

tiritar *vi* to shiver

tiroglobulina *f* thyroglobulin

tiroidectomía *f* thyroidectomy

tiroideo -a *adj* thyroid

tiroides *m&f* (*pl* -**des**) thyroid, thyroid gland

tiroiditis *f* thyroiditis; —— **de Hashimoto** Hashimoto's thyroiditis; —— **subaguda** subacute thyroiditis

tirón *m* muscle pull; **sufrir un** —— to pull a muscle

tirosina *f* tyrosine

tirotóxico -ca *adj* thyrotoxic

tirotoxicosis *f* thyrotoxicosis

tirotropina *f* thyrotropin (TSH)

tiroxina *f* thyroxine

título *m* titer

toalla *f* towel; —— **sanitaria** *or* **femenina** sanitary napkin

tobillera *f* ankle brace

tobillo *m* ankle

tocar *vt* to touch

tocino *m* bacon

tocoferol *m* tocopherol

tofo *m* tophus

tolazamida *f* tolazamide

tolbutamida *f* tolbutamide

tolerable *adj* bearable

tolerancia *f* tolerance

tolerante *adj* tolerant

tolerar *vt* to tolerate

tolueno *m* toluene

tomacorriente *m* electrical outlet

tomaína *f* ptomaine

tomar *vt* (*una bebida*) to drink; (*medicamentos, etc.*) to take; **Tome una pastilla en la mañana y una en la tarde**..Take one pill in the morning and one in the evening; —— **aire** (*fam*) to breathe in; to catch one's breath; —— **el sol** to get sun

tomate *m* tomato

tomografía *f* tomography; tomogram, (*fam*) CT scan; —— **axial computarizada (TAC)** computerized axial tomography (CAT); —— **computada (TC)** computed tomography (CT); —— **por emisión de positrones (TEP)** positron emission tomography (PET)

tomograma *m* tomogram

tónico -ca *adj* & *m* tonic

tonificador -ra *adj* toning

tonificar *vt* (*los músculos*) to tone

tono *m* tone; (*sonido*) tone, pitch; —— **muscular** muscle tone; **de** —— **alto** high-pitched; **de** —— **bajo** low-pitched

tonsilectomía *f* tonsillectomy

tonsilitis *f* tonsillitis

tópico -ca *adj* topical

torácico -ca *adj* thoracic

toracotomía *f* thoracotomy

tórax *m* thorax

torcedura *f* sprain

torcer *vt, vr* to sprain, twist, to get sprained *o* twisted; **¿Cuándo se torció el cuello?.. When did you sprain your neck?**

torcido -da *adj* crooked, twisted, bent

torniquete *m* tourniquet

toronja *f* grapefruit

torpe *adj* clumsy

torrente sanguíneo *m* bloodstream

torsión *f* torsion; —— **ovárica** ovarian torsion; —— **testicular** testicular torsion

torso *m* torso

tortícolis, torticolis *f* torticollis

tortura *f* torture

torturar *vt* to torture

torunda *f* cotton ball, wad of gauze

torus *m* torus; —— **palatino** torus palatinus

torzón *m* (*Mex, fam*) abdominal cramp

tos *f* cough; —— **chifladora** (*CA, fam*), —— **de perro** (*fam*), —— **ferina**, *or* —— **perruna** (*fam*) whooping cough; —— **seca** dry cough; **jarabe** *m* **para la** —— cough syrup; **pastilla para la** —— cough drop

toser *vi* to cough; **Tosa fuerte..Cough hard.**

tosferina *See* **tos ferina**.

tostado -da *adj* (*fam*) tan

tostarse *vr* (*fam*) to tan, to get a suntan

total *adj* & *m* total

toxemia *f* toxemia

toxémico -ca *adj* toxemic

toxicidad *f* toxicity

tóxico -ca *adj* toxic

toxicología *f* toxicology

toxicólogo -ga *mf* toxicologist

toxicomanía *f* drug addiction

toxicómano -na *mf* drug abuser

toxina *f* toxin

toxocariasis *f* toxocariasis

toxoide *m* toxoid; —— **diftérico** diphtheria toxoid; —— **tetánico** tetanus toxoid

toxoplasmosis *f* toxoplasmosis

trabajador -ra *mf* worker; —— **social** social worker

trabajar *vi* to work

trabajo *m* work, job

tracción *f* traction

tracoma *m* trachoma

tracto *m* tract; —— **digestivo** digestive tract; —— **respiratorio** respiratory tract; —— **urinario** urinary tract

traducir *vt* to translate

tragar *vt, vi* to swallow; —— **saliva** to swallow; **Debe chupar esta pastilla, no tragarla..You should suck on this pill, not swallow it.**

trancazo *m* (*fam*) flu; (*Mex, fam*) dengue fever

trance *m* trance

tranquilizante *adj* sedating, tranquilizing; *m* tranquilizer

tranquilizar *vt* to sedate, tranquilize; *vr* to calm down; **Ud. necesita tranquilizarse.. You need to calm down.**

tranquilo -la *adj* calm

transcurso *m* course

transcutáneo -nea *adj* transcutaneous

transexual *adj* & *mf* transsexual

transferencia *f* (*psych*) transference

transferrina *f* transferrin

transfundir *vt* (*form*) to transfuse

transfusión *f* transfusion; **hacer una** —— to

transfuse, to give a transfusion; **Tenemos que hacerle una transfusión de plaquetas**..We need to give you a transfusion of platelets.

transición *f* transition

transicional *adj* transitional

transitorio -ria *adj* transient, temporary

translocación *f* translocation

transmisible *adj* communicable

transmisión *f* transmission

transmitir *vt* to transmit

transparente *adj* transparent

transpiración *f* perspiration

transpirar *vi* to perspire

transportar *vt* to transport

transporte *m* transport

transuretral *adj* transurethral

transvestista *mf* transvestite

trapecio *m* (*anat*) trapezius

tráquea *f* trachea, windpipe (*fam*)

traqueítis *f* tracheitis

traqueobronquitis *f* tracheobronchitis

traqueostomía *f* tracheostomy

traqueotomía *f* tracheotomy

trasero *m* (*fam*) buttocks, bottom (*fam*)

trasladar *vt* (*un paciente*) to transfer, move

traspié *m* **dar un** —— to stumble, trip

trasplantar *vt* to transplant

trasplante *m* transplant

trastornado -da *adj* upset; crazy, mentally deranged

trastornar *vt* to upset; to drive (*someone*) crazy; *vr* to become upset; to go crazy

trastorno *m* disorder, disturbance; —— **bipolar** bipolar disorder; —— **de la personalidad** personality disorder; —— **del estrés postraumático** posttraumatic stress disorder; —— **del sueño** sleep disorder *o* disturbance

tratamiento *m* treatment

tratar *vt* (*una enfermedad, un paciente*) to treat

trauma *m* trauma

traumático -ca *adj* traumatic

traumatismo *m* trauma

traumatizar *vt* to traumatize

travieso -sa *adj* mischievous

trazas *fpl* trace(s)

trazo *m* (*de EKG, etc.*) tracing

trazodona *f* trazodone

trementina *f* turpentine

treonina *f* threonine

treponema *f* treponeme

tretinoína *f* tretinoin

triamcinolona *f* triamcinolone

triamtereno *m* triamterene

triazolam *m* triazolam

tríceps *m* (*pl* **-ceps**) triceps

Trichomonas Trichomonas

tricocéfalo *m* whipworm

tricomoniasis *f* trichomoniasis

tricúspide *adj* tricuspid

trifluoperacina *f* trifluoperazine

trigémino -na *adj* trigeminal

triglicérido *m* triglyceride

trigo *m* wheat; —— **integral** *or* **entero** whole wheat

trigueño -ña *adj* olive-skinned; *mf* olive-skinned person

trillizo -za *mf* triplet

trimestre *m* trimester

trimetoprim *m* trimethoprim

tripa *f* (*frec pl*) gut, bowel, intestine

tripanosomiasis *f* trypanosomiasis

tripsina *f* trypsin

triptófano *m* tryptophan

triquinosis *f* trichinosis

trismo *m* trismus, lockjaw

trisomía *f* trisomy; —— **21** trisomy 21

triste *adj* sad

triturar *vt* (*form*) to crush, grind

trivalente *adj* trivalent

trocánter *m* trochanter

trocisco *m* lozenge, troche

trombectomía *f* thrombectomy

trombo *m* thrombus

trombocitopenia *f* thrombocytopenia

trombocitosis *f* thrombocytosis

tromboembolia *f* thromboembolism

tromboflebitis *f* thrombophlebitis

trombolítico -ca *adj* & *m* thrombolytic

trombosis *f* thrombosis

trompa *f* tube; —— **de Eustaquio** Eustachian tube; —— **de Falopio** fallopian tube

tronado -da *adj* (*Mex, vulg*) high (*on drugs*)

tronar *vt* (*la columna, los huesos*) to adjust,

crack; **El quiropráctico me truena la columna**..The chiropractor adjusts my spine...¿**Es malo tronarse los dedos?**..Is it bad to crack your knuckles? *vi* (*las tripas*) to growl (*one's stomach*); *vr* (*una articulación*) to click, make a clicking sound; **Me truena el hombro cuando lo muevo**..My shoulder clicks when I move it; **tronárselas** (*esp Mex, vulg*) to get high, to use drugs

tronco *m* (*anat*) trunk

tropezar *vi* to stumble, trip; —— **con** to stub one's foot against

tropical *adj* tropical

trotar *vi* to jog

trusa *f* (*Mex*) (*men's*) underpants

tuberculosis *f* tuberculosis

tubería *f* tubing

tubo *m* tube; —— **de drenaje** drainage tube; —— **de ensayo** test tube; —— **de ventilación** ventilation tube; —— **digestivo** digestive tract; —— **endotraqueal** endotracheal tube

tubular *adj* tubular

túbulo *m* tubule

tuerto -ta *adj* one-eyed

tularemia *f* tularemia

tullido -da *adj* disabled

tumor *m* tumor, lump, bump; —— **benigno** benign tumor; —— **de Ewing** Ewing's tumor; —— **de Wilms** Wilms' tumor; —— **maligno** malignant tumor

tumorcito *m* small lump *o* bump

túnel *m* tunnel

tupido -da *adj* (*Carib, SA*) stuffed up, congested; **Tengo tupida la nariz**..My nose is stuffed up..I have a stuffy nose.

turbio -bia *adj* turbid, cloudy

tusílago *m* (*bot*) coltsfoot

tutor -ra *mf* guardian, legal guardian

U

úlcera *f* ulcer, sore; —— **de decúbito** decubitus ulcer, bedsore; —— **de estrés** stress ulcer; —— **duodenal** duodenal ulcer; —— **gástrica** gastric ulcer; —— **péptica** peptic ulcer; —— **por presión** pressure sore

ulceración *f* ulceration

ulcerado -da *adj* ulcerated

ulna *f* ulna

ulnar *adj* ulnar

últimamente *adv* recently

último -ma *adj* last; **su última evacuación**.. your last bowel movement

ultrasonido *m* ultrasound

ultrasonografía *f* ultrasonography

ultravioleta *adj* ultraviolet

umbral *m* threshold

uncinaria *f* hookworm

ungüento *m* ointment, salve

unidad *f* unit; —— **de cuidado coronario** coronary care unit; —— **de cuidados intensivos (UCI)** *or* **de terapia intensiva** intensive care unit (ICU); —— **internacional** international unit

uniforme *adj* uniform; *m* uniform

unión *f* union

unir *vt* to unite, join; *vr* to unite, join together

untar *vt* to apply, daub, paint on; *vr* to apply to oneself, daub on oneself

uña *f* nail; (*del dedo*) fingernail; (*del dedo del pie*) toenail; —— **enterrada** *or* **encarnada** ingrown nail

uñero *m* ingrown nail; (*fam*) hangnail

urbano -na *adj* urban
urea *f* urea
uremia *f* uremia
urémico -ca *adj* uremic
uréter *m* ureter
ureteral, uretérico -ca *adj* ureteral
uretra *f* urethra
uretral *adj* urethral
uretritis *f* urethritis; —— no gonocócica non-gonococcal urethritis
urgencia *f* emergency; sala de urgencias emergency room (ER)
urgente *adj* urgent
úrico -ca *adj* uric
urinálisis, urianálisis *f* urinalysis
urinario -ria *adj* urinary
urocultivo *m* urine culture
urodinámica *f* urodynamics
urogenital *adj* urogenital
urografía *f* urography; urogram; —— excretoria excretory urography; —— retrógrada retrograde urography

urograma *m* urogram, pyelogram
urokinasa *f* urokinase
urología *f* urology
urológico -ca *adj* urologic, urological
urólogo -ga *mf* urologist
urosepsis *f* urosepsis
urticaria *f* urticaria; —— marítima swimmer's itch
uruguayo -ya *adj* & *mf* Uruguayan
usar *vt* to use
uso *m* use; —— excesivo overuse; para —— repetido reusable
usual *adj* usual
usuario -ria *mf* user
uta *f* American *o* mucocutaneous leishmaniasis
útero *m* uterus
utilizar *vt* to use, utilize
uva *f* grape
úvea *f* uvea
uveítis *f* uveitis
úvula *f* uvula

V

vaca *f* cow
vaciar *vt* to empty, to drain; —— la vejiga to empty one's bladder
vacío -a *adj* empty; *m* vacuum
vacuna *f* vaccine; —— BCG, DPT, Salk, etc. BCG vaccine, DPT vaccine, Salk vaccine, etc.; —— contra las paperas, —— contra la rabia, etc. mumps vaccine, rabies vaccine, etc.
vacunación *f* vaccination
vacunar *vt* to vaccinate
vagal *adj* vagal
vagina *f* vagina
vaginal *adj* vaginal
vaginitis *f* vaginitis
vago *m* vagus

vagotomía *f* vagotomy; —— selectiva selective vagotomy
vahído *m* dizzy spell, spell of lightheadedness
valeriana *f* (*bot*) valerian
valgo -ga *adj* valgus
valgus *adj* valgus
valina *f* valine
valor *m* value
valoración *f* evaluation; —— Apgar Apgar score
valorar *vt* to evaluate
valproico -ca *adj* valproic
válvula *f* valve; —— aórtica aortic valve; —— mitral mitral valve; —— pilórica pyloric valve; —— pulmonar pulmonic

valve; —— **tricúspide** tricuspid valve
valvuloplastia *f* valvuloplasty
vancomicina *f* vancomycin
vapor *m* vapor, steam, fumes; **cocido al** —— steamed
vaporizador *m* vaporizer; sprayer
variable *adj* & *f* variable
variación *f* variation
variante *adj* & *f* variant
variar *vi* to vary
várice *f* varix (*en inglés se emplea casi siempre la forma plural*: varices)
varicela *f* varicella (*form*), chickenpox (*fam*)
varicocele *m* varicocele
varicoso -sa *adj* varicose
varo -ra *adj* varus
varón *adj* & *m* male; **La señora Lugo tuvo un varón**..Mrs. Lugo had a baby boy.
varus *adj* varus
vascular *adj* vascular
vasculitis *f* vasculitis; —— **necrosante** necrotizing vasculitis; —— **por hipersensibilidad** hypersensitivity vasculitis
vasectomía *f* vasectomy
vaselina *f* petroleum jelly
vasija *f* basin, bedpan
vaso *m* vessel; glass; **un vaso con agua**..a glass of water; —— **sanguíneo** blood vessel
vasoconstricción *f* vasoconstriction
vasoconstrictor *m* vasoconstrictor
vasodilatación *f* vasodilation
vasodilatador *m* vasodilator
vasopresina *f* vasopressin
vasospasmo, vasoespasmo *m* vasospasm
vasovagal *adj* vasovagal
VDRL *m* VDRL
vecindad *f* neighborhood
vecino -na *mf* neighbor
vector *m* vector
vegetación *f* vegetation; **vegetaciones adenoides** adenoids
vegetal *m* vegetable
vegetarianismo *m* vegetarianism
vegetariano -na *adj* & *mf* vegetarian
vegetativo -va *adj* vegetative
vehículo *m* vehicle
vejez *f* old age

vejiga *f* bladder; blister
vello *m* body hair
vena cava *f* vena cava; —— —— **inferior** inferior vena cava; —— —— **superior** superior vena cava
vena *f* vein; —— **antecubital** antecubital vein; —— **femoral** femoral vein; —— **porta** portal vein; —— **safena** saphenous vein; —— **subclavia** subclavian vein; —— **varicosa** varicose vein; —— **yugular externa** external jugular vein; —— **yugular interna** internal jugular vein
vencido -da *adj* (*medicamento, etc.*) outdated, out of date
venda *f* bandage(s), dressing material; —— **elástica** elastic bandage
vendaje *m* bandage
vendar *vt* to bandage, dress
veneno *m* poison, venom; —— **para hormiga**, —— **para rata, etc.** ant poison, rat poison, etc.
venéreo -a *adj* sexually transmitted, genital; **enfermedad venérea** sexually transmitted disease
venezolano -na *adj* & *mf* Venezuelan
venir *vi* —— **de familia** to run in one's family
venodisección *f* cutdown
venografía *f* venography; venogram
venograma *m* venogram
venoso -sa *adj* venous
ventaja *f* advantage
ventana, ventanilla *f* (*de la nariz*) nostril
ventilación *f* ventilation
ventilador *m* ventilator; (*abanico*) electric fan
ventilar *vt* to ventilate
ventosear *vi* to pass gas
ventral *adj* ventral
ventricular *adj* ventricular
ventrículo *m* ventricle
vénula *f* venule
ver *vt, vi* (*pp* **visto**) to see
verano *m* summer
verapamil *m* verapamil
verde *adj* green
verdoso -sa *adj* greenish
verdugón *m* welt, bruise

verdura _f_ vegetable; _fpl_ greens
vergüenza _f_ shame, embarrassment; shyness;
  Me da vergüenza..It makes me feel embarrassed...**Tiene vergüenza**..He's shy.
vermicida _m_ vermicide
vermífugo _m_ vermifuge
vérnix caseosa _f_ vernix caseosa
verruga _f_ wart; —— **genital** genital wart;
  —— **plantar** plantar wart
vértebra _f_ vertebra
vértigo _m_ vertigo
vesícula _f_ vesicle, blister; (_fam_) gallbladder;
  —— **biliar** gallbladder
vespertino -na _adj_ (_form_) pertaining to
  evening, evening
vestido _m_ dress
vestir _vt_ to dress; _vr_ to dress (_oneself_), get
  dressed
veterano -na _mf_ veteran
veterinario -ria _adj_ veterinary; _mf_ veterinarian; _f_ veterinary medicine
vez _f_ (_pl_ **veces**) time; **a veces** at times; **cada**
  —— each time, every time; **cuatro veces**
  al día four times a day; **de** —— **en**
  cuando from time to time; **la primera**
  —— the first time; **la próxima** —— the
  next time; **la última** —— the last time;
  muchas veces many times, often; **una**
  —— one time
vía _f_ tract; —— **aérea** airway; **vías biliares**
  biliary tract; —— **corticospinal** corticospinal tract; —— **espinotalámica** spinothalamic tract; —— **piramidal** pyramidal
  tract; —— **respiratoria** respiratory tract
viable _adj_ viable
víbora _f_ viper, (_fam_) poisonous snake
vibración _f_ vibration
vicio _m_ vice, bad habit
vicioso -sa _mf_ addict
víctima _f_ victim
vida _f_ life; —— **media** half-life; ——
  sexual sex life; **con** —— alive
vidrio _m_ glass; **un pedazo de vidrio**..a piece
  of glass
viejo -ja _adj_ old; _m_ old man, old person;
  _f_ old woman
viento _m_ wind; (_flatulencia_) gas; **tirar**
  vientos to pass gas

vientre _m_ belly, abdomen; womb
vigilancia _f_ monitoring, follow-up
vigor _m_ stamina
vigorizar _vt_ to invigorate; _vr_ to become
  invigorated
vigoroso -sa _adj_ vigorous, strong
VIH _abbr_ **virus de inmunodeficiencia hu-**
  mana. _See_ **virus**.
vinagre _m_ vinegar
vinblastina _f_ vinblastine
vincristina _f_ vincristine
vínculo _m_ (_psych, obst_) bond
vino _m_ wine; —— **blanco** white wine; ——
  tinto red wine
violación _f_ rape
violar _vt_ to rape
violencia _f_ violence
violento -ta _adj_ violent
violeta _adj_ violet
viral _adj_ viral
virgen _adj_ & _mf_ virgin
virginidad _f_ virginity
vírico -ca _adj_ viral
viril _adj_ virile
virilidad _f_ virility
virilización _f_ virilization
virología _f_ virology
viruela _f_ smallpox; **viruelas locas** (_esp Mex,_
  _CA_) chickenpox
virulencia _f_ virulence
virulento -ta _adj_ virulent
virus _m_ (_pl_ **virus**) virus; —— **de**
  Epstein-Barr Epstein-Barr virus (EBV);
  —— **de inmunodeficiencia humana**
  (VIH) human immunodeficiency virus
  (HIV)
visceral _adj_ visceral
vísceras _fpl_ guts, innards; organ meats
viscosidad _f_ viscosity
viscoso -sa _adj_ viscous
visible _adj_ visible
visión _f_ vision, sight, eyesight; **visiones**
  (_fam_) hallucinations, the d.t.'s; ——
  borrosa blurred vision; —— **doble** double
  vision; —— **en túnel** tunnel vision; ——
  nocturna nocturnal _o_ night vision; ——
  periférica peripheral vision; ——
  profunda depth perception

visita *f* visit; visitor; —— **domiciliaria** house call; *fpl* (*de los médicos*) rounds; **pasar** —— to make rounds

visitante *mf* visitor

visitar *vt, vi* to visit

vista *f* vision, sight, eyesight; —— **cansada** *or* **fatigada** eyestrain; —— **doble** double vision; —— **empañada** blurred vision; —— **nocturna** nocturnal *o* night vision

visto *pp of* **ver**

visual *adj* visual

vital *adj* vital

vitalidad *f* vitality

vitalizar *vt* to vitalize

vitamina *f* vitamin; —— A, B$_{12}$, etc. vitamin A, B$_{12}$, etc.; —— **hidrosoluble** water-soluble vitamin; —— **liposoluble** fat-soluble vitamin

vitamínico -ca *adj* vitamin, pertaining to vitamins; **contenido** —— vitamin content

vitíligo *m* vitiligo

vítreo -a *adj* vitreous

viudo -da *adj* widowed; *m* widower; *f* widow; **viuda negra** black widow

vivir *vi* to live

vivo -va *adj* alive, (*virus, vacuna*) live

vocal *adj* vocal

vocear *vt* to page (*overhead*)

voltearse *vr* to turn over, roll over; ¿**Me**

volteo?..Should I turn over?

voltio *m* volt

volumen *m* volume

voluntad *f* will; **contra la** —— **de uno** against one's will; **fuerza de** —— will power; **por** —— **propia** of one's own free will

voluntario -ria *adj* voluntary; *mf* volunteer

volver *vi* (*pp* **vuelto**) —— **el estómago** (*esp Mex, fam*) to vomit, throw up; **Volví el estómago**..I threw up; —— **en sí** to regain consciousness; *vr* **volverse loco** to go crazy, to lose one's mind

vólvulo *m* volvulus

vomitar *vt, vi* to vomit, throw up (*fam*); —— **en seco** to retch

vómito *m* (*frec pl*) vomit; vomiting; **vómitos del embarazo** morning sickness; **vómitos en seco** dry heaves, retching

voyeurismo *m* voyeurism

voz *f* (*pl* **voces**) voice; **decir en** —— **baja** to whisper

vudú *m* voodoo

vuelta *f* turn; **darse** —— to turn; to turn over, roll over; to turn around; **darse media** —— to turn around

vuelto *pp of* **volver**

vulnerable *adj* vulnerable

vulva *f* vulva

W

warfarina *f* warfarin

X

xantoma *m* xanthoma

Y

yema *f* (*del dedo*) pad; (*de huevo*) yolk
yerba *See* **hierba**.
yerno *m* son-in-law
yeso *m* (*ortho*) cast, plaster (*for a cast*)
yeyunal *adj* jejunal
yeyuno *m* jejunum
yo *m* (*psych*) ego
yodado -da *adj* iodized

yodo *m* iodine
yoga *f* yoga
yogur *m* yogurt
yohimbé *m* (*bot*) yohimbe
yohimbina *f* yohimbine
yuca *f* (*bot*) yucca
yugular *adj* jugular

Z

zafada *f* (*fam*) dislocation
zafar *vt, vr* (*fam*) to dislocate, to become
   dislocated; **Me zafé el hombro..I** dislocated my shoulder.
zalcitabina *f* zalcitabine
zambo -ba *adj* bowlegged
zanahoria *f* carrot
zancudo *m* mosquito
zapato *m* shoe
zapeta *f* (*Mex*) diaper
zarzaparrilla *f* (*bot*) sarsaparilla
zidovudina *f* zidovudine

zinc *See* **cinc**.
zona *f* zone, area; (*fam*) herpes zoster,
   shingles; —— **afectada** affected area
zorrillo *m* skunk
zorro *m* fox
zumaque venenoso *m* poison oak
zumba *f* (*Es, Guat; fam*) binge
zumbar *vi* (*los oídos*) to ring, hum
zumbido *m* (*de oídos*) ringing, humming
zumo *m* juice
zurdo -da *adj* left-handed

DIALOGUES

DIÁLOGOS

HISTORY AND PHYSICAL /
HISTORIA CLÍNICA Y EXAMEN FÍSICO

PRESENT ILLNESS / HISTORIA CLÍNICA ACTUAL

Good morning. I'm Dr. Jones. / Buenos días. Soy la Dra. Jones.
Good afternoon. I'm Dr. Smith. / Buenas tardes. Soy el Dr. Smith.
Have a seat, ma'am. / Tome asiento, señora.
How can I help you? / ¿En qué puedo servirle?
Why did you come to the hospital? / ¿Porqué vino al hospital?
You have pain? / ¿Tiene dolor?
Where is the pain exactly? / ¿Dónde es que le duele exactamente?
Can you show me? / ¿Puede enseñarme?
Does the pain move around? / ¿El dolor se le mueve a otros lados?
The pain stays here? / ¿El dolor se le queda aquí?
What is the pain like? / ¿Cómo es el dolor?
Sharp? / ¿Agudo?
Dull? / ¿Sordo?
Does it burn? / ¿Le arde?
Like quick jabs? / ¿Cómo piquetes?
Stabbing? / ¿Punzante?
Like pressure? / ¿Cómo presión?
Crushing? / ¿Aplastante?
Is it a severe pain? / ¿Es un dolor fuerte?
Moderate? / ¿Moderado?
Mild? / ¿Suave?
When did the pain begin? / ¿Cuándo le empezó el dolor?
When was the first time you ever had this pain? / ¿Cuándo fue la
   primera vez en su vida que sintió este dolor?
It went away for a while? / ¿Se le quitó por un tiempo?
By itself? / ¿Solo? (¿Solito?)
When did it begin again? / ¿Cuándo le empezó de nuevo?
Does the pain come and go? / ¿Le va y le viene el dolor?
Is it a constant pain? / ¿Es un dolor constante?
When it comes, how long does it last? / ¿Cuando le viene, cuánto

tiempo le dura?

How often do you get the pain? / ¿Qué tan seguido le viene el dolor?

In the last week, how many times have you had the pain? / ¿En la última semana, cuántas veces ha tenido el dolor?

What were you doing when the pain came on? / ¿Qué estaba haciendo cuando le vino el dolor?

What time of day does the pain come on? / ¿A qué hora del día le viene el dolor?

Do you get it more often in the morning? / ¿Le viene más en la mañana?

In the afternoon? / ¿En la tarde?

Anytime? / ¿A la hora que sea?

Does it have anything to do with eating? / ¿Tiene algo que ver con la comida?

With exertion? / ¿Al hacer esfuerzos?

Is there anything which makes the pain worse? / ¿Hay algo que le agrava el dolor?

Is there anything which makes the pain better? / ¿Hay algo que le alivia el dolor?

Does it get better with exercise? / ¿Se alivia con el ejercicio?

It gets worse? / ¿Se pone peor?

Have you tried medications? / ¿Ha tomado medicamentos?

Which medication? / ¿Cuál medicamento?

Did it help a little? / ¿Le alivió un poco?

Are there relatives or friends who have the same problem? / ¿Hay familiares o amigos que tienen el mismo problema?

What do you think is causing the problem? / ¿Qué es lo que cree que le está causando el problema?

Have you seen a doctor before for this problem? / ¿Ha visto a un médico por este problema antes?

What did he say you had? / ¿Qué le dijo que tenía?

Did he do any studies? / ¿Le hizo estudios?

Did he draw blood? / ¿Le sacó sangre?

When was this? / ¿Cuándo fue?

What's the name of the doctor? / ¿Cómo se llama el médico?

Do you know his telephone number? / ¿Sabe su número de teléfono?

Why did you come to the hospital today instead of some other day? / ¿Porqué vino al hospital hoy en vez de algún otro día?

Do you have any other problems? / ¿Tiene alguna otra molestia?

How long have you been in the United States? / ¿Hace cuánto que está aquí en los Estados Unidos?

When was the last time you left the country? / ¿Cuándo fue la última vez que salió del país?

Where did you go? / ¿A dónde fue?

By the way, how old are you? / ¿A propósito, cuántos años tiene Ud.?

PAST MEDICAL HISTORY / HISTORIA CLÍNICA PREVIA

Do you have any other medical problems? / ¿Tiene otros problemas médicos?

How long have you had diabetes? / ¿Desde cuándo tiene diabetes?

Who takes care of you for your diabetes? / ¿Quién le atiende la diabetes?

Do you have a regular doctor? / ¿Visita regularmente a algún médico?

Where is he located? / ¿Dónde está ubicado?

Is he a private doctor? / ¿Es un médico privado?

When was the last time you saw a doctor? / ¿Cuándo fue la última vez que vio a un médico?

Have you ever been hospitalized? / ¿Ha estado hospitalizado alguna vez?

Have you ever had surgery? / ¿Ha sido operado alguna vez?

Have you ever had any serious illness? / ¿Ha tenido alguna enfermedad grave?

Have you ever had emotional problems? / ¿Ha tenido alguna vez dificultades emocionales?

MEDICATIONS / MEDICAMENTOS

Are you taking any medications? / ¿Está tomando medicamentos?

Have you taken any over-the-counter medications? / ¿Ha tomado algún medicamento que se vende sin receta médica?

Are you taking birth control pills? / ¿Está tomando píldoras anti-conceptivas?

Do you have your medications with you? / ¿Trae sus medicamentos?

What color are the pills? / ¿De qué color son las pastillas?

Are they tablets or capsules? / ¿Son tabletas o cápsulas?

How many times a day do you take them? / ¿Cuántas veces al día las toma?

Who prescribed the pills for you? / ¿Quién le recetó las pastillas?

Do you take them every day or do you forget every now and then? / ¿Las toma todos los días o se le olvida de vez en cuando?

For example, in a week how many times do you forget to take the pills? / ¿Por ejemplo, durante una semana cuántas veces se le olvida tomar las pastillas?

When was the last time you took this pill? / ¿Cuándo fue la última vez que tomó esta pastilla?

How many of these did you take yesterday? / ¿Cuántas de estas tomó Ud. ayer?

Show me exactly which pills you took this morning. / Muéstreme exactamente cuales pastillas tomó Ud. esta mañana.

When did you run out of pills? / ¿Cuándo se le acabaron las pastillas?

ALLERGIES / ALERGIAS

Are you allergic to penicillin? / ¿Es Ud. alérgico a la penicilina?

Have you ever taken penicillin? / ¿Ha tomado penicilina alguna vez?

Are you allergic to any medication? / ¿Es Ud. alérgico a algún medicamento?

Have you ever had a bad reaction to a medicine? / ¿Ha tenido alguna vez una mala reacción después de tomar alguna medicina?

What happened? / ¿Qué le pasó?

Does codeine bother you? / ¿Le cae mal la codeína?

Can you tolerate aspirin? / ¿Puede tolerar la aspirina?

SOCIAL HISTORY / HISTORIA SOCIAL

What kind of work do you do? / ¿En qué trabaja Ud.?

How long have you been out of work? / ¿Desde cuándo no trabaja?

Why haven't you been able to work? / ¿Porqué no ha podido trabajar?

What kind of work did you use to do? / ¿Qué trabajo tenía?

Were there chemicals or other hazards where you worked? / ¿Había substancias químicas u otras cosas peligrosas donde trabajaba?

What do you do during the day? / ¿Qué hace Ud. durante el día?

Do you eat well? / ¿Come bien?

Do you sleep well? / ¿Duerme bien?

Do you have a place to live? / ¿Tiene donde vivir?

Who do you live with? / ¿Con quién vive Ud.?

Do you smoke? / ¿Fuma Ud.?

Did you used to smoke? / ¿Fumaba?

How many packs a day did you use to smoke? / ¿Cuántas cajetillas fumaba al día?

When did you quit smoking? / ¿Cuándo dejó de fumar?

Do you drink alcohol? / ¿Acostumbra tomar bebidas alcohólicas?

Wine? / ¿Vino?

Beer? / ¿Cerveza?

Did you used to drink? / ¿Tomaba?

How long has it been since you quit drinking? / ¿Hace cuánto que no toma?

When was the last time you had a drink? / ¿Cuándo fue la última vez que tomó un trago?

How much can you drink when you have a mind to? / ¿Cuánto puede tomar cuando tiene ganas?

Do your hands ever shake when you quit drinking? / ¿Le tiemblan las manos a veces cuando deja de tomar?

Have you ever had the d.t.'s when you quit drinking? / ¿Ha tenido alguna vez visiones al dejar de tomar?

Have you ever had seizures when you quit drinking? / ¿Ha tenido alguna vez convulsiones (ataques) al dejar de tomar?

Have you tried to quit drinking? / ¿Ha tratado de dejar de tomar?

What happened? / ¿Qué pasó?

Have you ever used drugs? / ¿Ha usado drogas alguna vez?

Have you ever used I.V. drugs? / ¿Se ha inyectado drogas alguna vez?

Which drug? / ¿Cuál droga?

Do you have a habit or do you only use it occasionally? / ¿Tiene un hábito o la usa sólo de vez en cuando?

How often do you use it? / ¿Cada cuánto la usa?

Do you share needles? / ¿Comparte agujas con otros?

Have you had relations with other men? / ¿Ha tenido relaciones con otros hombres?

With prostitutes? / ¿Con prostitutas?

Did you use condoms? / ¿Usó condones?

Have you ever received a blood transfusion? / ¿Ha recibido alguna vez una transfusión de sangre?

Have you been tested for the AIDS virus? / ¿Le han hecho la prueba para el virus que causa el SIDA?

What was the result? / ¿Cuál fue el resultado?

FAMILY HISTORY / HISTORIA FAMILIAR

Are there any family members who have the same problem you have? / ¿Hay familiares que tienen el mismo problema que Ud.?

Are there any diseases which run in the family? / ¿Hay enfermedades que vienen de familia?

Are there family members who have had colon cancer? / ¿Hay familiares que han tenido cáncer del colon?

Are your parents still living? / ¿Todavía viven sus padres?

Does your mother have any medical problems? / ¿Tiene algún problema médico su madre?

What did your father die of? / ¿De qué murió su papá?

How old was he when he died? / ¿Qué edad tenía cuando murió?

REVIEW OF SYSTEMS / REVISIÓN DE APARATOS Y SISTEMAS

General / General:

Has your weight changed recently? / ¿Ha cambiado de peso últimamente?

How many kilos have you gained? / ¿Cuántos kilos ha ganado?

How many pounds have you lost? / ¿Cuántas libras ha perdido?

Over what period of time? / ¿En cuánto tiempo?

Do you have as much energy as usual? / ¿Tiene la misma energía de siempre?

How long have you felt tired? / ¿Desde cuándo se siente cansado?

Have you had fever? / ¿Ha tenido fiebre?

Night sweats? / ¿Sudores durante la noche?

Skin / Piel:

Do you have problems with your skin? / ¿Tiene problemas con la piel?

Rash? / ¿Erupción? (¿Salpullido?)

Itching? / ¿Picazón?

Sores? / ¿Úlceras? (¿Llagas?)

Has your skin changed color anywhere? / ¿Ha cambiado el color de su piel en alguna parte?

Head / Cabeza:

Do you have headaches? / ¿Tiene dolores de cabeza?
Have you hurt your head recently? / ¿Se ha lastimado la cabeza últimamente?

Eyes / Ojos:

Can you see well? / ¿Puede ver bien?
Do you wear glasses? / ¿Usa lentes?
Does your vision get blurry at times? / ¿Ve borroso a veces?
Do you ever see double? / ¿Ve doble a veces?
Do your eyes get red? / ¿Se le ponen rojizos los ojos?
Do you have cataracts? / ¿Tiene cataratas?
Glaucoma? / ¿Glaucoma?
Do you see halos around lights at night? / ¿Ve Ud. halos (círculos) alrededor de las luces en la noche?
Have you ever had your vision tested? / ¿Le han revisado la vista alguna vez?
When was the last time you saw an eye doctor? / ¿Cuándo fue la última vez que vio a un médico de los ojos?

Ears / Oídos:

Do you hear well? / ¿Oye bien?
Do you hear equally well in both ears? / ¿Oye igual en los dos oídos?
Do you hear less with one ear? / ¿Oye menos con uno de los oídos?
Has your hearing gotten worse recently? / ¿Oye menos últimamente?
Do you have an earache? / ¿Tiene dolor de oído?
Have you had ear infections? / ¿Ha tenido infecciones del oído?
Is there liquid draining from your ear? / ¿Le sale líquido del oído?
Do you feel as though the room were spinning around you? / ¿Siente como si el cuarto le estuviera dando vueltas?

Nose / Nariz:

Do you get a lot of nosebleeds? / ¿Le sale sangre de la nariz frecuentemente?
Are you allergic to pollen? / ¿Es Ud. alérgico al polen?

Do you have sinusitis? / ¿Tiene sinusitis?
Do you get a lot of colds? / ¿Le dan resfriados muy seguido?
Can you smell all right? / ¿Puede distinguir bien los olores?

Oropharynx / Orofaringe:

Do any of your teeth hurt? / ¿Le duele algún diente?
Do you have false teeth? / ¿Tiene dientes postizos?
How often do you brush your teeth? / ¿Qué tan seguido se cepilla los dientes?
Do your gums bleed easily? / ¿Le sangran fácilmente las encías?
When was the last time you saw a dentist? / ¿Cuándo fue la última vez que vio a un dentista?
Is your throat sore? / ¿Le duele la garganta?
Do you get canker sores frequently? / ¿Le salen pequeñas úlceras en la boca frecuentemente?
Has your voice changed recently? / ¿Le ha cambiado la voz últimamente?

Neck / Cuello:

Is your neck sore? / ¿Le duele el cuello?
Do you have any lumps in your neck? / ¿Tiene algunas bolas (bolitas) en el cuello?

Breasts / Senos:

Do you have any lumps in your breasts? / ¿Tiene algunas bolas (bolitas) en los senos?
Have you ever had a mammogram? / ¿Le han hecho un mamograma alguna vez?
Do your nipples ever secrete milk? / ¿Le sale leche de los pezones a veces?
Any kind of liquid? / ¿Algún líquido?
Blood? / ¿Sangre?

Lungs / Pulmones:

Do you have trouble breathing? / ¿Tiene dificultad para respirar?

Are you short of breath? / ¿Le falta aire?

Can you climb stairs? / ¿Puede subir escaleras?

Do you have to stop to catch your breath? / ¿Tiene que parar para recobrar el aliento?

How may blocks can you walk without stopping? / ¿Cuántas cuadras puede caminar sin parar?

Do you use oxygen at home? / ¿Usa oxígeno en casa?

Do you have a cough? / ¿Tiene tos?

Are you bringing up phlegm? / ¿Le sale flema?

What does it look like? / ¿Cómo se ve?

Is it thick? / ¿Es espesa?

What color is it? / ¿De qué color es?

Is it like saliva? / ¿Es como saliva?

Have you coughed up blood? / ¿Le ha salido sangre cuando tose?

Do you have wheezing? / ¿Tiene chillidos en el pecho?

Do you have asthma? / ¿Tiene asma?

Is there anything that brings on the asthma attacks? / ¿Hay algo que le provoca los ataques de asma?

Would it have anything to do with the time of year? / ¿Tendrá algo que ver con las estaciones del año?

Do you have allergies? / ¿Tiene alergias?

Is there a lot of dust in your home? / ¿Hay mucho polvo en su casa?

Are there animals in your home? / ¿Hay animales en la casa?

Have you ever had pneumonia? / ¿Ha tenido pulmonía alguna vez?

Tuberculosis? / ¿Tuberculosis?

Have you ever had a TB test? / ¿Le han hecho alguna vez la prueba para la tuberculosis?

What was the result? / ¿Cuál fue el resultado?

Have you ever had a chest x-ray? / ¿Le han tomado una radiografía del pecho alguna vez?

Heart / Corazón:

Do you have heart problems? / ¿Tiene problemas con el corazón?

High blood pressure? / ¿Presión alta?

How do you know you have high blood pressure? / ¿Cómo sabe que tiene la presión alta?

Do you ever have chest pain? / ¿Tiene dolor de pecho a veces?

Do you use pillows when you sleep? / ¿Usa Ud. almohadas cuando duerme?

What happens when you don't use pillows? / ¿Qué le pasa cuando no usa almohadas?

Have you ever woken up in the middle of the night with a smothering sensation? / ¿Alguna vez se ha despertado durante la noche con una sensación de ahogo?

Have you ever been told you had a heart murmur? / ¿Le han dicho alguna vez que tiene un soplo cardiaco?

When you were a child, did you have a disease called rheumatic fever? / ¿Cuando era niño, le dio una enfermedad que se llama fiebre reumática?

Were you sick with a fever and joint pains or rash? / ¿Le dio una fiebre con dolores en las articulaciones (coyunturas) o con una erupción (salpullido)?

Gastrointestinal / Gastrointestinal:

Do you have trouble swallowing? / ¿Tiene dificultades para tragar (pasar alimentos)?

Does food stick in your throat? / ¿Se le atora la comida?

Do you have trouble swallowing liquids too? / ¿Tiene dificultades para tragar (pasar) líquidos también?

Do you have heartburn? / ¿Tiene agruras?

Nausea? / ¿Náusea?

Vomiting? / ¿Vómito(s)?

Were you actually vomiting or did you just feel like it? / ¿Vomitaba algo o sólo tenía ganas?

Did you vomit blood? / ¿Vomitó sangre?

Do you have a stomachache? / ¿Tiene dolor de estómago?

Are there certain foods that bring on the pain? / ¿Hay ciertas comidas que le provocan los dolores?

Do you have trouble going to the bathroom? / ¿Tiene problemas para ir al baño?

Do you have constipation? / ¿Tiene estreñimiento?

Diarrhea? / ¿Diarrea?

Have you noticed blood in your stool? / ¿Ha notado sangre en el excremento?

Have you had stools that were black like asphalt? / ¿Ha tenido excremento negro como el asfalto de la calle?

Do you have hemorrhoids? / ¿Tiene hemorroides?

Have you had your gallbladder taken out? / ¿Le han sacado la vesícula?

Have you had hepatitis? / ¿Ha tenido hepatitis?

Has your skin ever turned yellow? / ¿Se le ha puesto amarilla la piel alguna vez?

Your eyes? / ¿Los ojos?

Genitourinary / Genitourinario:

Do you have problems urinating? / ¿Tiene problemas para orinar?

Are you urinating more often than usual? / ¿Orina más que de costumbre?

Do you have to get up in the middle of the night to urinate? / ¿Tiene que levantarse durante la noche para orinar?

Does it burn when you urinate? / ¿Le arde al orinar?

Have you ever had a urinary tract infection? / ¿Ha tenido alguna vez una infección de la orina?

Have you ever noticed blood in your urine? / ¿Ha notado sangre en la orina alguna vez?

Have you ever passed a stone? / ¿Ha eliminado una piedra en la orina alguna vez?

Have you ever had a sexually transmitted disease? / ¿Ha tenido alguna vez una enfermedad venérea?

That is, a disease you get from having sexual relations? / ¿Es decir, una enfermedad que se transmite por tener relaciones sexuales?

Were you treated by a doctor? / ¿Recibió tratamiento de un médico?

Do you have any sexual problems? / ¿Tiene alguna dificultad sexual?

(**Males** / Hombres)

Do you have to strain to get your urine out? / ¿Tiene que esforzarse para que salga la orina?

How is your stream? / ¿Cómo es el chorro?

Do you have problems with dribbling? / ¿Siguen saliendo gotas después de que haya terminado?

Do you have sores on your penis? / ¿Tiene úlceras (heridas) en el pene?

Do you have a discharge from your penis? / ¿Le sale una secreción del pene?

(**Females** / Mujeres)

Do you ever lose your urine accidentally? / ¿Se le sale la orina a veces sin querer?

When you laugh or cough? / ¿Cuándo se ríe o tose?

Do you still have periods? / ¿Todavía le viene la regla?

When was your last period? / ¿Cuándo fue su última regla?

Was it normal? / ¿Fue normal?

Do you have pain with your periods? / ¿Tiene dolores con la regla?

Do you bleed a lot during your periods? / ¿Sangra mucho durante la regla?

How many sanitary napkins do you use? / ¿Cuántas toallas usa?

Do you use tampons? / ¿Usa tampones?

Are your periods regular? / ¿Vienen a tiempo sus reglas?

Have you had bleeding between periods? / ¿Ha sangrado entre las reglas?

How old were you when you had your first period? / ¿A qué edad le vino la regla por primera vez?

When did you go through menopause? / ¿Cuándo le vino la menopausia?

Have you had bleeding since then? / ¿Ha sangrado desde entonces?

Do you get hot flashes? / ¿Le vienen calores (bochornos)?

How many children have you had? / ¿Cuántos niños ha tenido?

Did you have problems with any of your pregnancies? / ¿Tuvo problemas con alguno de los embarazos?

Have you had any abortions or miscarriages? / ¿Ha tenido abortos?

An abortion or a miscarriage? / ¿Con intención o natural?

When was the last time you had sexual relations? / ¿Cuándo fue la última vez que tuvo relaciones?

Are you using any birth control? / ¿Usa algún método anticonceptivo?

The pill? / ¿La píldora?

The diaphragm? / ¿El diafragma?

An IUD? / ¿Un dispositivo intrauterino (aparato)?

Condoms? / ¿Condones (preservativos)?

Could you be pregnant? / ¿Podría estar embarasada?

Do you have a vaginal discharge? / ¿Tiene secreción (desecho, flujo) vaginal?

As usual or different? / ¿Cómo siempre o diferente?

What is it like? / ¿Cómo es?

Do you have sores on your genitals? / ¿Tiene úlceras (heridas) en los genitales?

Do you have itching? / ¿Siente picazón (comezón)?

Does it hurt when you have intercourse? / ¿Le duele cuando tiene relaciones?

Musculoskeletal / Musculoesquelético:

Do you have joint pains? / ¿Tiene dolores de las articulaciones (coyunturas)?

Do your joints swell up? / ¿Se le hinchan las articulaciones (coyunturas)?

Do you feel stiff in the morning? / ¿Se siente tieso en la mañana?

Does your back hurt? / ¿Le duele la espalda?

Do you feel weak? / ¿Se siente débil?

Do you have trouble climbing stairs? / ¿Le dificulta subir escaleras?

Getting up from a chair? / ¿Levantarse de una silla?

Combing your hair? / ¿Peinarse?

Neurological / Neurológico:

Which hand do you write with? / ¿Con cuál mano escribe Ud.?

Have you had a stroke? / ¿Ha tenido un derrame cerebral (embolia)?

Has a single part of your body ever turned weak, like your arm or your leg? / ¿Se le ha puesto débil una sola parte del cuerpo alguna vez, como el brazo o la pierna?

Has your vision in one eye ever gone black? / ¿Se le ha puesto negra la vista en un solo ojo alguna vez?

Does any part of your body feel numb? / ¿Siente dormida alguna parte del cuerpo?

Do you have tingling? / ¿Tiene hormigueo?

Do you have trembling? / ¿Tiene temblores?

Do you have trouble remembering things? / ¿Tiene dificultades para recordar cosas?

Do you get dizzy at times? / ¿Siente mareos a veces?

As if you were going to faint? / ¿Como si fuera a desmayarse?

Have you fainted? / ¿Se ha desmayado?

Have you ever had a seizure? / ¿Ha tenido alguna vez una convulsión (ataque)?

Mental status / Estado mental:

What's your name? / ¿Cómo se llama Ud.?

Do you know where you are? / ¿Sabe donde está?
What type of building are we in? / ¿En qué tipo de edificio estamos?
What's the date? / ¿Cuál es la fecha?
What year is it? / ¿Qué año es?
Do you know who I am? / ¿Sabe quien soy yo?

Psychiatric / Psiquiátrico:

Would you say you are a nervous person? / ¿Diría que Ud. es una
persona nerviosa? (¿Tiene nervios?)
Is something bothering you? / ¿Hay algo que le molesta?
Would you say you suffer from depression at times? / ¿Diría que
padece a veces de la depresión?
Have you ever seen a psychiatrist? / ¿Ha visto alguna vez a un
psiquiatra?
Did it help? / ¿Le ayudó?
Have you ever thought of killing yourself? / ¿Ha pensado alguna vez
en suicidarse?
Have you thought about how would you do it? / ¿Ha pensado en
como lo haría?
Have you thought of hurting someone else? / ¿Ha pensado en hacerle
daño a otra persona?
Do you think you can take care of yourself? / ¿Puede valerse por sí
mismo?
Are you going to be able to manage? / ¿Podrá arreglárselas?

Endocrine / Endocrino:

Do you have thyroid problems? / ¿Tiene problemas con la tiroides?
Did a doctor tell you? / ¿Se lo dijo un médico?
Do you feel hot a lot? / ¿Siente calor muy seguido?
More than usual? / ¿Más que de costumbre?
Do you feel cold a lot when others don't? / ¿Siente frío muchas veces
cuando los demás no lo sienten?
Are you thirsty a lot? / ¿Tiene mucha sed?
Have you always been thirsty or is this something new? / ¿Siempre
ha tenido sed o es algo nuevo?
Do you have to get up in the middle of the night to urinate? /
¿Tiene que levantarse durante la noche para orinar?
Are you eating a lot? / ¿Está comiendo mucho?

PHYSICAL EXAMINATION / EXAMEN FÍSICO

GENERAL EXAMINATION / EXAMEN GENERAL

Have a seat on the exam table. / Siéntese en la mesa de exploración (mesa de exámenes).

Take off your jacket. / Quítese la chaqueta.

I need to take your blood pressure. / Necesito tomarle la presión.

Roll up your sleeve, please. / Súbase la manga, por favor.

Let your arm fall, I will hold it up. / Deje caer el brazo, yo lo sostengo.

Your blood pressure is one hundred thirty over seventy. / Su presión es ciento treinta sobre setenta.

Take off your clothes from the waist up, please. / Desvístase, por favor, de la cintura hacia arriba.

Take off all your clothes except your underwear. / Quítese toda la ropa menos la ropa interior.

Take off all your clothes and put on this gown. / Quítese toda la ropa y póngase esta bata.

Including your underwear. / Incluyendo su ropa interior.

You can use the curtain. / Puede usar la cortina.

Sit facing this wall, please. / Siéntese de frente a esta pared, por favor.

Sit with your legs dangling. / Siéntese con las piernas colgando.

Let me take your pulse. / Déjeme tomarle el pulso.

Follow my finger with your eyes without moving your head. / Siga mi dedo con los ojos sin mover la cabeza.

Look at my nose. / Míreme la nariz.

Stare at that point on the wall. / Fije la vista en aquel punto en la pared.

Keep staring at the point on the wall. / Siga mirando el punto en la pared.

Try not to move your eyes. / Trate de no mover los ojos.

Now look directly at the light. / Ahora mire directamente a la luz.

Raise your eyebrows. / Levante las cejas.

Frown. / Frunza el entrecejo.

Wrinkle your nose. / Arrugue la nariz.

Smile. / Sonría.

Show me your teeth. / Enséñeme los dientes.

Clench your teeth. / Apriete los dientes.

Push against my hand with your face. / Empuje mi mano con su cara.

Raise your shoulders against my hands. / Levante sus hombros contra mis manos.

Look up at the ceiling. / Mire al techo.

Open your mouth. / Abra la boca.

Lift your tongue up. / Levante la lengua.

Stick your tongue out. / Saque la lengua.

Move it from side to side. / Muévala de lado a lado.

Say "Ah." / Diga "A."

Swallow. / Trague (Pase) saliva.

I'm going to examine your heart. / Le voy a examinar el corazón.

Don't talk for a moment. / No hable por un momento.

Lean forward. / Inclínese hacia adelante.

I'm going to examine your lungs. / Le voy a examinar los pulmones.

Cross your arms. / Cruce los brazos.

Breathe deeply with your mouth open. / Respire profundo con la boca abierta.

Out. / Afuera.

Again. / Otra vez.

I need to examine your breasts. / Necesito examinarle los senos.

Take off your brassiere, please. / Quítese el brassiere (sostén), por favor.

Place your hands on your hips and push inward. / Ponga las manos en la cadera y empuje hacia dentro.

Lift your arms above your head like this. / Levante los brazos arriba de la cabeza así.

Now lie down. / Ahora acuéstese.

I'm going to examine your abdomen. / Le voy a examinar el abdomen (la barriga).

Arrange yourself straight on the table. / Acomódese recto en la mesa.

Relax your muscles. / Relaje los músculos.

Don't lift your head. / No levante la cabeza.

Tell me if it hurts. / Dígame si le duele.

I have to do a rectal examination. / Es necesario hacer un tacto rectal.

Do you know what a rectal exam is? / ¿Sabe que es un tacto rectal?

I need to examine your rectum with my finger, using a glove. / Necesito examinar su recto con mi dedo, usando un guante.

Roll over onto your left side. / Voltéese a su lado izquierdo.

Bend your knees toward your chest. / Doble las rodillas hacia el pecho.

Bear down as if you were having a bowel movement. / Puje como si estuviera defecando.

Squeeze my finger. / Apriete mi dedo.

I need to examine you for a hernia. / Necesito examinarle a ver si tiene una hernia.

Cough, please. / Tosa, por favor.

PELVIC EXAMINATION / EXAMEN GINECOLÓGICO

I need to do a pelvic examination. / Necesito hacerle un examen ginecológico.

Put your feet in the stirrups. / Ponga los pies en los estribos.

Move forward. / Muévase hacia adelante.

Toward me. / Hacia mí.

Separate your legs. / Separe las piernas.

I'm going to insert the speculum. / Voy a introducirle (meterle) el espéculo.

I'm going to do a Pap test. / Voy a hacerle un examen de Papanicolaou (prueba del cáncer).

The exam is almost over. / Falta poco para terminar el examen.

I need to examine you with my fingers, using a glove. / Necesito examinarla con mis dedos, usando un guante.

Now I am going to examine your vagina and rectum and the tissue in between. / Ahora le voy a examinar la vagina y el recto y el tejido entre ellos.

NEUROLOGICAL EXAMINATION / EXAMEN NEUROLÓGICO

Close your eyes. / Cierre los ojos.

Do you smell anything? / ¿Huele algo?

What does it smell like? / ¿A qué huele?

I am going to examine your peripheral vision. / Voy a examinarle la visión periférica.

Cover this eye and with your other eye look in my eye. / Tápese este ojo y con el otro mire a mi ojo.

Now tell me "Yes" the moment you see my finger wiggling. / Ahora diga "Sí" al momento que vea menear mi dedo.

Don't look at my finger. / No mire mi dedo.

Keep looking at my eye. / Siga mirando mi ojo.

Close your eyes and don't let me open them. / Cierre los ojos y no deje que se los abra.

Can you hear the sound of my fingers rubbing? / ¿Escucha el sonido de mis dedos frotando?

Close your eyes and tell me the moment you hear my fingers rubbing. / Cierre los ojos y dígame al momento que escuche mis dedos frotando.

On which side does the tuning fork sound louder? / ¿En cuál lado suena más fuerte el diapasón?

Or does it sound the same on both sides? / ¿O suena igual en los dos lados?

Which sound seems louder, this? / ¿Cuál sonido le parece más fuerte, este?

Or this? / ¿O este?

(For additional dialogue concerning the cranial nerves see GENERAL EXAMINATION above. Para diálogos adicionales sobre los nervios craneales, vea el EXAMEN GENERAL arriba.)

Stand, please. / Póngase de pie, por favor.

Walk toward the door. / Camine hacia la puerta.

Now walk to me. / Ahora camine hacia mí.

Walk on your toes. / Camine de puntillas.

Walk on your heels. / Camine con los talones.

Walk in a straight line, putting one foot directly in front of the other, like this. / Camine en una línea recta, poniendo un pie directamente enfrente del otro, así.

Hop on one foot. / Brinque en un pie.

Now on the other one. / Ahora en el otro.

Squat down. / Póngase en cuclillas.

Now get up without using your arms. / Ahora levántese sin usar los brazos.

Stand with your feet together and your arms extended in front of you, palms up, like this. / Párese con los pies juntos y los brazos extendidos enfrente, las palmas hacia arriba, así.

Close your eyes. / Cierre los ojos.

Keep your arms extended. / Mantenga los brazos extendidos.

I'm going to push you lightly to test your sense of balance. / Voy a empujarlo un poco, para revisar su equilibrio.

I won't let you fall. / No lo voy a dejar caer.

Sit here, please. / Siéntese aquí, por favor.

Squeeze my fingers as hard as you can. / Apriete mis dedos lo más fuerte que pueda.

Separate your fingers like this and don't let me close them. / Separe los dedos de la mano así y no deje que se los cierre.

Make a circle like this and don't let me break it. / Haga un círculo así y no deje que se lo rompa.

Pull against my hand. / Jale contra mi mano.

Push against my hand. / Empuje contra mi mano.

Harder. / Más fuerte.

Make a fist. / Haga un puño.

Flex your wrist against my hand. / Doble la muñeca contra mi mano.

Raise your arms against my hands. / Levante los brazos contra mis manos.

Extend your leg against my hand. / Extienda la pierna contra mi mano.

Pull it back. / Jálela hacia atrás.

Push your foot against my hand. / Empuje el pie contra mi mano.

Bend your foot upward. / Doble el tobillo hacia arriba.

Raise your leg against my hand. / Levante la pierna contra mi mano.

Touch your nose with your finger. / Tóquese la nariz con el dedo.

Now touch my finger. / Ahora toque mi dedo.

Keep on touching your nose and my finger, back and forth, rapidly. / Siga tocando su nariz y mi dedo, uno y otro, rápido.

Touch your knee with the heel of your other leg. / Toque la rodilla con el talón de la otra pierna.

Now slide your heel down your shin to your foot. / Ahora con el talón recorra la espinilla hasta el pie.

Can you feel the tuning fork vibrating? / ¿Siente vibrar el diapasón?

Now it isn't vibrating. / Ahora no está vibrando.

Can you tell the difference? / ¿Siente la diferencia?

Close your eyes. / Cierre los ojos.

Is it vibrating or not? / ¿Está vibrando o no?

Now? / ¿Ahora?

Can you feel when I touch you with this piece of cotton? / ¿Puede sentir cuando le toco con este algodón?

Close your eyes and tell me "Yes" each time you feel the cotton. / Cierre los ojos y diga "Sí" cada vez que sienta el algodón.

The moment you feel it, tell me. / Al momento que lo sienta, me dice.

I'm going to use this pin to test your sensations. / Voy a usar este alfiler para examinar sus sensaciones.

This is sharp. / Esto es agudo.

This is dull. / Esto es sordo (romo).

Can you feel the difference? / ¿Siente la diferencia?

Close your eyes and tell me "Sharp" or "Dull" each time I touch you. / Cierre los ojos y dígame "Agudo" o "Sordo" ("Romo") cada vez que lo toco.

Did you feel anything? / ¿Sintió algo?

Do you feel this point? / ¿Siente esta punta?

Do you feel these two separate points? / ¿Siente estas dos puntas por separado?

Close your eyes and tell me "One" or "Two" according to how many points you feel. / Cierre los ojos y dígame "Una" o "Dos" según las puntas que sienta.

I am going to check your reflexes. / Voy a examinar sus reflejos.

Relax. / Relájese.

Relax your leg. / Relaje la pierna.

NURSING / ENFERMERÍA

Orientation / Orientación:

Hello. I'm Lee. I'll be your nurse today. / Hola. Me llamo Lee. Hoy voy a ser su enfermera (enfermero).

Let me show you how your bed works. / Permítame mostrarle como funciona su cama.

This button here raises your head and this other one raises your legs. / Este botón aquí eleva su cabeza y este otro eleva sus piernas.

This works the T.V. / Esto hace funcionar la televisión.

If you need me, press this button here. / Si me necesita, oprima este botón aquí.

If you want to make a call, dial nine first. / Si quiere hacer una llamada, marque el nueve primero.

You need to put on this gown. / Tiene que ponerse esta bata.

You can put your clothes in this drawer. / Puede poner su ropa en este cajón.

Do you have any valuables with you? / ¿Lleva algo valioso?

Do you want us to lock it up? / ¿Quiere que se lo guardemos bajo llave?

I need to take your vital signs. / Necesito tomarle sus signos vitales.

Relax your arm. / Relaje su brazo.

Hold this thermometer under your tongue. / Mantenga este termómetro bajo su lengua.

Please step over to this scale; I need to weigh you. / Por favor, párese sobre esta báscula; necesito pesarlo.

I need to start an IV on you. / Necesito ponerle suero.

Make a fist. / Haga puño.

You're going to feel a stick. / Va a sentir un pinchazo (piquete).

Don't forget you're attached to this IV now. / No olvide que ahora está conectado a este suero.

If you want to walk around, I can get you an IV pole. / Si quiere pasearse, puedo conseguirle un tripíe para el suero.

Visiting hours are from nine in the morning to eight in the evening. / Las horas de visita son de las nueve de la mañana a las ocho de la noche.

Comfort / Comodidad:

Are you cold? / ¿Tiene Ud. frío?
Would you like an extra blanket? An extra pillow? / ¿Quisiera otra cobija más? ¿Otra almohada más?
Are you too warm? / ¿Tiene demasiado calor?
Are you comfortable? / ¿Está cómodo?
Are you having pain? / ¿Tiene dolor?
Where is the pain? / ¿Dónde tiene el dolor?
What do you usually take for the pain? / ¿Qué es lo que toma de costumbre para el dolor?
I'll call your doctor and see if he can prescribe something for the pain. / Voy a llamar a su médico para ver si le puede recetar algo para el dolor.

Nourishment / Alimentación:

Here's a menu showing your choices for dinner. / Aquí tiene un menú de lo que puede escoger para cenar.
You can order something from the cafeteria if you like. / Puede ordenar algo de la cafetería si gusta.
Are you on any kind of special diet? / ¿Está Ud. en alguna dieta especial?
Are you diabetic? / ¿Es diabético?
Do you have high blood pressure? / ¿Padece de presión alta?
Do you need help eating? / ¿Necesita Ud. ayuda para comer?
After midnight you won't be able to eat or drink anything because of the study they are doing in the morning. / Después de la medianoche no va a poder comer ni tomar nada debido al estudio que le van a hacer en la mañana.
Try to drink more fluids. / Trate de tomar mas líquidos.
Your doctor doesn't want you to eat in case you need surgery. / Su médico no quiere que coma en caso de que necesite cirugía.
Would you like ice chips? / ¿Quisiera pedacitos de hielo?
You're getting plenty of fluids through your IV. / Está recibiendo suficientes líquidos a través del suero.
Here's a basin in case you need to throw up. / Aquí tiene un riñón en caso de que necesite vomitar.
I need to pass a tube through your nose down into your stomach. / Necesito pasarle un tubo por la nariz hasta el estómago.
It will be a little uncomfortable but not painful. / Le será un poco

incómodo, pero no doloroso.

When I tell you, I'm going to want you to swallow. / Cuando yo le avise, quiero que trague.

Swallow. / Trague.

Good. / Bien.

Elimination / Eliminación:

Do you have diarrhea? / ¿Tiene Ud. diarrea?

Do you want something for constipation? / ¿Quiere Ud. algo para el estreñimiento?

I need to give you an enema. / Necesito ponerle un enema (lavativa).

Roll over onto your left side, please. / Voltéese a su lado izquierdo, por favor.

Are you going to be able to walk to the bathroom? / ¿Va a poder caminar al baño?

Do you want me to bring you a bedpan? / ¿Quiere que le traiga una bacinilla (cómodo)?

I can bring you a urinal. / Puedo traerle un orinal (pato).

You need to urinate in this container. / Necesita orinar en este recipiente.

I'm going to need a sample of your stool. / Necesito una muestra de su excremento.

Let me close the curtain. / Déjeme cerrar la cortina.

Your doctor has ordered a catheter. / Su médico le ha indicado un catéter.

I'm going to pass this tube through your urethra, that is, through the opening just above your vagina. / Le voy a pasar este tubo por su uretra, o sea, por la abertura justo arriba de su vagina.

I'm going to pass this tube through your penis into your bladder. / Voy a pasar este tubo por su pene hasta la vejiga.

It's not as bad as it sounds. / No está tan malo como parece.

Just relax. / Tránquilizese.

Be sure not to pull this out. / Asegúrese de no sacarse esto.

Medication / Medicamentos:

What medications do you normally take at home? / ¿Qué medicamentos normalmente toma Ud. en casa?

Are you allergic to any medicines? / ¿Es alérgico a alguna medicina?

Here are your medicines. / Aquí están sus medicinas.

Drink this liquid, please. / Tome este líquido, por favor.

Would you like a pill to help you sleep? / ¿Quisiera una pastilla que le ayude a dormir?

Would you like another injection for the pain? / ¿Quisiera otra inyección para el dolor?

I need to give you a suppository. / Necesito darle un supositorio.

It's a medicine that goes up your rectum. / Es una medicina que se pone en el recto.

Activity / Actividad:

You need to walk around in order to get back your strength. / Necesita caminar para que recupere las fuerzas.

I'll help you. / Yo le ayudaré.

Your doctor wants you to sit up in a chair for a while. / Su médico quiere que se siente en una silla por un rato.

Ask for help before getting out of bed. / Pida ayuda antes de levantarse de la cama.

Do you feel dizzy when you stand up? / ¿Se siente mareado cuando se levanta?

Your doctor doesn't want you to get out of bed. / Su médico no quiere que Ud. se levante de la cama.

You need to rest. / Necesita descansar.

I will be coming in every couple hours to turn you. / Estaré viniendo cada dos horas para voltearlo.

Hygiene / Higiene:

Would you like to take a shower? / ¿Quisiera tomarse una ducha (baño de regadera)?

I'm going to give you a sponge bath. / Voy a darle un baño de esponja.

Here's a toothbrush and toothpaste. / Aquí tiene un cepillo de dientes y pasta dental.

Here's a washcloth and towel. / Aquí tiene una toallita para lavarse y una toalla.

Here is a container for your dentures. / Aquí tiene un recipiente para su dentadura.

Respiratory / Respiratorio:

Are you short of breath? / ¿Se le hace difícil respirar?
You need to keep your oxygen mask on. / Necesita mantener su máscarilla de oxígeno puesta.
Take a deep breath. / Haga una respiración profunda.
You're due for another breathing treatment. / Es hora para otro tratamiento respiratorio.
Put this mouthpiece in your mouth and suck in air. / Póngase esta boquilla en la boca y chupe aire.
Make the ball go as high as you can. / Haga que la bolita suba lo más alto que pueda.
You need to do this every hour or so. / Tiene que hacer esto cada hora más o menos.
I need you to spit into this container. / Es necesario que escupa en este recipiente.
There's no smoking in the hospital. / Está prohibido fumar en el hospital.
If you need to smoke, you can use the patio on the second floor. / Si tiene que fumar, puede usar el patio en el segundo piso.

Discharge Planning / Planes Para Dar De Alta:

Who do you live with? / ¿Con quién vive Ud.?
Is there someone who can help you? / ¿Hay alguien que pueda ayudarle?
Do you have a wheelchair at home? / ¿Tiene una silla de ruedas en su casa?
A hospital bed? / ¿Una cama de hospital?
Who prepares your meals? / ¿Quién le prepara la comida?
Your doctor says you can go home now. / Su doctor dice que ya puede regresar a su casa.
You can call your family and tell them to come pick you up. / Puede llamar a su familia y decirles que vengan a recogerlo.

Miscellaneous / Misceláneas:

You better ask your doctor the next time you see her. / Es mejor que le pregunte a su médico la próxima vez que la vea.
Sr. Gomez, can you hear me? / ¿Sr. Gomez, puede oírme?

Open your eyes. / Abra sus ojos.

Squeeze my hand. / Apriete mi mano.

Push against my hand. / Empuje contra mi mano.

I'm sorry to wake you up, but I need to take your blood pressure and temperature. / Disculpe que lo despierte, pero necesito tomarle la presión sanquínea y temperatura.

I need to prick your finger to measure your sugar. / Necesito pincharle (picarle) el dedo para medirle el azúcar.

Would you like the hospital priest to visit you? / ¿Quisiera que el sacerdote del hospital lo visite?

PEDIATRICS / PEDIATRÍA

Your baby is fine. / Su bebé está bien.

He's a little jaundiced, but we can fix that with light treatments. / Está un poco amarillento, pero podemos arreglarlo con unos tratamientos de luz.

Are you going to breast-feed or use a bottle? / ¿Va a darle pecho o le va a dar biberón (mamadera)?

You need to burp him after each feeding. / Necesita hacerlo eructar después de cada alimento.

Don't dilute the formula. / No le agregue más agua a la fórmula.

It's not good to put your baby to bed with a bottle of milk. / No es bueno que acueste a su bebé con un biberón con leche.

Have you weaned her yet? / ¿La ha destetado ya?

She is ready to eat solids. / Ya puede comer alimentos sólidos.

Don't give her food that could make her choke, like beans or peanuts. / No le de comida que pueda asfixiarla, como frijoles o cacahuates.

Make sure your children aren't eating chips of paint off the walls. / Asegúrese de que sus niños no estén comiendo pedacitos de pintura de las paredes.

Who cares for your baby when you are at work? / ¿Quién cuida a su bebé cuando Ud. está en el trabajo?

Does your son coo? Squeal? Laugh? Babble? Say any words? Talk? / ¿Su hijo arrulla? ¿Chilla? ¿Ríe? ¿Balbucea? ¿Dice algunas palabras? ¿Habla?

Can he lift his head up? Sit up? Crawl? Walk? / ¿Puede levantar la cabeza? ¿Sentarse? ¿Gatear? ¿Caminar?

Don't worry, he's developing fine. / No se preocupe, se está desarrollando bien.

Many children his age can't talk yet. / Muchos niños a su edad no pueden hablar todavía.

Tantrums are normal at this age. / Los berrinches a esta edad son normales.

There's nothing wrong; she's just teething. / Nada está mal. Solamente que le están saliendo los dientes.

Does she get a lot of colds? / ¿Se resfría seguido?

Has she been pulling on her ear lately? / ¿Ha estado jalándose la oreja últimamente?

Ear infections are common among children her age. / Las infecciones del oído son comunes en niños de su edad.

Does she have asthma? Allergies? A heart murmur? / ¿Tiene ella asma? ¿Alergias? ¿Un soplo cardiaco?

Has he ever had seizures? Eye problems? Pneumonia? / ¿Ha tenido alguna vez convulsiones (ataques)? ¿Problemas de los ojos? ¿Pulmonía?

Do you have a record of your child's immunizations? / ¿Tiene una tarjeta de vacunas de su niño?

You need to lower the temperature of the water coming out of your faucets. / Necesita bajar la temperatura del agua que sale de la llave (grifo).

You need to put all poisons out of reach of your children. / Necesita poner todos los venenos fuera del alcance de sus niños.

Do you have a car seat for your child? / ¿Tiene un asiento de seguridad en el carro para su niño?

Is there a working smoke alarm on each floor of your house? / ¿Hay un detector de humo que funciona en cada piso de su casa?

Would you like to attend a class on parenting? A class on cardiopulmonary resuscitation (CPR)? / ¿Quisiera asistir a una clase para padres? ¿Una clase de resucitación cardiopulmonar (RCP)?

Does your daughter know her street address? / ¿Sabe su hija la dirección de su casa?

Can she brush her own teeth? Dress herself? Comb her hair? / ¿Puede cepillarse los dientes ella misma? ¿Vestirse? ¿Peinarse?

She will probably quit sucking her thumb on her own eventually. / Con el tiempo, probablemente dejará de chuparse el dedo gordo.

I wouldn't worry about it. / Yo no me preocuparía por eso.

How long has she been acting listless? / ¿Desde cuándo ha estado decaída?

Do you think she has been molested? / ¿Cree que la han abusado?

How often does your son wet the bed at night? / ¿Cada cuánto se orina en la cama su hijo por las noches?

It's normal for him to feel jealous of his younger brother. / Es normal que su hijo tenga celos de su hermanito.

Have you had trouble disciplining him? / ¿Ha tenido problemas disciplinándolo?

How do you punish him? / ¿Cómo lo castiga?

Has he been missing school a lot? / ¿Ha faltado mucho a la escuela?

To patient / Para el paciente:

How are you doing in school? / ¿Cómo te va en la escuela?

Do you have trouble paying attention? / ¿Se te hace difícil poner atención?

What grade are you in? / ¿En qué grado estás?

Do you smoke cigarettes? / ¿Fumas cigarros?

Have you tried any drugs? / ¿Has probado alguna droga?

Are you sexually active? / ¿Estás teniendo relaciones sexuales?

Do you use birth control? / ¿Usas algún método anticonceptivo?

Do you have any questions regarding sexual matters? / ¿Tienes algunas preguntas sobre asuntos sexuales?

Are you unhappy about your appearance in any way? / ¿Por algún motivo te sientes descontento con tu apariencia?

Do you get along with your parents? / ¿Te llevas bien con tus padres?

Do you feel you can talk to them about personal things? / ¿Sientes que puedes hablar con ellos acerca de cosas personales?

What do they do that bothers you? / ¿Qué es lo que te molesta de ellos?

What do you do that makes them upset? / ¿Que haces que los hace enojar?

What do you do during your free time? / ¿Qué haces en tu tiempo libre?

Do you spend a lot of time alone? / ¿Pasas mucho tiempo solo?

Are you involved in sports? / ¿Participas en los deportes?

Do you belong to a gang? / ¿Eres miembro de una pandilla?

Have you had any trouble with the law? / ¿Has tenido problemas con la ley?

What do you plan to do after high school? / ¿Qué piensas hacer después de terminar la preparatoria?

DENTISTRY / ODONTOLOGÍA

When was the last time you saw a dentist? / ¿Cuándo fue la última vez que vio a un dentista?

Do you brush your teeth after each meal? / ¿Se cepilla los dientes después de cada comida?

Do you floss regularly? / ¿Usa hilo dental regularmente?

You need to brush more along the gum line. / Necesita cepillarse más en la linea de la encía.

Open really wide now. / Ahora abra bien la boca.

Open part way. / Ábrala un poco.

Bite down. / Muerda.

Close your mouth around this as though it were a straw. / Cierre la boca alrededor de esto como si fuera un popote.

Rinse your mouth and spit. / Enjuáguese la boca y escupa.

Turn your head toward me. / Voltée la cabeza hacia mí.

Turn away. / Voltéese hacia allá.

Are you feeling any pain? / ¿Está sintiendo algún dolor?

You have a loose filling. / Ud. tiene un empaste suelto.

I'm going to replace it with an acrylic filling. / Se lo voy a reemplazar con un empaste acrílico.

You need a root canal. / Necesita una endodoncia.

I need to remove one of your teeth and put in a bridge. / Necesito sacarle uno de los dientes y ponerle un puente.

Is there someone who can drive you home afterward? / ¿Hay alguien que lo pueda llevar a su casa después?

Have you ever had to take antibiotics before a dental procedure? / ¿Alguna vez ha tenido que tomar antibióticos antes de un procedimiento dental?

The only part that hurts is when I give you the numbing medication. / La única parte que le dolerá es cuando le ponga el anestésico.

It will only hurt for a minute or so. / Le va a doler solamente por un minuto más o menos.

You're going to feel a little stick. / Va a sentir un pequeño piquete.

You may feel a little burning. / Puede sentir un ardorcito.

Bite down hard. / Muerda fuerte.

Does your bite feel normal or does it feel as though your tooth is too high? / ¿Al morder, siente normal o siente como si su diente está demasiado alto?

You have some staining on your front teeth. / Tiene un poco manchados los dientes de enfrente.

Would you be interested in a treatment which would make your teeth whiter? / ¿Estaría interesado en un tratamiento que le pondría los dientes más blancos?

Swish this around for a minute and then spit it out. / Mueva este líquido dentro de la boca por un minuto y luego escúpalo.

You shouldn't eat, drink or rinse your mouth for half an hour. / No debe comer, beber, ni enjuagarse la boca por media hora.

NOTES / NOTAS

NOTES / NOTAS

NOTES / NOTAS

NOTES / NOTAS

NOTES / NOTAS

NOTES / NOTAS

NOTES / NOTAS

NOTES / NOTAS

NOTES / NOTAS

NOTES / NOTAS

ISBN 0-07-053680-5